CLINICAL VECTORCARDIOGRAPHY

CLINICAL VECTORCARDIOGRAPHY

Second Edition

Te-Chuan Chou, M.D.

Professor of Medicine
University of Cincinnati College of Medicine

Robert A. Helm, M.D.

Professor of Medicine
University of Cincinnati College of Medicine

Samuel Kaplan, M.D.

Professor of Pediatrics
Associate Professor of Medicine
University of Cincinnati College of Medicine

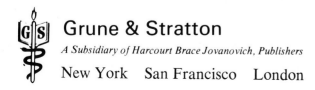

Grune & Stratton
A Subsidiary of Harcourt Brace Jovanovich, Publishers
New York   San Francisco   London

Library of Congress Cataloging in Publication Data

Chou, Te-Chuan, 1922–
    Clinical vectorcardiography.

    Includes bibliographies.
    1. Vectorcardiography.   I. Helm, Robert A., joint
author.   II. Kaplan, Samuel, 1922–   joint author.
III. Title. [DNLM: 1. Vectorcardiography. WG140
C552c 1974]
RC683.5.V4C45   1974   616.1'2'0754   74-3202
ISBN 0-8089-0838-3

Grune & Stratton, Inc.
111 Fifth Avenue
New York, New York 10003

Library of Congress Catalog Card Number 74-3202
International Standard Book Number 0-8089-0838-3
Printed in the United States of America

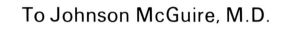

To Johnson McGuire, M.D.

Contents

conventional electrocardiogram. Vectorcardiographic criteria for the diagnosis of left ventricular hypertrophy. Genesis of the vectorcardiographic pattern of left ventricular hypertrophy.

Some Specific Pediatric Problems
    Counterclockwise superior frontal QRS loop
    Initial QRS forces
    Complete right bundle branch block

SECTION III

**Exercises in Vectorcardiographic Interpretation and Correlation
with the Clinical and Anatomical Findings**
    Fifty vectorcardiograms recorded from patients with various
disease entities are presented for the reader to interpret. The
conventional electrocardiogram, the author's interpretation, the
clinical information and, in most instances, the anatomical findings
are given for reference.

Index

Foreword

I am pleased to write the Foreword to this revised edition of CLINICAL VEC-
TORCARDIOGRAPHY. The authors, Drs. Chou, Helm and Kaplan bring to this
task unique qualifications in cardiology, and especially in vectorcardiography. Drs.
Chou and Helm have published widely in the field of vectorcardiography, and have
studied specifically comparisons of various vectorcardiographic lead systems, the
TsÊ loop of the vectorcardiogram, and the vectorcardiogram in certain varieties of
congenital heart disease. They have done much experimental work on dipole theory.
Dr. Helm's system of precordial lead placement has been widely recognized and applied. Both Drs. Chou and Helm are full Professors of Medicine in the University of
Cincinnati College of Medicine. Dr. Kaplan has had extensive experience in heart
disease of children spanning a period of several decades in his capacity as Professor
of Pediatrics and Director of the Division of Cardiology at the Children's Hospital in
Cincinnati.

The previous edition of this textbook, CLINICAL VECTORCARDIO-
GRAPHY, has become widely known and has been well received. It has been among
the most popular books on clinical vectorcardiography. The topic of vectorcardiography is especially timely in view of the recent increase in the application and useful-
ness of noninvasive methods of cardiac study, including vectorcardiography. This
text can be recommended because of the clarity of the presentations and its practical
approach, as exemplified by the excellence of the illustrations and the exercises in interpretation which are offered.

The revision of this popular text offers several important new features. These include a more specific statement of the vectorcardiographic criteria for the diagnosis
of myocardial infarction; a study of the vectorcardiogram in ventricular hypertrophy;
the application of the vectorcardiographic concept in hemiblock, and an extensive
section on pediatric vectorcardiography written by Dr. Kaplan.

I predict that this new edition will be a welcome addition to this important area
of cardiology.

Noble O. Fowler, M.D.
Professor of Medicine
Director, Division of Cardiology
University of Cincinnati College of Medicine

Acknowledgments

The many suggestions from the fellows and staff members of the Division of Cardiology, University of Cincinnati College of Medicine, and the Childrens' Hospital, Cincinnati, have been most helpful in the revision of this volume. Mrs. Esther Schumacher and Mr. Robert Schwemberger have recorded the majority of vectorcardiograms. Their effort to obtain good quality tracings is appreciated. Mrs. Laura Hanson was responsible for typing most of the manuscript and has patiently carried out many other secretarial tasks. Mrs. Linda DiMuzio has helped with the proof reading.

Dr. Gene Conway, Chief of Cardiology Service at the Veterans Administration Hospital has kindly made available materials from the V.A. Hospital for inclusion in this text.

We also appreciate the cooperation and patience of our publisher, the Grune and Stratton Company, and especially Mr. John de Carville.

A substantial portion of the data presented was obtained from investigations supported in part by funds received from the Heart Association of Southwestern Ohio, the Mabel Stonehill Fund for Electrocardiographic Research, and the Children's Heart Association of Cincinnati.

Te-Chuan Chou, M.D.
Robert A. Helm, M.D.
Samuel Kaplan, M.D.

SECTION I

1

The Vector Concept

During each cardiac cycle the heart generates potentials which produce an electrical field in the surrounding tissues extending to the body surface. The heart acts as a generator and the body behaves as a volume conductor. If the heart is considered to be quite small in proportion to the size of the volume conductor, it may be looked on as a point generator of successive instantaneous electromotive forces. Each such force can then be considered to have the properties of a vector and can be represented by an arrow (Fig. 1.1). The length of the arrow indicates the magnitude of the force and the direction of the arrow depicts the spatial direction of the force. The electrical field of the heart can be represented graphically by an infinite number of arrows, arising from the location of the point generator, depicting the infinite number of successive instantaneous electromotive forces developed during the cardiac cycle. This graphic representation may be greatly simplified by merely joining the termini of each of the successive arrows by a continuous line, the time course of which depicts the continuously changing magnitude and direction of the electrical field from instant to instant (Fig. 1.2).

One of the objects of spatial vectorcardiography is to record accurately the electrical field of the heart by means of electrodes placed on the body surface. Such a recording presents several difficulties:

1. The body constitutes a volume conductor with an irregular limiting boundary surface.
2. The electrical conductivities of the various tissues of the body are not uniform.
3. The heart is a relatively large organ in proportion to the size of the thorax in which it is embedded. Electromotive forces are generated simultaneously within multiple regions of the heart. Therefore, the representation of the heart as a point generator can only be an approximation.

These three factors would seem to preclude the development of a practical method of obtaining a reasonably accurate representation of the electrical field generated by the heart. However, certain conceptual approaches to this problem

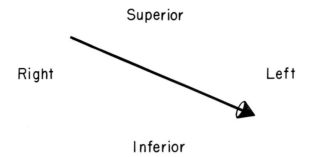

Fig. 1.1. A spatial electromotive force may be represented in the form of a vector by means of an arrow. The length of the arrow indicates the magnitude of the force. The direction of the arrow represents the direction in which the force is applied. The vector which is illustrated indicates that the force is directed inferiorly, to the left, and posteriorly. The latter direction is indicated by the shading of the point of the arrow.

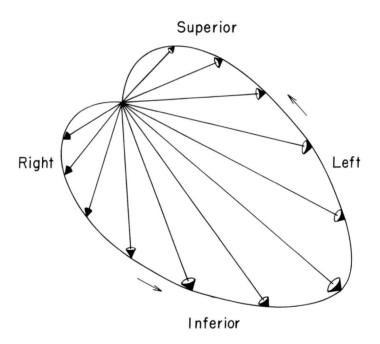

Fig. 1.2. A spatial vector loop can be formed by joining the termini of the infinite number of successive instantaneous vectors. (For simplicity only 12 of these vectors are illustrated.) The vector loop is directed initially to the right and anteriorly. As the efferent limb of the loop sweeps inferiorly, the pathway of its inscription indicates that the vectorial forces are increasing in magnitude and are changing their directions from right to left and from anterior to posterior. The afferent limb of the loop is formed by instantaneous forces which remain oriented leftward and posteriorly, but they successively diminish in magnitude and change in direction from inferior to superior.

have evolved, beginning with Einthoven's suggestion of using a dipole to represent
the electrical activity of the heart. A dipole is the simplest possible generator, one
which has a single pair of positively and negatively charged poles. In a physical
dipole the poles are separated by a finite distance. Decreasing the distance between
the poles reduces the strength of the dipole. The dipole strength is commonly
expressed in milliampere-centimeters (mA–cm). In a mathematical dipole the
distance between the poles is considered to approach zero, whereas the pole strength
in milliamperes concomitantly increases so that the strength of the dipole in
milliampere–centimeters remains constant. The strength of a dipole can change from
instant to instant, and the spatial orientation of the axis between the poles of a
dipole, physical or mathematical, can also vary from instant to instant. Einthoven,
Fahr, and deWaart postulated that the heart could be represented by a single
mathematical dipole of variable strength and variable axial orientation and that the
sites of the attachments of the extremities to the torso were, in an electrical sense,
equally distant from the dipole and equally distant from each other. Standard leads
I, II, and III were then represented as an equilateral triangle with the dipole located
at its geometric center. At any instant the strength and orientation of the dipole was
depicted by a vector, and the magnitudes of the projections of this vector on the sides
of the triangle represented the scalar voltages recorded with each lead at that instant
(Fig. 1.3).

Burger and van Milaan modified the concept of the Einthoven equilateral
triangle. These investigators constructed a model of a human torso, filled it with a
conducting solution, and placed a physical dipole with a small pole separation in the
region of the model which would be occupied by the central portion of the heart. The
difference in potential between the sites where the right arm, left arm, and left leg
would attach to the torso were measured when the axis of the dipole was successively
oriented in transverse and longitudinal directions. From such measurements they

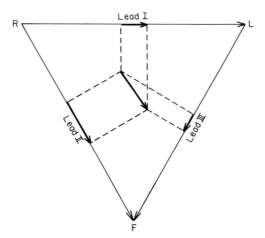

Fig. 1.3. The attachments of the right arm (R), left arm (L), and left leg (F) to the torso
form the equilateral triangle of Einthoven. An instantaneous electromotive force, depicted as
a vector at the center of this triangle, is projected upon each of the three sides representing
leads I, II, and III. The scalar deflection recorded by each lead is directly proportional to the
magnitude of the projected vector.

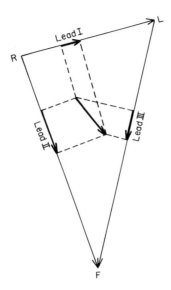

Fig. 1.4. The attachments of the right arm (R), left arm (L), and left leg (F) to the torso form a nonequilateral triangle, often referred to as a Burger triangle. As in Figure 1.3 the vector at the center of the triangle, representing an instantaneous electromotive force, is projected on each of the three sides of the triangle. However, the scalar deflection recorded by each lead is dependent not only on the magnitude of the projected vector but also on the magnitude of the lead vector. If the length of lead II is taken as unity, the magnitude of the projected vector on lead I is reduced by a factor equal to the ratio of the length of lead I to the length of lead II. Similarly, the magnitude of the projected vector on lead III is increased by a factor equal to the ratio of the length of lead III to the length of lead II.

constructed three vectors to form a triangle which had a configuration similar to that illustrated in Figure 1.4. Unlike the Einthoven triangle, the Burger triangle does not possess sides of equal length. At any instant the strength and orientation of a dipole located at the geometric center of the triangle* can be represented by a vector. When this vector is projected on each of the sides of the triangle, the scalar voltages recorded by each lead at that instant are not equal to the magnitudes of the projections. The scalar voltage recorded by a lead is equal to the product of the magnitude of the projected vector and the length of the lead. In Figure 1.4 lead II is arbitrarily assigned a length of unity; the magnitude of the projected vector on this lead will be equal to the voltage which it records, but the voltage recorded by lead I would be considerably smaller than the magnitude of the vector projected on it, and the voltage recorded by lead III would be somewhat larger than the vector projected upon this lead. In the Einthoven equilateral triangle the projected vector need not be multiplied by the length of any lead since each of three sides is considered to have lengths of unity.

The concept of Burger and van Milaan that an electrocardiographic lead has both magnitude and direction and is, therefore, a vector quantity represents a very significant contribution. These authors used the term *lead vector* to signify that a lead is a vector quantity. (Other terms sometimes used in place of lead vector are

*The geometric center of a triangle is located at the intersection of lines drawn from each of the three apices to the midpoints of the respective opposite sides.

Frank's image vector and *Schmitt's transfer impedance*). A lead vector is commonly expressed in ohms per centimeter. Since this is equivalent to millevolts per milliampere–centimeter (mV/mA–cm), the product of a lead vector and a dipole vector (in mA–cm) is a scalar quantity expressed in millivolts (mV). Lead vector measurements have been made by a number of investigators by immersing dipoles in human torso models. The publications of Frank are noteworthy in that data are available not only for numerous points on the surface of his model for a single dipole location but also for 16 points at the periphery of a transverse plane of his model for 71 dipole locations on this transverse plane. Although there is a great need for more complete data on a variety of torso models constructed from both children and adults, male and female, with varying physiques, the early work of Burger and van Milaan pointed the way to the solution of the problem related to the irregularity of the bounding surface of the body. These authors also approached the problem of tissue inhomogeneity by introducing internal structures into their model to simulate a nonhomogeneous medium. They found that similar results were obtained with the homogeneous and the heterogeneous models, suggesting that for the fronta . plane, tissue inhomogeneity may not play a very important role in modifying body surface potentials. The studies of den Boer, who used a fresh cadaver in place of a model, lead to a similar conclusion. A number of investigators have measured the conductivity of various tissues; although there is some discrepancy in the interpretation of findings, there is agreement that blood is a much better conductor than any other tissue. The influence of intracardiac blood probably plays an important role in modifying the distribution of cardiac potentials. Therefore, any final conclusions on the influence of electrical inhomogeneity of body tissues would be premature at the present time.

The problem related to the relatively large size of the heart in proportion to the size of the body, particularly the anteroposterior and transverse diameters of the chest, has been attacked more recently by means of the *multiple* lead vector concept. As an approach to understanding this concept, two dipoles on a plane are considered in Figure 1.5A and B. Dipole number 1 (Fig. 1.5A) produces a vector force which is directed toward the left and bottom of the page, and dipole number 2 yields a vector force in a right and (Fig. 1.5B) downward direction. If these two electromotive forces are generated simultaneously, they would combine to produce a deflection in a lead recorded by a galvanometer. The principles underlying the proper method of summing these two dipole forces are illustrated in Figure 1.5A and B. For each of the two points, point **A** and point **B**, a separate lead vector exists for the single arbitrary lead under consideration. These separate lead vectors are not identical.* The dipole vector of dipole number 1 is projected on its corresponding lead vector and the dipole vector of dipole number 2 is similarly projected on its lead vector as

* Each lead vector could be obtained experimentally by placing a single dipole *of unit magnitude*, that is, 1 mA–cm at point **A** and subsequently at point **B**. If the unit dipole is oriented horizontally at point **A**, the measurement of the voltage in millivolts recorded by the lead under consideration yields the *x* component for the lead vector of point **A** in ohms per centimeter. If the unit dipole is then oriented vertically at point **A**, the *y* component in ohms per centimeter is equal to the voltage in millivolts which is recorded by the lead. From these *x* and *y* components (which are 3 and 2 ohms/cm, respectively in Figure 1.5), the lead vector for point **A** can be drawn on the plane. In like manner, by subsequently recording the voltages in millivolts obtained with the lead in question when the unit dipole is oriented horizontally and then vertically at point **B**, the *x* and *y* components of the lead vector in ohmg per centimeter for point **B** are obtained. (In Figure 1.5 these are 2 and 5 ohms/cm, respectively).

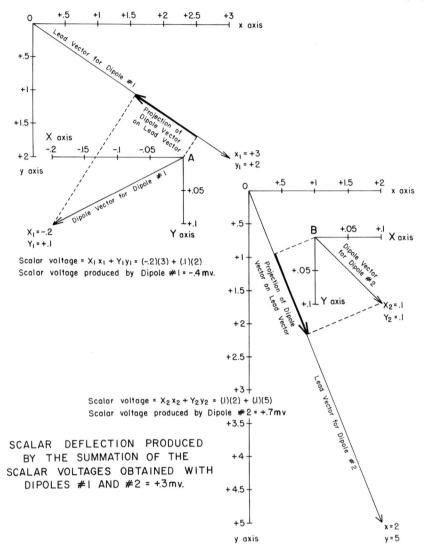

Fig. 1.5. For explanation, see text. The *X* and *Y* coordinate scales are in milliampere–centimeters (mA–cm), and the *x* and *y* coordinate scales are in ohms per centimeter (ohm/cm). The product of (mA–cm) (ohm/cm) is millivolts (mV).

depicted by the dotted lines in Figure 1.5. The scalar voltages produced by each dipole may be determined in a number of ways. For example, the length of the lead vector in ohms per centimeter may be multiplied by the length of the projected vector in milleampere–centimeters. (The projected vectors for points **A** and **B** are depicted by the darker lines in Fig. 1.5.) A second, simpler method of determining these scalar voltages is the calculation of the sum of the products of the corresponding horizontal and vertical components of the dipole vector and lead vector as illustrated in Figure 1.5. In this illustration the scalar voltage produced by dipole number 1 is −0.4 mV and the scaler voltage produced by dipole number 2 is +0.7 mV. Since the dipoles are considered to be generating their respective electromotive forces simultaneously, the scaler deflection recorded by the lead is the algebraic sum of the voltages produced by the two dipoles. This is the sum of -0.4 and $+0.7$ mV which is $+0.3$ mV.

This method of dealing with multiple dipoles has been illustrated in detail by means of the simplest possible situation, that is, by the use of only two dipoles which produce electromotive forces in a two-dimensional plane rather than in three-dimensional space. However, the proper method of determining the voltages produced by multiple spatially located dipoles, the axes of which may point in any direction in space, is entirely analogous to the two-dimensional procedure illustrated in Figure 1.5. In the three-dimensional situation each dipole is represented by a dipole vector which has three components, X, Y, and Z, rather than only the two components X and Y. For each dipole location a separate lead vector is postulated to exist for any given lead, and each of these lead vectors can be obtained experimentally by measuring the voltages recorded by the lead in question when a dipole of unit magnitude is oriented successively in the x, y, and z directions. Each of the multiple spatial lead vectors can be expressed in terms of its x, y, and z components. The voltage produced by each of the dipole vectors is then most easily obtained by the addition of the products of the corresponding components of the dipole vector and the lead vector, that is, by calculating $Xx + Yy + Zz$. Finally, the scalar voltage produced by each of the separate dipoles is added algebraically to yield the scalar deflection which the lead records from the simultaneously acting multiple-dipole aggregate.

Such a concept can be applied to the heart. The heart need not be represented as a point generator, that is, as a single dipole. Rather an almost infinite number of spatially oriented dipoles can be considered to be located at all points within the myocardial tissue where electromotive forces are generated. Then, for any given lead, there are likewise an almost infinite number of lead vectors, one for every myocardial point where a dipole is postulated to exist. If it were possible to know the X, Y, and Z components of each of the dipole vectors at each instant, and if it were possible to obtain experimentally, for any given lead, the x, y, and z components of each of the corresponding lead vectors (and if these were postulated to remain constant from instant to instant*), then the voltage produced at each instant by each dipole could be calculated, and the deflection recorded by the lead at each instant would represent the algebraic sum of these voltages.

We recognize that such a formidable task is manifestly impossible. However, before considering a practical and valid method of simplifying the entire procedure, it would be illuminating to discuss and illustrate an alternate but invalid method of dealing with multiple dipoles which is described in many publications and books devoted to spatial vectorcardiography. This approach involves the summing of multiple dipole vectors to obtain a single resultant vector. Figure 1.6 depicts the methods involved. In the lower left portion of the illustration the dipole vectors of dipoles number 1 and number 2 (at points **A** and **B**, respectively, in Fig. 1.5) are brought to a single point of intersection at their origins. The resultant dipole vector may be obtained by completing the parallelogram with the dotted lines as illustrated. An alternate method of finding the resultant vector is the simple addition of the X

---

* The mechanical movement of the heart during systole and the changing character of tissue conductance resulting from respiration and pulsatile blood flow makes this a theoretical concept.

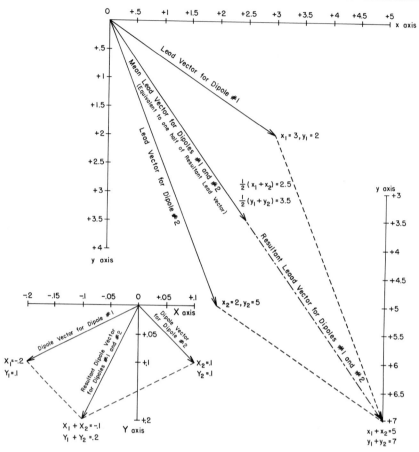

Fig. 1.6. For explanation, see text. The X and Y coordinate scales are in milliampere–centimeters (mA–cm), and the x and y coordinate scales are in ohms per centimeter (ohm/cm). The product of (mA–cm) (ohm/cm) is millivolts (mV).

and Y components of the two dipole vectors to obtain the resultant components of -0.1 and 0.2 mA–cm, respectively. (When the resultant of more than two vectors is desired, the addition of the components is certainly the preferable and much less involved method of calculating it). In the upper right diagram the resultant of the two lead vectors for points **A** and **B** of Figure 1.5 is obtained either by the parallelogram method or by the addition of the lead vector components. Either method produces x and y components of 5 and 7 ohms/cm, respectively. To obtain the mean lead vector, the resultant lead vector is divided by the number of vectors forming the resultant, which, in this case, is two. Therefore, one-half of the resultant lead vector represents the mean lead vector with x and y componets of 2.5 and 3.5 ohms/cm, respectively. The mean lead vector is displayed with a solid line, and the remaining portion of the resultant lead vector is depicted with alternate dots and dashes.

In Figure 1.7 the resultant dipole vector for dipoles number 1 and number 2 of Figure 1.5 and the mean lead vector for these dipole locations are illustrated. The scalar deflection produced by the resultant dipole vector is obtained either by multiplying the length of its projection by the length of the mean lead vector or by summing the products of corresponding horizontal and vertical components. Either method yields a value of +0.45 mV as the scalar deflection produced by the resultant dipole. When this is compared with the value of +0.3 mV obtained in Figure 1.5, the marked difference in the results is apparent. The discrepancy has its origin in the summing of the multiple dipole vectors to form a single resultant dipole. These dipoles do not contribute identical voltages to the recording lead, not only because of differences in their strengths and orientations but also because of differences in their lead vectors which are dependent on the factor of dipole locations and also on other factors such as tissue inhomogeneity and irregularity of the bounding surface of the volume conductor.

If it is invalid to sum into a single resultant vector the almost infinite number of dipole vectors postulated to arise from an almost infinite number of myocardial

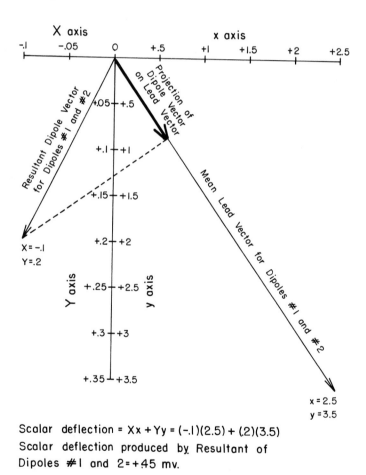

Scalar deflection = Xx + Yy = (−.1)(2.5) + (.2)(3.5)
Scalar deflection produced by Resultant of
Dipoles #1 and 2 = +45 mv.

Fig. 1.7.   For explanation, see text. The X and Y coordinate scales are in milliampere–centimeters (mA–cm), and the x and y coordinate scales are in ohms per centimeter (ohm/cm). The product of (mA–cm) (ohm/cm) is millivolts (mV).

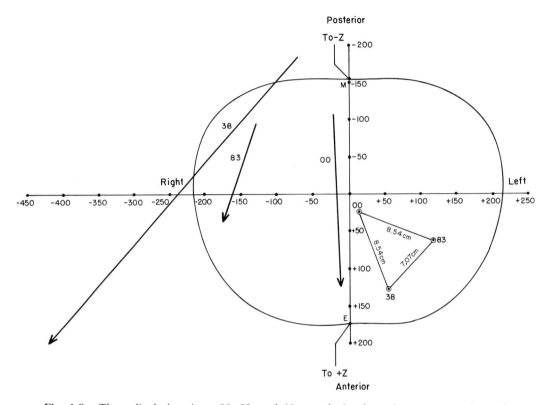

Fig. 1.8.   Three dipole locations, 00, 83, and 38, are depicted on the transverse plane of Frank's torso model, which has a transverse width of 33 cm and an anteroposterior width of 25 cm. The distances between the dipole locations are shown. The lead vectors for a lead taken between anterior point **E** and posterior point **M** are depicted by arrows, each labeled to correspond to its respective dipole location. The scales are in arbitrary units defined by Frank. The marked variation in the magnitudes and directions of the three lead vectors is readily apparent. This finding indicates that the influence which an electromotive force has on a lead may be greatly modified by the location of the force. For example, an anteriorly and rightward directed electromotive force arising at point 38 would produce a deflection approximately four times as large as the deflection produced by a similar force located only 7 cm away at point 83.

points, how can the study of these numerous dipole forces be simplified? An approach to this problem lies in the development of leads possessing multiple lead vectors which are uniform in magnitude and direction for each of the dipole locations in the myocardial tissue. If this ideal could be realized, the entire heart would, in effect, be functioning electrically as a single dipole for the leads in question. An approach to the development of such leads is illustrated by contrasting Figure 1.8 with Figure 1.9. In Figure 1.8 an anatomically anteroposterior lead can be obtained by measuring the differences in potential between points E and M, located in the midline on opposite sides of the transverse plane of Frank's torso model. Three widely separated dipole sites in the region of the heart are considered, and these are designated as 00, 83, and 38 in accordance with the nomenclature of Frank's publication. The three arrows represent the lead vectors of lead **E–M** for each of the three dipole locations. The marked disparity in both magnitude and direction of the three lead vectors is readily apparent.

In Figure 1.9 an anteroposterior lead is formed by substituting networks of points joing through unequal resistors for the single points, **E** and **M**, of Figure 1.8. With such a strategic selection of points and with the calculation of the appropriate values for the resistors, it is possible to obtain absolutely uniform lead vectors for the dipole locations 00, 38, and 83. Thus an electromotive force would make the same contribution to this lead regardless of whether it arose at point 00, point 38, or point 83. This would not be true of the leads shown in Figure 1.8.

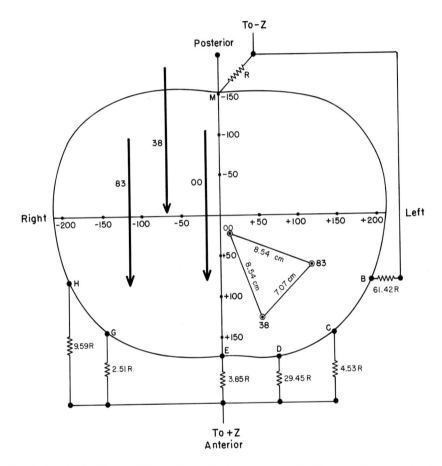

Fig. 1.9. As in Figure 1.8 the three dipole locations, 00, 83, and 38 are depicted on the transverse plane of Frank's model. The lead is now formed by networks of points joined through resistors before being connected to the poles of a glavanometer or electrocardiograph. Because of the suitable selection of points on the body surface and the calculation of appropriate values for the resistors, the lead vectors for this lead not only are strictly anteroposterior in direction but also are identical in magnitude for all three dipole locations. This means that the lead would be influenced in an identical manner by a given electromotive force arising at any of the three dipole locations.

Making use of data obtained from models, the multiple lead vector concepts* provides a method for the synthesis and analysis of leads having characteristics desirable for spatial vectorcardiography. In the development of such vectorcardiographic leads, the problems related to the complicated form of the body's bounding surface and to the relatively large volume of the heart in proportion to the size of the thorax can be effectively attacked by the application of this concept. The problem created by tissue inhomogeneity can likewise be approached. However, an adequate solution of this latter problem depends on the availability of complete data collected from more complicated models constructed in accordance with known and yet-to-be-learned facts concerning the conducting properties of body tissues.

References

1. Burger HC, van Milaan JB: Heart vector and leads. I. Br Heart J 8:157, 1946
2. Burger HC, van Milaan JB: Heart vector and leads. II. Br Heart J 9:154, 1947
3. Burger HC, van Milaan JB: Heart vector and leads. III. Br Heart J 10:229, 1948
4. den Boer, W: The clinical value of vectorcardiography. Acta Med Scand 144:217, 1952
5. Einthoven W, Fahr G, deWaart A: Uber die Richtung und die Manifeste Grosse der Potential-Schwankungen im Menschlichen Herzen und uber den Einfluss der Herzlage auf die Form des Electrokardiogramms. Arch Ges Physiol 150:275, 1913. Translation: Hoff HE, Sekelj P: On the direction and manifest size of the variations of potential in the human heart and on the influence of the position of the heart on the form of the electrocardiogram. Am Heart J 40:163, 1950
6. Frank E: The image surface of a homogeneous torso. Am Heart J 47:757, 1954
7. Frank E: Determination of the electrical center of ventricular depolarization in the human heart. Am Heart J 49:670, 1955
8. Helm RA: The lead vectors of multiple dipoles located on an electrically homogeneous circular lamina. Am Heart J 50:883, 1955
9. Helm RA: The lead vectors of multiple dipoles located on a transverse plane of Frank's homogeneous torso model. Am Heart J 52:323, 1956
10. Helm RA: Mathematical methods for analyzing leads. Am Heart J 57:149, 1959
11. McFee R, Johnston FD: Electrocardiographic leads. I. Introduction. Circulation 8:554, 1953
12. McFee R, Johnson FD: Electrocardiographic leads. II. Analysis. Circulation 9:255, 1954
13. McFee R, Johnson FD: Electrocardiographic leads. III. Synthesis. Circulation 9:868, 1954
14. Schmitt OH, Simonson E: The present status of vectorcardiography. Arch Intern Med 96:574, 1955

* Closely related to the concept that a lead may be considered to be constructed of multiple lead vectors, one for each of the postulated dipole locations in the heart where electromotive forces are generated, is the lead field concept. If a galvanometer measuring the voltage of a lead is temporarily replaced by a generator which introduces a current into the lead, the voltage between the poles of any of the postulated intracardiac dipoles would be identical with the voltage which would have been measured by the galvanometer if the same current had been introduced between the poles of the postulated dipole in question, providing that the directional orientation of the dipole remains constant during both of these maneuvers. It follows that if a current of unit magnitude is introduced into a lead, the densities and directions of this current at each of the points within the myocardium where a dipole is postulated to exist will be equivalent, respectively, to the magnitudes and directions of the lead vectors for each of these dipole locations.

2
Vectorcardiographic Lead Systems

A perfect lead system for vectorcardiography would consist of three leads with the following characteristics:

1. The three leads would be mutually perpendicular and each would be parallel to one of the rectilinear coordinate axes of the body. These axes are the horizontal or x axis (right-left axis), the longitudinal or y axis (superior-inferior or head-foot axis), and the sagittal or z axis (posteroanterior axis).
2. The three leads would be of equal amplitude from a vectoral standpoint.
3. The lead vectors of the three leads would not only be of equal amplitude and mutually perpendicular for a single point within the heart but also would retain the same magnitude and the same direction for all points where cardiac electromotive forces are generated.

Vectorcardiographic leads which purportedly meet conditions (1) and (2) are referred to as orthogonal leads. If, in addition, such leads also reasonably meet condition (3), they are called *corrected orthogonal leads*.

Certain lead systems such as the tetrahedron, the cube, and the rectilinear trihedron or "double cube" are approximately orthogonal in an anatomic sense. These leads do not use the lead vector concept of Burger and van Milaan and therefore are not necessarily orthogonal in an electrical sense. The tetrahedron was first described by Wilson, Johnston, and Kossmann, and represents an extension of Einthoven's frontal plane triangle. In addition to electrodes on the right arm, left arm, and left leg, a fourth electrode is placed on the posterior thorax just to the left of the midline at the level of the spinous process of the seventh dorsal vertebra (Fig. 2.1). Three leads which are anatomically approximately perpendicular are formed with these four electrodes: lead I, lead aVF (or VF), and lead VB. The connections of the first two leads are identical with the corresponding leads of the electrocardiogram. Lead VB represents the difference in potential between the back electrode and the Wilson central terminal, which is an averaging network of the electrodes of the three extremities. Two forms of the tetrahedron have been used as illustrated in Figures 2.2 and 2.3. In the equilateral tetrahedron (Fig. 2.2), the four faces of the

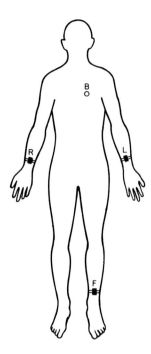

Fig. 2.1. The placement of electrodes for either the equilateral or the isosceles tetrahedron.

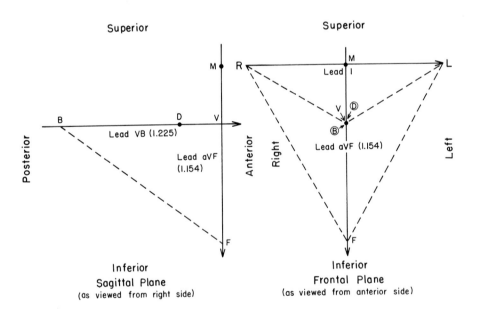

Fig. 2.2. The equilateral tetrahedron. The four faces of tetrahedron are considered to be identical equilateral triangles. The assumed dipole center of the heart, D, is located equally distant from the apices of the tetrahedron. The Wilson central terminal, V, is located in the frontal plane and does not coincide with point D. Leads aVF and VB are amplified by Factors of 1.154 and 1.225, respectively, the amplification of lead I being unity.

tetrahedron are theoretically identical equilateral triangles. To achieve this configuration this configuration lead aVF is amplified by a factor of $2/3\sqrt{3}$ or 1.154, and lead VB is amplified by a factor of $\sqrt{3/2}$ or 1.225, the amplification of lead I being kept at unity. In the isosceles tetrahedron (Fig. 2.3), a point on the frontal plane representing the Wilson central terminal is considered to be equally distant from the four apices of the tetrahedron. To achieve this configuration, lead VB is amplified by a factor of $\sqrt{3}$ or 1.732, whereas the standardization factors of leads I and aVF are the same as those used for the equilateral tetrahedron. Thus, the tetrahedron provides three anatomically orthogonal leads which are equalized by appropriate standardization factors. The tetrahedron in its equilateral form has been used extensively by Burch and his associates.

Although the three leads of the tetrahedron are anatomically orthogonal, they are not orthogonal from an electrical standpoint. In Figure 2.4 the lead vectors of the tetrahedron leads are plotted from data published by Frank. The variation of the electrical configuration from the anatomical forms of the tetrahedron (Figs. 2.2 and 2.3) is readily apparent.

Another lead system which is anatomically orthogonal is the cube (Fig. 2.5). Three electrodes are located in the left posterior axillary line, in the right posterior axillary line, and in the right anterior axillary line, all at the level of the first or second lumbar vertebra; a fourth electrode is placed in the right posterior axillary line over the right scapula. Closely related to the cube is the rectilinear trihedron or "double cube," in which the lower three electrodes have more caudad positions (Fig. 2.6). Equal standarization factors are used for all three leads of the cube and also for all three leads of the "double cube," despite the fact that the vertical lead of the

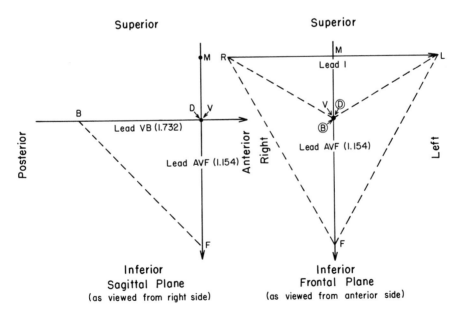

Fig. 2.3. The isosceles tetrahedron. The assumed dipole center of the heart, D. and the Wilson central terminal, V, coincide and lie on the frontal plane. Points D and V are considered to be equally distant from the apices of the tetrahedron. Leads aVF and BV are amplified by factors of 1.154 and 1.732, respectively, the amplification of lead 1 being unity.

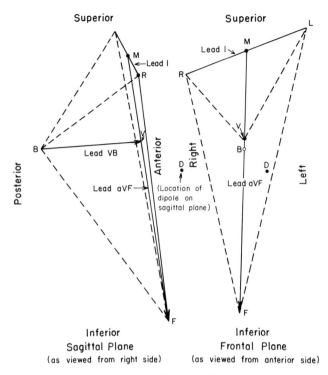

Fig. 2.4. The points of electrode attachment of the tetrahedron are plotted in space according to data published by Frank. The solid lines represent leads I, aVF, and VB, and should be compared with corresponding lines representing these leads in Figures 2.2. and 2.3. In an electrical sense the tetrahedral leads are neither orthogonal nor of equal length. (V represents the central terminal. It does not coincide with D, the dipole location for which the leads are constructed. M represents the midpoint of lead I.)

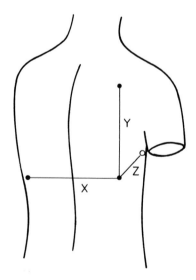

Fig. 2.5. The placement of electrodes for the cube.

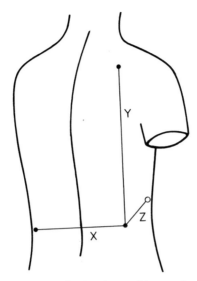

Fig. 2.6. The placement of electrodes for the rectilinear trihedron or "double cube."

latter system is anatomically considerably longer than the horizontal and sagittal leads. In both systems the leads are mutually perpendicular anatomically. However, there is considerable discrepancy between the anatomic locations of the lead axes and the corresponding electrical configurations of these axes based on Frank's published data and illustrated in Figure 2.7.

Because of the discrepancies between anatomic and electrical lead axes, other systems have been devised which not only are orthogonal, in an electrical sense, for a

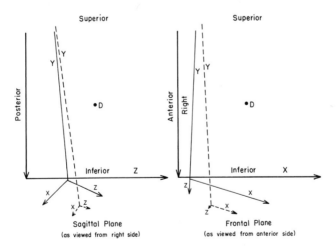

Fig. 2.7. The heavy solid lines delineate, in the frontal and sagittal planes, the assumed equality of magnitude and orthogonality of direction of the three leads of the cube and "double cube." These leads are to be compared with their lead vector counterparts, plotted in space from Frank's data, with respect to the dipole center, D. The lighter solid lines represent the cube, and the dotted lines represent the "double cube." The marked discrepancies between the assumed leads and their electrical counterparts are striking and are even more marked than those illustrated for the tetrahedron (Figs. 2.2, 2.3, and 2.4).

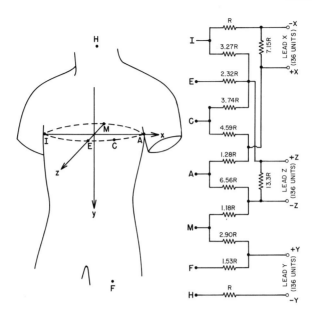

Fig. 2.8.   The seven-electrode vectorcardiographic lead system described by Frank. The exact electrode placement is described in the text. The constant values of R for the resistors should be preferably 100,000 ohms and not less than 25,000 ohms to prevent errors resulting from differences in electrode skin resistance.

single dipole location, but also are approximately orthogonal for a cluster of dipole locations. Such lead systems are referred to as corrected orthogonal systems. At the present time most vectorcardiography is being carried out with one of these corrected systems. A description of several of these will be given.

In 1956 Frank described a seven-electrode system; five electrodes are placed on the trunk and the remaining two are located on the back of the neck and on the left leg. Four of the five thoracic electrodes are placed at the level of the intersection of the fifth interspaces with the parasternal lines* where the plane formed by this transverse level intersects the left and right midaxillary lines, the sternal line and the vertebral line. These points on the transverse plane are designated by the letters A, E, I, and M in Figure 2.8. The fifth thoracic electrode is located on the same transverse plane at point C. Frank indicated that the angle formed by points A and E with the center of the chest should be bisected by the line drawn between point C and the center of the chest. From a practical standpoint, we locate point C midway between points A and E as measured on the surface of the chest. The electrodes are joined through resistors, as shown in Figure 2.8 and in more detail in Figure 2.9, to form leads, X, Y, and Z. (R stands for any convenient but adequate resistance such as 50,000 or 100,000 ohms). The natural magnitudes of leads X, Y, and Z are 174, 136, and 156 units,† respectively. The magnitudes of leads X and Z are equalized

---

* Langner and his associates showed a better correlation of the Frank system with other corrected orthogonal systems if the fourth interspace was selected.

† These are arbitrary units often referred to as Frank units.

with that of lead Y by the shunt resistances of $7.15R$ and $13.3R$, respectively, across the terminals of leads X and Z as shown in Figure 2.8. In Figures 2.8 and 2.9 the polarity of lead Z is the reverse of that originally published by Frank in order that the sagittal plane may be conveniently visualized from the right side as discussed subsequently in this chapter.

The advantages of the Frank system are its relatively few electrodes and that the electrode placement is fairly simple and reproducible. The placement of the electrode at point C in the region of the left breast may be rather inexact in female subjects. However, the contributions of the C electrode are only 22 percent to the left terminal of lead X and 27 percent to the anterior terminal of lead Z. A disadvantage of the Frank system is the difficulty of always placing the five-chest electrodes at that transverse level of the thorax where Y components of the cardiac electromotive forces are minimal. The elaborate and time-consuming technique which Frank described to determine this level experimentally has not generally been adopted.

The Frank system has become increasingly popular; it has been used in many clinical studies described in more recent publications. All the vectorcardiograms illustrated in this book were taken with the Frank system.

Another excellent set of leads formed by nine electrodes is the so-called axial system described by McFee and Parungao and illustrated in Figure 2.10. Point A is located in the fifth interspace 2 cm lateral to the left parasternal line. The anterior terminal of lead Z is formed by a network of three electrodes (#'s 1, 2, and 3) joined

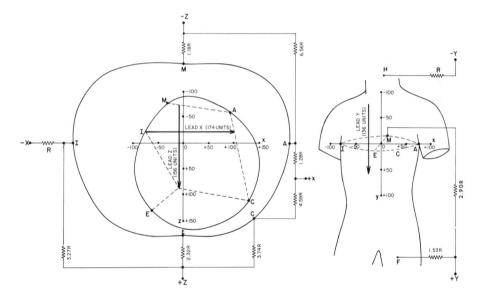

Fig. 2.9. Another illustration of the Frank system. The lead vectors for leeds X, Y, and Z are depicted on the transverse and frontal planes for the presumed electrical center of the heart. The natural lengths of leads X, Y, and Z are respectively, 174, 156, and 136 Frank units. (These are equalized to be 136 Frank units by means of the shunt resistors of $7.15\,R$ and $13.3\,R$ across the terminals of leads X and Z, respectively, as shown in Fig. 2.8.) The polarity of lead Z has been reversed when compared with the originally suggested by Frank. This has been done to allow the sagittal plane to be viewed from the right as in Figure 2.12, rather than from the left as illustrated in Figure 2.13.

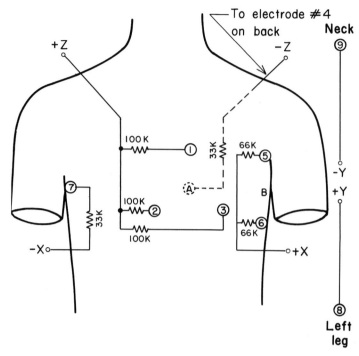

Fig. 2.10. The nine-electrode vectorcardiographic lead system described by McFee and Parungao. The numbered electrode placements are described in detail in the text. (In the original description of McFee and Parungao the 33,000-ohm resistors in the negative terminals of leads X and Z were not described or illustrated. We believe that such resistors should be inserted to aid in the rejection of 60-Hz interference.)

through 100,000-ohm resistors and arranged in an equilateral triangle about point **A** in such a manner that each electrode is 6 cm from point **A** and the base of the triangle is closest to the subject's feet. The posterior terminal of lead Z is formed by a single electrode (#4) placed on the back directly behind point **A**. Point **B** is located on the left side of the thorax one-third of the way from the anterior surface to the posterior surface of the chest at the same transverse level as point **A**. The left terminal of lead X is formed by a network of two electrodes (#'s 5 and 6) located 5.5 cm above and below point **B** and joined through 66,000-ohm resistors. The right terminal of lead X is attached to a single electrode (#7) located in a position on the right side of the chest corresponding to the location of point B on the left side. Lead Y is simply formed by electrode 8 on the left leg and electrode 9 on the left side of the neck. This description of the McFee–Parungao system applies to adult individuals with a height of 170 ± 30 cm. For children the 6-and 5.5-cm measurements are reduced in proportion to the ratio of the child's height in centimeters divided by 170 cm.

Duchosal has described a simplified method for applying the electrodes of the McFee–Parungao system. Duchosal has also indicated that inverting the triangle formed by the three anterior electrodes (#'s 1, 2, and 3) so that the horizontally oriented base of the triangle is closest to the head and the apex of the triangle is closest to the feet produces no significant change in the potentials recorded by lead Z. Such an alteration in electrode positioning warrants further investigation since it would provide a practical way to avoid the difficulty of exact electrode placement in the region of the left breast in female subjects.

Schmitt and Simonson described a group of leads generally known as the SVEC-III system, referring to its being the third system which these investigators have used for spatial vectorcardiography. Figure 2.11 illustrates the placement of the 14 electrodes. The anterior terminal of lead Z is formed by four electrodes located at the levels of the intersections of the third interspaces (#'s 1 and 2) and the sixth interspaces (#'s 3 and 4) with the parasternal lines. Electrodes 1 and 2 on the right side of the chest and electrodes 2 and 4 on the left side of the chest are all located 30° from the midline. Electrodes 2, 3, and 4 are joined together through 100,000-ohm resistors and electrode 1 is joined to the other three electrodes through a 70,000-ohm resistor. The posterior terminal of lead Z is formed by electrodes 5, 6, 7, and 8 which have positions on the back directly behind electrodes 1, 2, 3, and 4, respectively.

Electrodes 10 and 12 are located 60° from the midline on the left and right sides of the chest at the level of the intersections of the fifth intercostal spaces with the parasternal lines. The left terminal of lead X is formed by joining through equal resistors electrode 10 with electrode 9 placed on the left wrist or at any convenient position on the left arm. Electrodes 12 and 11 are similarly joined through equal

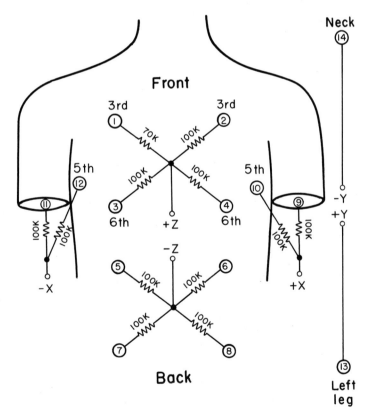

Fig. 2.11. The 14-electrode vectorcardiographic lead system described by Schmitt and Simonson. This system is generally known as the SVEC-III system. The numbered electrode placements are described in detail in the text.

resistors to form the right terminal of lead X. Electrode 13 on the left leg and electrode 14 on the neck form lead Y.

The major disadvantage of the SVEC-III system is the large number of electrodes which must be applied. The four-electrode network forming the posterior terminal of lead Z and the two-electrode network used for the right terminal of lead X could probably each be replaced by a single electrode without significant reduction in the correction of the system.

Another type of lead designed to achieve a reasonable degree of uniformity of its lead vectors for all myocardial points is that which utilizes grids formed by a large number of metal screwtype electrodes mounted on flexible plastic sheets. The electrodes on such a sheet are joined through resistors to a common terminal. These grids were originally developed by Johnston and his group at Ann Arbor. For the sagittal lead two grids are used, one on the anterior surface of the chest and one posteriorly. For the transverse lead two grids are placed on the left and right sides of the chest. The number of electrodes on each grid is not critical, except that Reynolds and his coworkers showed that 16 or more electrodes are desirable for the anterior grid of the sagittal lead. It is probable that single small electrodes can replace the posterior grid of the sagittal lead and the right grid of the transverse lead without any significant reduction in the uniformity of the multiple lead vectors of these leads. Barber and Fischmann have ingeniously modified the flexible grids by using balsa wood electrodes attached to a solid flat platform by means of spring mounts which hold the electrode tips firmly against the chest. The balsa wood electrodes are impregnated with lithium chloride which eliminates the need for using electrode paste.

In 1957 Helm described the use of large saline-containing sponge electrodes to replace (on the anterior and left regions of the thorax) the less convenient grid electrodes then available. The assumption was made that the resistance at the interface of the sponge and skin is sufficiently uniform that individual electrodes connected through resistors are not necessary to achieve uniformity. Comparison of the saline-containing sponge leads with leads formed by electrode grids verified this assumption for practical purposes. Sangiorgi and his associates suggested that the sponges could be replaced by large saline-moistened gauze flats. These are convenient in that, folded to the proper size, they adhere closely to the chest wall and, being inexpensive, can be discarded after each use. Either the sponge or the gauze flat is attached to a vectorcardiographic lead wire by means of a small, light-weight battery clip.

Complete descriptions of the various grid electrode systems and of the sponge electrode system are given in Reference 12 as well as in the individual papers of the various authors listed in the references.

VECTORCARDIOGRAPHIC DISPLAY

The voltages recorded by any system of vectorcardiographic leads can, after amplification, be displayed on the face of a cathode-ray tube. The tube has two sets of plates which control the horizontal and vertical deflections of the electron beam. When the frontal plane projection of the spatial vectorcardiogram is to be displayed, the left and right terminals of the transverse (or x) lead are attached, respectively, to the left and right plates controlling the horizontal deflections of the electron beam, and the inferior and superior terminals of the longitudinal (or y) lead are connected, respectively, to the lower and upper plates controlling the beam's vertical deflections. These connections allow the frontal (xy) plane projection of the spatial vectorcardiogram to be viewed as an observer would view an upright subject from the front (Figs. 2.12, 2.13, and 2.14).

For the display of the transverse (xy) plane projection of the spatial vectorcardiogram, the left and right terminals of the transverse (or x) lead are attached, respectively, to the left and right plates of the cathode-ray tube just as in the frontal plane. The anterior and posterior terminals of the sagittal (or z) lead are customarily connected to the lower and upper plates controlling the vertical deflections of the cathode-ray beam. With such connections the transverse plane of the spatial vectorcardiogram is viewed as if the observer were facing the head of a subject who is reclining on his abdomen (Figs. 2.12 and 2.13).

An alternate method of observing the transverse (xz) plane is depicted in Figure 2.14. This plane is viewed as if the observer were facing the foot end of a subject who is reclining on his back. In our opinion, the method described below would be the preferable way of displaying the transverse plane, but the alternate method illustrated in Figures 2.12 and 2.13 is so ingrained in vectorcardiography that it may not now readily be changed.

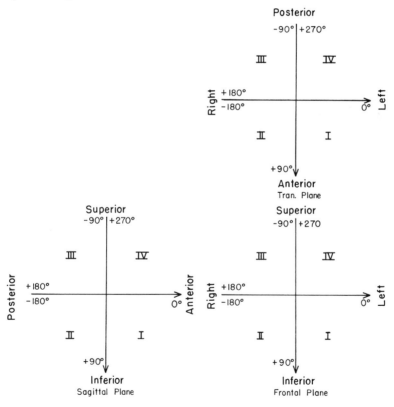

Fig. 2.12. The frontal, sagittal, and transverse planes are displaced in the manner in which they are viewed for all vectorcardiograms illustrated in this book.

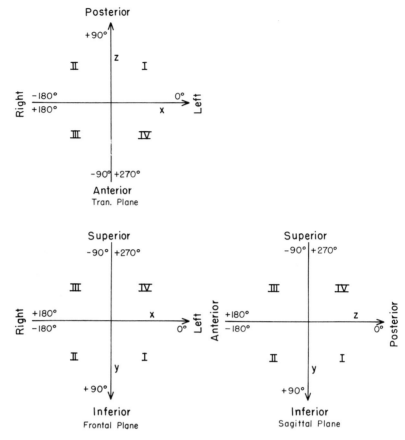

Fig. 2.13. The frontal, sagittal, and transverse planes are displayed in the manner recommended by the committee on Electrocardiography of the American Heart Association in 1967.

There is no general agreement as to whether the sagittal (zy) plane projection of the spatial vectorcardiogram should be viewed by an observer from the right (Fig. 2.12) or from the left (Figs. 2.13 and 2.14) of the upright subject. In 1954, the Committee on Electrocardiography of the American Heart Association recommended that this plane should be viewed from the left as depicted in Figure 2.13. However, in 1956 Helm pointed out that this method of observing the sagittal plane prevents measurement of angles in a uniform manner in the three planes. Thus, Figure 2.13 illustrates that it is impossible to maintain, in both the transverse and sagittal planes, the well-established frontal plane convention of Einthoven who designated the left end of the transverse (x) axis as 0° and the right end as $\pm180°$ and measured angles in a clockwise direction of rotation. If the left and inferior ends of the x and y axes bound the first quadrant of the frontal plane, and the left and posterior ends of the x and z axes bound the first quadrant of the transverse plane, then the left, inferior, and posterior ends of the x, y, and z axes, respectively, must be positive, since first quadrant coordinates are positive in accordance with well-established trigonometric convention. When such positive polarity is maintained in the transverse plane for the left end of the x axis and the posterior end of the z axis,

Figure 2.13 shows that the numbered quadrants of the transverse plane are incongruous with the sequence of the corresponding quadrants of the other two planes. Despite this incongruity in the measurement of angles in the three planes, the Committee on Electrocardiography of the American Heart Association in 1967 recommended not only the display but also the method of measuring the angles as illustrated in Figure 2.13. These 1967 recommendations specifically stated that the polarity of the sagittal (z) lead should be such that the posterior end of this lead should be chosen as positive. This polarity was selected because the mean direction of the excitation of the ventricles in normal subjects is usually predominantly posterior. The selection of posterior positivity for the z lead on the basis of such a consideration is justifiable on the basis that the polarities of the x and y leads are similarly correlated with the mean direction of excitation of the ventricles along these axes in normal subjects. Thus the direction of the mean QRS vector in a normal subject is usually to the left, downward, and posterior. The positive ends of the x, y, and z axes would then likewise be left, inferior, and posterior, if the 1967 recommendations of the Committee on Electrocardiography of the American Heart Association are accepted.

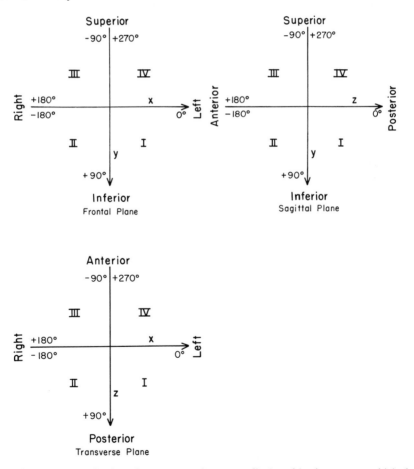

Fig. 2.14. The frontal, sagittal, and transverse planes are displayed in the manner which the authors consider to be ideal and which they are advocating for future adoption.

The authors would like to make a strong plea that the method of display depicted in Figure 2.14 be given serious consideration in the future. At the present time, practically all vectorcardiographers display the transverse plane as if the observer were viewing the prone subject in a head-to-foot direction. This method of viewing has become so customary that it does not seem propitious at present to adopt the method of displaying the transverse plane illustrated in Figure 2.14. However, such a display in which the observer views the supine subject in a foot-to-head direction would have several advantages:

1. It would make Einthoven's conventional method of making angular measurements in the frontal plane applicable to the other two planes.
2. A subject is always reclining on his back in the supine position and is never in the prone position when a vectorcardiogram (as well as an electrocardiogram) is recorded. (It seems strange indeed that early workers in vectorcardiography should have chosen the prone position for the transverse plane when a subject is almost always in the supine rather than in the prone position for all forms of cardiac examination.)
3. The leftward, inferior, and posterior directions of the mean spatial vector in normal subjects would correlate completely with the polarities of the x, y, and z leads, respectively, with this method of display.

At the present time, the authors are unwilling to accept the compromise of making counterclockwise angular measurements in the transverse plane and clockwise angular measurements in the frontal and sagittal planes; therefore the display depicted in Figure 2.13 is not being used in the present edition of this text. As in the first edition, all of the illustrations will be presented in accordance with Figure 2.12 in which the sagittal plane is viewed from the right side of the upright subject and the transverse plane is viewed from the head of the prone subject. We realize that this display forces the sagittal (z) axis to have its positive polarity directed anteriorly rather than posteriorly and thus to be incongruous with the usual posterior direction of mean QRS forces. However, we consider this incongruity to be more desirable than the confusing method of making angular measurements in the three planes as illustrated in Figure 2.13. It is for this reason that we are not following the current (1967) recommendation of the Committee on Electrocardiography of the American Heart Association. We might mention that electrocardiographers are, at the present time, about equally divided in viewing the sagittal plane from the right (Fig. 2.12) or from the left (Fig. 2.13). We feel that this dichotomy of opinion will never be resolved satisfactorily until the much more desirable method of display illustrated in Figure 2.14 is universally adopted. If the reader wishes to view the illustrations in this book in the manner advocated by the 1967 Committee on Electrocardiography of the American Heart Association, he should reverse the polarity of the z axis in the sagittal and transverse planes and should "flip over" the right sagittal view so that it becomes a left sagittal display. If, in addition, the reader would then "flip over" the transverse plane, the vectorcardiographic presentation would be that depicted in Figure 2.14. It is this latter display for which we are making a strong plea for the future but which is too unconventional at the present time for the illustrations in this text.

INSTRUMENTATION

The instrumentation used in the recording of the vectocardiograms illustrated in this book will be described.

The vector loops are displayed on and photographed from a 5-in. (12.5-cm) flat cathode-ray screen having a short persistance phosphor. The photographs are made with a Polaroid camera on film having rated speed of ASA 3000. The paper print depicting a white trace on a black background is developed in 10 sec.

The horizontal and vertical deflection plates of the cathode-ray tube are connected to two identical amplifiers. The maximum sensitivity of the amplifiers is such that a 1-cm deflection on the screen will result from 0.02 mV. (Thus, 1 mV would theoretically produce a maximum deflection of 50 cm or four times the diameter of the screen). The common sensitivity control has 11 steps for gain control so that each step simultaneously increases the sensitivity of both amplifiers by a factor of $\sqrt{2}$ or 1.41. The gain of each amplifier can also be adjusted individually. It is important that the amplifiers controlling the horizontal and vertical deflections have no phase shift; if equal voltages are applied to the deflection plates simultaneously, a straight line deflection at a 45° angle should occur.

The maximum spectrum of the frequency response of our instrument's amplifiers is 0.1 to 1500 Hz (hertz-cycles per second) with an error not exceeding 10 percent. Cut-off points are provided at 1500, 300, and 60 Hz. Many recordings illustrated in subsequent chapters were made at 300 Hz. However, the upper frequency response was often set at 60 Hz, especially when this was necessary to clarify the T and P loops. The amplifier noise is typically 0.003 mV, peak-to-peak, over the full spectrum of 0.1 to 1500 Hz with a maximum of 0.005 mV. The noise is less than 0.001 mV when the spectrum is restricted to 0.1 to 60 Hz.

The vectorcardiographic loops can be interrupted at any desired frequency from 0.5- to 20-msec periods for timing purposes. The dash intervals of the vectorcardiograms illustrated in this book are 2 msec unless otherwise stated. The dashes can be adjusted to have a "comet" or "tear-drop" appearance. The brighter, broader portion of such dashes indicates the advance of the loop in that direction. An important provision for greatly improving the quality of vectorcardiographic recordings is automatic trace brightening. This feature is highly desirable because of the marked differences in the rate of movement of the cathode-ray beam during various phases of the cardiac cycle. With appropriate circuitry for continuously variable brightness control, the beam becomes brighter as it moves faster, and it becomes quite dim when it is motionless. This effectively prevents the initial and terminal portions of the QRS loop, as well as the P and T loops, from being obscured by a meaningless "blob" of light.

The automatic brightness control is not effective if there is much extraneous muscle tremor. Since this produces movement of the beam which in turn increases its brightness, these undesirable deflections are superimposed on and obscure the desired cardiac deflections. In such a circumstance it is possible with our instrument to use an internal sweep generator which can be connected to either the horizontal or vertical amplifier, or to both, to sweep the vector loop across the screen in any desired direction. In this manner, random, nonrepetitive extraneous deflections can be separated from repetitive cardiac deflections.

To facilitate photography of the rapidly moving beam, it is desirable to use appropriate beam blanking. Such blanking can be adjusted so that the beam is continually off and continually on for alternating complete cardiac cycles. The operator simply opens the camera shutter while the beam is off, holds it open while the beam traces the events in one cardiac cycle, and then closes the shutter when the beam again goes off. For recording only certain portions of the events within a single cardiac cycle, the beam can be turned off and on for the desired period by means of internal, trace-derived triggers and adjustable delay timers.

It is highly desirable that the amplifiers, power pack, and cathode-ray tube be housed in a single, sturdy, but relatively light-weight container which can be moved easily to a patient's bedside. The camera should be accurately and securely attached to the housing so that the focus of the image of the cathode-ray beam on the focal plane of the camera need only rarely be checked. Depending on the type of camera setup used, some method of preventing ambient light from falling on the cathode-ray screen in sufficient quantity to reduce the contrast of the blue vectrocardiographic trace is a necessity. This can be simply but effectively accomplished by placing a transparent, folding hood of deep amber color in such a way as to surround the conical area subtended by the camera lens. The operator can view the screen continuously through this amber hood as the photographic records are made with a blue filter placed over the camera lens.

References

1. Barber MR, Fischmann EJ: A lead system recording total outward cardiac dipole strength. Br Heart J 23:649, 1961
2. Burch GE, Abildskov JA, Cronvich JA: *Spatial Vectorcardiography*. Philadelphia, Lea & Febiger, 1953
3. Committee on Electrocardiography, American Heart Association: Recommendations for standardization of electrocardiographic and vectorcardiographic leads. Circulation 10:564, 1954
4. Committee on Electrocardiography, American Heart Association: Recommendations for standardization of leads and of specifications for instruments in electrocardiography and vectorcardiography. Ciruclation 35:83, 1967
5. Duchosal PW, Sulzer R: La Vectorcardiographie. Basel, S Karger, 1949
6. Duchosal PW: Practical remarks on the McFee and Parungao VCG lead system. Am Heart J 72:287, 1966
7. Frank E: The image surface of a homogeneous torso. Am Heart J 47:757, 1954
8. Frank E: An accurate, clinically practical system for spatial vectorcardiography. Circulation 12:737, 1956
9. Grishman A, Scherlis L: Spatial Vectorcardiography. Philadelphia, Saunders Co, 1952
10. Helm RA: An accurate lead system for spatial vectorcardiography. Am Heart J 53:415, 1957
11. Helm RA: Vectorcardiographic notation. Circulation 13:581, 1956
12. Helm RA, Chou TC: Electrocardiographic leads. Am J Cardiol 14:317, 1964
13. Johnston FD: The clinical value of vectorcardiography. Circulation 23:297, 1961
14. Langner PH Jr, Okada RH, Moore SR, Fies HL: Comparison of four orthogonal systems of vectorcardiography. Circulation 17:46, 1958

15. McFee R, Parungao A: An orthogonal lead system for clinical electrocardiography. Am Heart J 62:93, 1961

16. Reynolds EW Jr, Cordes JF, Willis PW, Johnston FD: The use of the lead-field concept in the development of leads satisfactory for vectorcardiography. I. The sagittal lead. Circulation 14:48, 1956

17. Sangiorgi M, Corsi V, Cofano L, Salvo E, Coppolino L: A comparative study of some vectorcardiographic methods based on the use of unipolar leads, bipolar leads between electrically symmetrical points and bipolar leads with multiple electrodes. Acta Cardiol 15:101, 1960

18. Schmitt OH, Simonson E: The present status of vectorcardiography. Arch Int Med 96:574, 1955

19. Wilson FN, Johnston FD, Kossmann CE: The substitution of a tetrahedron for the Einthoven triangle. Am Heart J 33:594, 1947

3

The Sequence of Cardiac Activation and the Derivation of the P, QRS, and T Vector Loops

The knowledge of the sequence of cardiac activation is most valuable for understanding and interpreting normal and abnormal electrocardiograms and vectorcardiograms. In this chapter the histoanatomy of the cardiac pacemaker and of the specialized conduction system are described, and the normal sequence of atrial and ventricular activation are outlined. The activation potentials are represented by mean vectors, from which the **P, QRS,** and **T** vector loops are derived. Their general characteristics are correlated with the sequence of activation and the proportional contribution of the various regions of the cardiac chambers.

ATRIAL ACTIVATION AND THE P VECTOR LOOP

The atrial activation begins in the SA node which is located at the junction of the superior vena cava and the right atrium (Fig. 3.1). Three specialized tracts containing Purkinje fibers have been identified to connect the SA node to the AV node. They are called the *anterior*, the *middle*, and the *posterior internodal pathways*. An interatrial pathway, the Bachmann bundle, has also been described to connect the right atrium and the left atrium. However, the role of these fibers in human atrial impulse conduction under normal circumstances has not been defined clearly. Direct epicardial mapping in isolated human hearts and experimental animals indicates that the atrial excitation proceeds in a radial fashion (Fig. 3.2). In the initial period only the right atrium is activated but soon the activation process also involves the interatrial septum and the left atrium. During the later period the left atrium alone is depolarized. According to Lewis the last region of the left atrium to be activated is the tip of the left atrial appendage but Puech et al found it to be the posteroinferior portion of the left atrium near the insertion of the inferior pulmonary veins. More recent data tend to support Lewis' findings. The wave of atrial depolarization has been estimated to have a velocity of slightly less than 1 meter/sec.

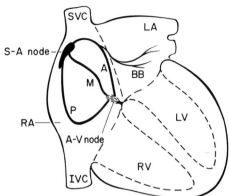

Fig. 3.1. Schematic diagram of the heart to illustrate the anterior (A), the middle (M), and the posterior (P) internodal pathways connecting the SA node with the AV node. The Bachmann bundle (BB) connects the right and the left atrium.

Anatomically, the right atrium is located anteriorly and the left atrium posteriorly. Since the SA node is situated more or less at the right upper posterior portion of the right atrium, the direction of the spread of the wave is thus mainly from above downward, from the right toward the left, and at first toward the front (when the right atrium is activated) and then toward the back (when the left atrium is activated). If the initial right atrial forces are represented by a mean spatial vector, P_1 (Fig. 3.3A), the vector will be directed inferiorly, slightly toward the left and anteriorly. If the combined right and left atrial force which follows is represented by the spatial vector P_2, the vector will be pointed inferiorly, more to the left, either slightly anteriorly or slightly posteriorly. The late left atrial force may be represented by the spatial vector P_3, which is directed inferiorly, further to the left and posteriorly. It is to be emphasized that there are actually numerous vectors at any given time and the activation process is continuous. Only three vectors are described here for the sake of simplicity. The changing course of the vectors inscribe a loop which is the spatial P loop, or PsÊ loop.

In the transverse plane projection (Fig. 3.3B), the anteroposterior and right–left components of the spatial vectors are viewed. Since all the vectors are oriented to the

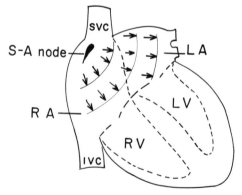

Fig. 3.2. Simplified diagram of the heart viewed from the front. From the SA node, the radial spread of the waves of atrial activation, and the vectors representing the activation potentials are indicated.

left and the early vector is anterior and the late vector is posterior, the course of the vectors inscribes a counterclockwise loop. In the right sagittal plane projection the anterposterior and the superior–inferior components of the vectors are viewed. The early anterior and inferior and the late posterior and inferior directions of the vectors inscribe a clockwise loop. In the frontal plane the superior–inferior and right–left components are viewed. Since all the vectors are directed inferiorly, the increasing leftward direction of the successive vectors results in a counterclockwise loop.

VENTRICULAR ACTIVATION AND THE QRS VECTOR LOOP

The activation process in the ventricles is closely related to a specialized conduction system (Fig. 3.4). The system consists of the atrioventricular node (AV node), atrioventricular bundle (bundle of His), the bundle branches, and the peripheral Purkinje fibers. The AV node lies in the lower and distal part of the floor of the right atrium between the orifice of the coronary sinus and the medial leaflet of the tricuspid valve. From the AV node the fibers of the bundle of His proceed

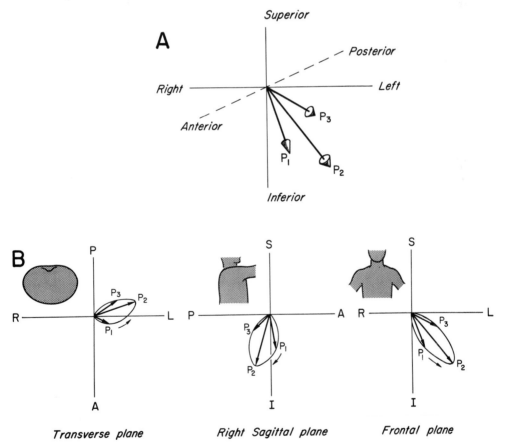

Fig. 3.3.   The P_1, P_2, and P_3 represent the three mean spatial vectors of the atrial activation potentials as described in the text.   (B)   The planar projections of the spatial vectors and the P loops they inscribe are shown.

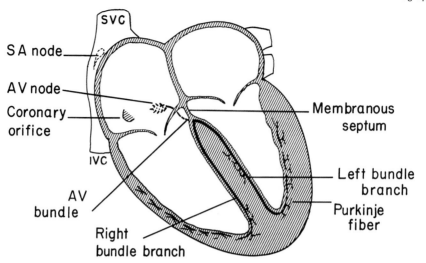

Fig. 3.4. Schematic diagram of the atrioventricular conduction system as viewed in the frontal section.

anteriorly and inferiorly and can be divided into two portions. The proximal segment is called the *penetrating portion*. It penetrates the central fibrous body which is an area of fibrous tissue bounded by the left and right atrioventricular annuli and the aortic annulus. The distal segment is called the *branching portion* which travels along the lower edge of the membranous interventricular septum to its distal angle. From this portion the fibers of the left and right bundle branches are given off and descend subendocardially on each side of the muscular interventricular septum. The right bundle branch remains as a distinct cord until it reaches the base of the anterior papillary muscle of the right ventricle, where it begins to arborize (Fig. 3.5). Its

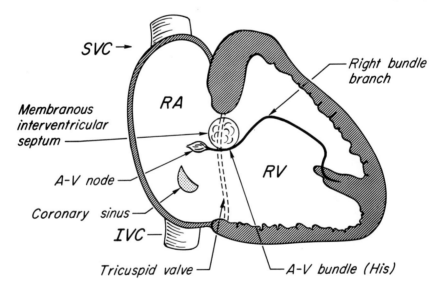

Fig. 3.5. Schematic diagram of the heart opened from the right to depict the AV node, the AV bundle, the right bundle branch and their relation to the other structures of the heart.

branches supply the subendocardial Purkinje fibers to the lower portion of the right septum and the right ventricular wall. The left bundle branch, in contrast, gives rise to two divisions soon after its origin (Fig. 3.6). They are called the *anterior* (or superior) and *posterior* (or inferior) *divisions*. In some cases the main left bundle branch cannot be identified and the two divisions branch off from the bundle of His directly. Both divisions are actually radiations consisting of fine fasciculi which fan out beneath the endocardium and become continuous with the network of Purkinje fibers. The anterior division sweeps across the outflow tract of the left ventricle toward the base of the anterior papillary muscle. Its fibers supply the myocardium of the anterolateral wall of the left ventricle. The posterior division proceeds posteriorly and inferiorly toward the base of the posterior papillary muscle. Its fibers are continuous with the Purkinje network which supplies the myocardium of the posterior and inferior wall of the left ventricle. It is believed that there is rather deep penetration of the Purkinje fibers into the inner part of the ventricular wall. The left ventricular septum is supplied by fibers from both the anterior and posterior divisions as well as some fibers directly from the bundle of His. However, very few Purkinje fibers have been demonstrated in the basal portion of the septum and the posterobasal portion of the left ventricle. This finding is quite significant in view of the sequence of the ventricular activation.

The atrial activation impulse is received at the AV node and travels rapidly through the AV conduction system to the subendocardial layer of the ventricles. The conduction through the Purkinje fibers is estimated to have a speed of 2.5 meters/sec. In the area of the myocardium where the Purkinje fibers are absent, the spread of excitation has a much slower speed of about 0.3 meter/sec.

It has been generally agreed that the ventricular activation begins at the middle third of the left septal surface (Fig. 3.7A). From there the impulse spreads in a rightward direction. Shortly afterwards the activation also begins on the right septal

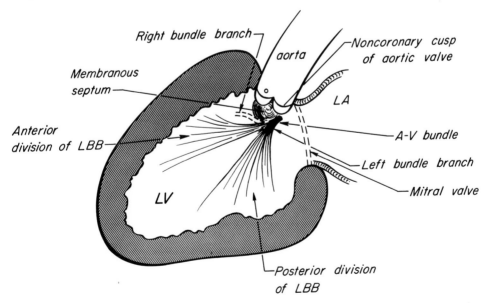

Fig. 3.6. The heart is opened from the left to depict the two divisions of the left bundle branch.

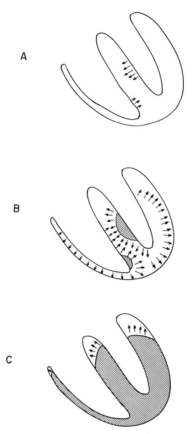

Fig. 3.7. Sequence of the ventricular activation and the vectors representing the activation potentials (see text).

surface near the base of the anterior papillary muscle, and the impulse spreads leftward. Since a much larger area of the left septum is depolarized in comparison to that of the right septum, the net effect of the septal activation is from the left toward the right.

Recent investigation by Durer and associates in isolated human hearts has given further details in regard to the initial ventricular activation. According to their data three endocardial areas are synchronously excited at the beginning of the left ventricular activation (Fig. 3.8):

1. An area high on the anterior paraseptal wall just below the attachment of the mitral valve extending toward the apex into the region of the anterior papillary muscle.
2. The central area on the left surface of the interventricular septum.
3. The posterior paraseptal area at about one-third of the distance from apex to base.

They believe that fibers from the anterior division of the left bundle branch are probably responsible for the excitation of the anterior paraseptal region as well as the mid septum. The activation of the posterior paraseptal region is provided by fibers from the posterior division of the left bundle branch. The upper part of the anterior wall of the left ventricle near the septum is oriented anteriorly, leftward, and superiorly (Fig. 3.9). The posterior paraseptal area is directed posteriorly, rightward, and inferiorly. The forces generated from the endocardial to epicardial activation of these two areas are therefore in the opposite directions and are mostly neutralized by each other. The net effect of early left ventricular excitation is determined, in most instances, by the midseptal region.

Soon after the beginning of the septal and paraseptal activation, the impulse arrives at most of the subendocardial layer of the myocardium of the apical and free wall of both ventricles through the Purkinje network (Figs. 3.7B and 3.8). Within the inner layers of the ventricular wall, because of the deep penetration of the Purkinje fibers into the myocardium, the activation waves spread in all directions. Consequently, their effects cancel each other and very little potential can be detected outside the area. The thickness of the layers to be activated in this manner has been

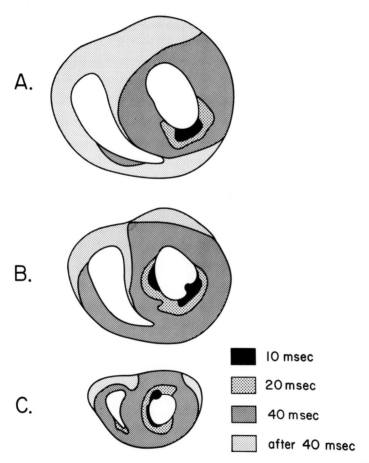

■ 10 msec

▒ 20 msec

▨ 40 msec

□ after 40 msec

Fig. 3.8. Sequence of the ventricular activation in isolated human heart as viewed in sections perpendicular to the long axis of the heart. Section B is at the level of midseptum; A, upper part of the septum toward the base; C, lower part of the septum toward the apex. (Adapted from Durrer et al.)

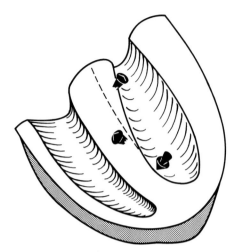

Fig. 3.9. Spatial vectors representing the initial activation potentials in the three areas of the left ventricle described in the text.

estimated to be one-third to two-thirds of the entire wall. In the outer layers of the ventricles the impulse spreads uniformly in the endocardial to epicardial direction. Because of the much larger muscle mass of the left ventricle, the result of its activity dominates that of the right ventricle.

The last regions of the ventricle to be depolarized are the basal portion of the septum and the posterobasal portion of the free wall of the left ventricle (Figs. 3.7C and 3.8). The late arrival of the impulse can easily be explained by the rarity of the Purkinje fibers in these areas. The general direction of the spread of the impulse in the ventricular wall is outward and backward. In the basal septum the wave proceeds toward the base and is from the left to the right.

If the sequence of ventricular activation is simplified and arbitrarily divided into three phases, it can be represented by three vectors. The initial phase, which is represented by vector 1 in Figure 3.10A, concerns the early septal and paraseptal activation. As stated previously, the effect of early left ventricular excitation is essentially determined by the forces from the midseptum. The interventricular septum has an anatomical position such that its right septal surface is facing the front and the right side. Depending on whether the heart is in a vertical or horizontal position, the right septal surface may be oriented either slightly upward or downward. Thus, the essentially left-to-right activation of the septum results in a vector which is directed anteriorly, to the right, either slightly superiorly or inferiorly (vector 1). Vector 2 represents the second phase which is the activation of the free wall of the ventricles. Since the left ventricle lies in a more posterior and inferior position than the right ventricle, a normally dominant left ventricular force would result in a vector (vector 2) which is directed to the left, inferiorly, and posteriorly. Vector 3 represents the terminal phase of the activation of the basal portion of the heart. The vector is oriented posteriorly, either slightly to the left or to the right, because of the generally apex-to-base direction of movement of the activation impulse in this region.

If the course of the successive vectors representing the ventricular depolarization (only three of which are described above) is traced, a spatial loop is formed which is the QRSsÊ loop. Except for its early and terminal portions, the great majority of the QRSsÊ loop occupies a leftward, inferior, and posterior position in the three-dimensional space. When the spatial loop is projected on the transverse plane, the early anterior, then leftward, followed by the later posterior directions of the vectors inscribe a counterclockwise loop (Fig. 3.10B). In the right sagittal plane, the early anterior, then inferior, followed by the late posterior directions of the vectors result in a loop which is inscribed clockwise. In the frontal plane the direction of inscription of the QRS loop may be either clockwise or counterclockwise and usually depends on whether the heart is in a vertical or a horizontal position.

VENTRICULAR REPOLARIZATION AND THE T VECTOR LOOP

The sequence of ventricular repolarization has not been elucidated in detail because of technical difficulties. Normally, it is probably not a uniformly propagated phenomenon. Several local factors, such as pressure and temperature, have been thought to control the rate and sequence of repolarization. From indirect evidence

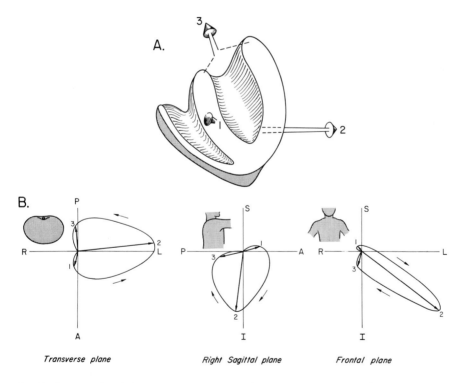

Fig. 3.10. (A) Spatial vector 1 represents the resultant force of the initial septal and paraseptal activation; vector 2, the resultant force of the activation of the free wall of the ventricles; and vector 3, the basal portions of the ventricles. (B) The planar projections of the spatial vectors and the QRS loop they inscribe are shown.

the overall direction of "pathway" of the normal repolarization is from the epicardium toward the endocardium, opposite to that of the depolarization. Since the direction of the vector representing the potential of repolarization is opposite to that of the movement of the repolarization process, the **T** vectors of ventricular repolarization are thus oriented in an endocardium-to-epicardium direction. In fact, the **T** vector loop normally has a spatial orientation quite similar to that of the QRS loop. In the plane projections the direction of inscription of the QRS and T loops in the three planes are usually the same.

References

1. Amer NS, Stuckey JH, Hoffman BF, Cappelletti RR, Domingo RT: Activation of the interventricular septal myocardium studied during cardiopulmonary bypass. Am Heart J 59:224, 1960
2. Durrer D, vanDam RT, Freud GE, Janse MJ, Meijler FL, Arzbaecher RC: Total excitation of the isolated human heart. Circulation 41:899, 1970
3. Hudson REB: Surgical pathology of the conducting system of the heart. Br Heart J 29:646, 1967
4. James TN, Sherf L: Specialized tissues and preferential conduction in the atria of the heart. Am J Cardiol 28:414, 1971
5. Kennamer R, Bernstein JL, Maxwell MH, Prinzmetal M, Shaw CM: Studies on the mechanism of ventricular activity. V. Intramural depolarization potentials in the normal heart with a consideration of currents of injury in coronary artery disease. Am Heart J 46:379, 1953
6. Lev M: Anatomic basis for atrioventricular block. Am J Med 37:742, 1964
7. Lewis T, Meakins J, White PD: The excitatory process in the dog's heart. Part I: The auricles. Phil Trans R Soc 205B:375, 1914
8. Lewis T, Rothschild MA: The excitatory process in the dog's heart. II. The ventricles. Philos Trans R Soc Lond 206B:181, 1915
9. Puech P, Esclavissat M, Sodi-Pallares D, Cisneros F: Normal auricular activation in the dog's heart. Am Heart J 47:175, 1954
10. Rosenbaum MB, Elizari MV, Lazzari JO: The Hemiblocks. Oldsmar, Florida, Tampa Tracings, 1970 p 18
11. Scher AM: Excitation of the heart, in Hamilton WF (ed): Handbook of Physiology, Section 2: The Ciruclation, vol. 1., Washington, D.C., American Physiological Society, 1962, p 287
12. Scher AM: The sequence of ventricular excitation. Am J Cardiol 14:287, 1964
13. Sodi-Pallares D, Calder RM: New Bases of Electrocardiography. St. Louis, Mosby, 1956, p 388
14. Van Dam RT, Durrer D: The T wave and ventricular repolarization. Am J Cardiol 14:294, 1964

4

Terminology and Method of Analysis
Derivation of the Scalar Leads

As in the conventional electrocardiogram, systematic analysis of the vectorcardiogram is important in making a correct interpretation. In this chapter some of the frequently used terminologies and measurements will be defined and the method of their determination described. Many of the less frequently used terms will be mentioned later when the abnormalities in which they are useful are discussed. A complete description and measurement of all the characteristics is time consuming and often unrewarding for clinical purpose. However, it is very useful for the beginners to be familiar with them, and as one gains experience, many of the characteristics can be obtained by a simple glance, and only a very few measurements actually have to be quantitated.

E POINT (ISOELECTRIC POINT, NULL POINT) (FIG. 4.1,B)

The E point on the vectorcardiogram is that point where the electron beam of the oscilloscope remains stationary for a period of time before it begins to inscribe the P loop. It corresponds to the isoelectric line between the T (or U) wave and the succeeding P wave in the scalar electrocardiogram. The coordinate axes X, Y, and Z pass through the E point. The three perpendicular planes—transverse, sagittal, and frontal—intersect at the E point and form eight octants in three-dimensional space.

Since the electron beam of the oscilloscope remains stationary at the E point for a much longer time than is required for the inscription of the other portions of the vectorcardiogram, its photographed image is often very bright and obscures the adjacent part of the P, QRS, and T loops. The difficulty can be partly avoided either by magnifying the E point area or by shifting the E point electronically during the isoelectric period. Most commercially available vectorcardiographs have incorporated a circuit which automatically adjusts the brightness of the electron beam according to its speed of movement. The intensity of the beam decreases as the velocity of the beam diminishes and increases as the beam travels more rapidly. The design substantially improves the clarity of the records.

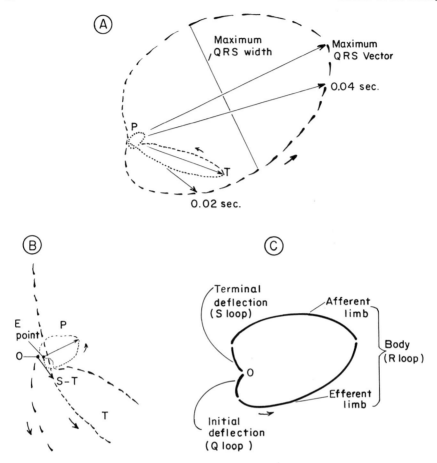

Fig. 4.1. (A) Schematic diagram of the P, QRS and T loops illustrating some of the parameters mentioned in the text. (B) Enlargement of the area surrounding the E point of (A). (C) The various portions of the QRS loop.

The beam is usually interrupted at a certain interval so as to provide a means of timing. As a result of the interruptions, dashes or tear drops are formed. In this text the tear drops appear at intervals of either 2 or, less often, 2.5 msec. The blunt end of the tear drop indicates the leading end and provides a means for determining the direction of the inscription of the loops.

P VECTOR LOOP (FIG. 4.1,A,B)

The spatial loop of atrial activation is usually called the *Ps$\hat{E}$ loop:* E equals equivalent cardiac dipole; $\hat{E}$ equals E expressed as vector quantity; s$\hat{E}$ equals $\hat{E}$ expressed as spatial vector quantity. Its planar projections are called the *P loops*, such as the transverse plane P loop, right sagittal plane P loop or frontal plane P loop.

The information obtained from the P loop includes the configuration and direction of inscription of the P loop, the magnitude and direction of the maximum **P** vector, and the location of the major portion of the loop. Because of the small magnitude of the P loop, detailed information is difficult to obtain, and great magnification is usually necessary. The methodology of obtaining some of the above measurements is similar to that applied to the QRS loop, which will be described later.

The effect of atrial repolarization is manifested by the failure of the P loop to close. It is represented by the *atrial T* (**Ta**) *vector.* A straight line drawn from the beginning of the P loop to the end of the P loop gives the magnitude and direction of the **Ta** vector. Depending on the duration of the PR interval, part of the atrial repolarization potential may be obscured by the much larger initial QRS forces.

The *PR interval* cannot be measured in the vectorcardiogram since most of the PR segment is isoelectric, and the beam remains stationary during that period.

QRS VECTOR LOOP (FIG. 4.1,A,B,C)

The spatial loop of ventricular depolarization is called the $QRSs\hat{E}$ *loop.* Its planar projections are called the QRS *loops,* such as the transverse plane QRS loop, right sagittal plane QRS loop, and frontal plane QRS loop.

Analysis of the QRS loop may begin with the general morphology of the loop, such as its configuration, contour, and the presence or absence of distortion. Its orientation and direction of inscription (clockwise or counterclockwise) are determined. The speed of inscription is indicated by the distance between the tear drops. Closely spaced tear drops indicate a slow rate of inscription, and widely spaced and elongated tear drops mean that the speed of inscription is rapid. However, a definite conclusion as to the speed of inscription cannot be made until all the three planes have been studied, since a normally inscribed loop may appear to be slowly inscribed in a plane which is perpendicular to the direction of the movement.

The QRS loop may be divided into several portions for the convenience of description. The *initial deflection,* inscribed by the initial vectors or forces, is sometimes also called the *Q loop* and is arbitrarily defined as the very first deflection of the QRS loop before the loop changes its direction. It usually represents the first 10 to 15 msec of the QRS interval. The *body* of the QRS loop constitutes the major portion of the loop and is sometimes called the *R loop.* It consists of the efferent (centrifugal) and the afferent (centripetal) limbs. These two parts of the body are usually separated by an easily recognizable turning point. The *terminal deflection* (terminal forces, terminal appendage, S loop) refers to the last portion of the QRS loop when it returns toward its origin. It ends at the J point from where the T loop begins. The J point may or may not coincide with the origin of the QRS loop.

After the morphologic characteristics of the QRS loop are obtained, the interpreter may proceed with some quantitative measurements. The *maximum* **QRS** *vector* is sometimes called the *long axis of the QRS loop.* It is the vector which is drawn from the point of origin of the QRS loop (point O) to its most remote point. Although the maximum **QRS** vectors in the three planes usually represent the planar projections of the same maximum *spatial* **QRS** vector, this is by no means always true. If the maximum spatial vector is more or less perpendicular to the plane on which the projection is made, the vector will be foreshortened and may not appear to be the long axis of the loop in that particular plane. Thus it is important to

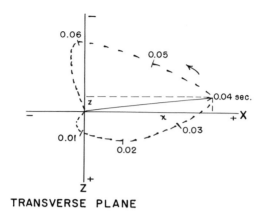

TRANSVERSE PLANE

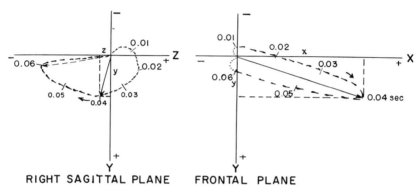

RIGHT SAGITTAL PLANE   FRONTAL PLANE

Fig. 4.2. Diagrams illustrating the methods to identify the same vector in the three planes by either the time of occurrence of the vector or by the magnitude of its projections on the X, Y, and Z axes.

distinguish between the planar projection of the maximum spatial **QRS** vector and the maximum vector of the given planar projection. Since our aim is to study the spatial vector, effort should be directed toward identifying the projections of the same maximal spatial vector in all three planes. Throughout the text the term *maximum* **QRS** *vector* will be used, unless otherwise specified, to indicate the projection of the maximum spatial vector in a plane.

Accurate identification of the maximum spatial vector or its projection is sometimes difficult from the clinical vectorcardiogram. The use of a lead resolver as designed by Schmitt, or a rather complicated mathematical calculation, may be necessary for such a purpose. However, in the great majority of instances, the largest **QRS** vector among the three planes does represent or approximate the projection of the maximum spatial vector. The corresponding vectors in the other two planes can be identified by noting the time of occurrence of the vector, or by measuring the magnitudes of their projections on the X, Y, and Z axes. If the vectors in the planar projections represent the same spatial vector, the magnitude of their X, Y, or Z component in one plane should be identical to that obtained from another plane. An example is given in Figure 4.2. The largest **QRS** vector in the three planar projections is the 0.04-sec vector in the transverse plane, which is also found to be the projection of the maximum spatial QRS vector by the more elaborate methods mentioned above. Thus the same vector can easily be identified in the other two planes by determining the time interval. It is apparent that although the 0.04-sec vector is also the largest QRS vector in the frontal plane, such is not the case in the right sagittal plane. In the latter projection the 0.06-sec vector is the largest one, instead. This is because the maximum spatial vector (i.e., 0.04-sec vector) is more perpendicular to the right sagittal plane and is foreshortened to a much greater extent than the 0.06-sec vector. A measurement of the X, Y, and Z components of the planar vectors x, y, and z also shows that the 0.04-sec vector in the right sagittal plane has a y identical to the y of the 0.04-sec vector in the frontal plane, and a z identical to the z of the 0.04-sec vector in the transverse plane.

The instantaneous vectors at various intervals (e.g., 0.02, 0.04, or 0.06-sec vector) can be measured by joining the origin of the QRS loop (O point) with the distal end of the dash corresponding to the end of the period (Fig. 4.1A). Great care should be exercised in the determination of the initial vectors. The dashes usually travel slowly and may not be clearly separated from each other. Any error in the determination would propagate itself and affect the rest of the measurements. It is usually advisable to examine all of the planes to be certain that the X, Y, or Z component of the instantaneous vector in the different projections has the same magnitude.

The magnitude of a *spatial vector* can be calculated from the Pythagorean formula

$$s\hat{E} = \sqrt{E_x^2 + E_y^2 + E_z^2}$$

in which $s\hat{E}$ is the magnitude of the spatial vector and E_x, E_y, and E_z are the magnitudes of the projections of the spatial vector on leads X, Y, and Z.

The *half-area vector* represents the vector that divides the planar QRS loop into equal half-areas through the O point in each projection. It may be estimated by planimetry through trial and error. The half-area vector has been claimed to approximate closely the *mean* **QRS** *vector* (**ÂQRS**), which is the average direction and magnitude of all the instantaneous vectors during the QRS interval.

The *maximum QRS width* is obtained by drawing lines perpendicular to the maximum QRS vector. The longest distance between the two points of intersection of the QRS loop with the perpendicular line is the maximum width of the loop.

ST VECTOR (FIG. 4.1B)

The **ST** vector is the vector joining the origin of the QRS loop to the beginning of the T loop (J point). Unless the magnitude of the **ST** vector is abnormally increased, the vector can only be identified after great amplification.

T VECTOR LOOP (FIG. 4.1,A)

The spatial loop of the ventricular repolarization is called the *Ts$\hat{E}$ loop*. Its planar projections are called the *T loops*. The configuration, the direction and speed of inscription of the loop, the direction and magnitude of the maximum **T** vector, and the maximum width of the loop are determined by the method described for the QRS loop. In the determination of the direction and magnitude of the maximum **T** vector the E point instead of the beginning of the T loop (J point) is used because the latter is often displaced by the **ST** vector.

The *QRS-T angle* theoretically should represent the angle subtended by the mean **QRS** and **T** vectors (**ÂQRS, ÂT**). Because of the difficulty in obtaining the values for the mean vectors, the maximum **QRS** and **T** vectors are often used to calculate the angle. The spatial QRS-T angle may be determined by using the table prepared by one of the authors (Helm).

Although the U wave of the vectorcardiogram can occasionally be seen as a small loop after the T loop, in the great majority of instances it cannot be clearly identified.

DERIVATION OF THE SCALAR ELECTROCARDIOGRAM FROM THE VECTORCARDIOGRAM

The scalar leads that are commonly recorded can be derived from the vectorcardiogram with a reasonable degree of accuracy. After a little practice this can be accomplished readily. The exercise not only serves to correlate the vectorcardiogram with the scalar electrocardiogram but also promotes the understanding of both. One who is more experienced in the interpretation of the scalar electrocardiogram can often improve his ability in the interpretation of the spatial vectorcardiogram by means of the analysis. In the following paragraphs the method of the derivation of the QRS complex from the QRS loop will be illustrated. The same method can be applied to derive the P and T waves from the P and T loops.

The derivation of any given scalar lead contained in a given plane may begin by drawing the lead axis through the origin (point O) of the QRS loop (Fig. 4.3). Another line (zero line) is then drawn through the point O perpendicular to the lead axis.* The polarity of the lead axis is noted. The origin of the loop corresponds to a point on the isoelectric line of the scalar lead. Any portion of the loop which is on the positive side of the axis of derivation will inscribe a positive deflection in the scalar electrocardiogram, and any portion which is on the negative side of the axis will give a negative deflection. As the instantaneous vectors inscribe the loop, their projections on the lead axis give the magnitude of the deflection of the QRS complex in the scalar lead. If the magnitude of the deflection is plotted on an ordinate against its time of occurrence indicated on an abscissa, a QRS complex will be formed. Thus in Figure 4.3 the projections of the instantaneous vectors **OQ, OR,** and **OS** (i.e., **Oq, Or,** and **Os** respectively) are used sequentially to outline the scalar lead QRS complex. The accuracy of the derivation will be improved as more points on the vector loop are transplanted on the scalar lead.

The method described above can readily be applied to derive the orthogonal leads, *X, Y,* and *Z* from the planar projections of the spatial loop. The procedure is actually the dissolution of the vector loop into its component parts. The transverse

---

*Strictly speaking, point O is slightly separated from the isoelectric point (E point) because of the atrial **T** vector, but the displacement is small and can therefore be ignored for this purpose.

plane is the vectorial sum of leads X and Z, the sagittal plane, the sum of leads Y and Z, and the frontal plane X and Y. Since the corrected orthogonal lead systems, such as the Frank system, are so designed that their X, Y, and Z leads are nearly perpendicular to each other and are of uniform strength, it is thus justifiable to use the geometrically orthogonal axes as the lead axes of derivation. An example is given in Figure 4.4. Since the X, Y, and Z components are all used twice in the formation of the transverse, sagittal, and frontal planes, only two planes are needed to obtain the three orthogonal leads.

The standard and unipolar limb leads (leads I, II, III, aVL, aVR, and aVF) can be approximately derived from the frontal plane projection of the spatial loop.

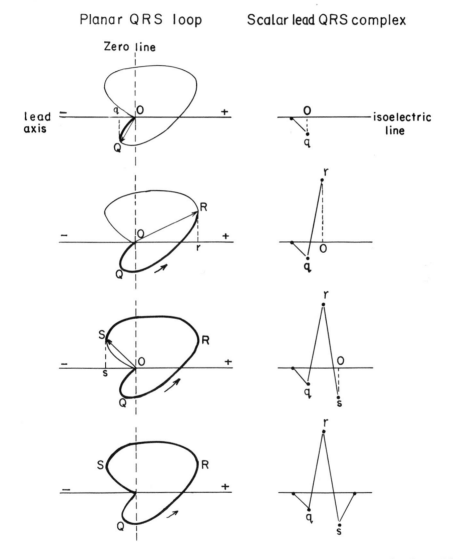

Fig. 4.3. The derivation of the scalar QRS complex in any given lead from the planar QRS loop.

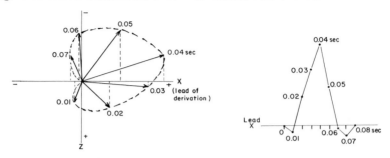

Ⓐ Derivation of the Orthogonal lead X from the Transverse Plane QRS loop

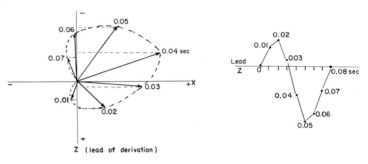

Ⓑ Derivation of the Orthogonal lead Z from the Transverse Plane QRS loop

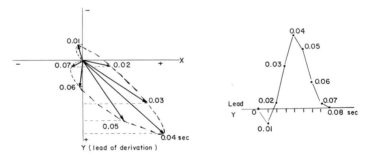

Ⓒ Derivation of the Orthogonal lead Y from the Frontal Plane QRS loop

Fig. 4.4. The derivation of the orthogonal leads X, Y, and Z from the planar loops.

Customarily, the hexaxial reference system based on Einthoven's equilateral triangle with the addition of the unipolar limb leads has been used (Fig. 4.5). The lead axes are equally separated from each other by 30°, and the lead axes are assumed to possess equal strength. However, since the advent of the concept of lead vectors by Burger and Van Milaan, it has generally been recognized that the scalene triangle, as they have defined it, more accurately represents the lead axes of the standard limb leads. Thus it becomes apparent that better results can be obtained for the lead derivation by using a reference system which is based on the Burger triangle (Fig. 4.6 A and B). Langner, taking into consideration both the direction and the magnitude of the lead vectors, has devised a hexaxial system based on the Burger's triangle with the addition of the "proportionality factors" (Fig. 4.6 C). The use of the "proportionality factors" is necessary to compensate for the unequal strength of the various leads. For example, when the same unit potential is applied to lead I and lead III, the magnitude of the deflection in lead III is twice of that in lead I. In the reference system the lead axes are scaled according to the "proportionality factors" so that the different degrees of amplification in the various leads can be realized. Thus, if the length of the scale unit on lead I is 1.0, the length of the unit on lead III is 0.5. The factors for the other leads are lead II = 0.6, lead aVL = 0.8, lead aVR = 1.1, and lead aVF = 0.6. Figure 4.7 gives an example in which the standard unipolar limb leads are derived from a normal frontal plane QRS loop using the improved hexaxial reference system. As can be seen, the configuration and relative magnitude of the deflections in the derived complexes are quite similar to those actually recorded.

The lead axes corresponding to the precordial leads are indicated in Figure 4.8 and are based on the study of Abildskov and Wilkinson. The lead axes actually are not in the same plane. Lead V_1 is directed slightly upward, and the axes gradually shift downward from V_1 through V_6. However, none of the axes deviates signifi-

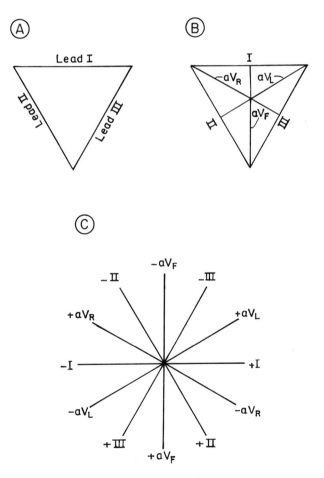

Fig. 4.5. (A) Einthoven's equilateral triangle formed by leads I, II, and III. (B) The unipolar limb leads are added to the equilateral triangle. (C) The hexaxial reference system derived from (B).

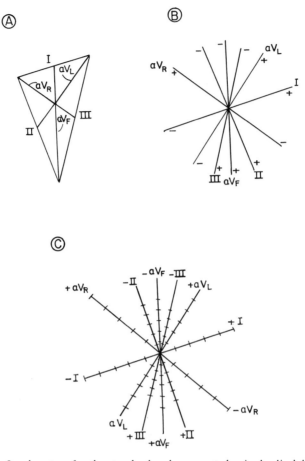

Fig. 4.6. (A) Lead vectors for the standard and augmented unipolar limb leads. (B) The lead vectors in (A) are rearranged in the form of a hexaxial reference system. (C) The hexaxial reference system with the addition of the units according to the "proportionality factors" for vector projection (after Langner)

cantly from the transverse plane, and for practical purpose the precordial leads can be derived with a reasonable degree of accuracy from the transverse plane loop by using the lead axes as shown.

DERIVATION OF THE VECTORCARDIOGRAM FROM THE SCALAR LEADS

The derivation of the vectorcardiogram from the orthogonal leads X, Y, and Z may be accomplished easily as the planar vectors are merely the vectoral sum of their orthogonal components. The transverse, sagittal, and frontal plane vector loops are the result of interaction of leads X and Z, Y and Z, and X and Y, respectively. However, the orthogonal leads should be recorded simultaneously and preferably with rapid paper speed. Otherwise the temporal relationship of the various portions of the scalar complexes in the two component leads cannot be determined accurately and the vector loop so derived may differ significantly from the vectorcardiogram obtained by electronic synthesis.

The plotting of vector loop from the conventional scalar electrocardiogram may also be done but usually with much less accuracy. For example, leads V_2 and V_6 may be used for the transverse plane as they resemble the orthogonal leads Z and X, respectively. Similarly, leads I and aVF, V_2 and aVF may be used for the construction of the frontal and sagittal planes as lead I also resembles lead X, and

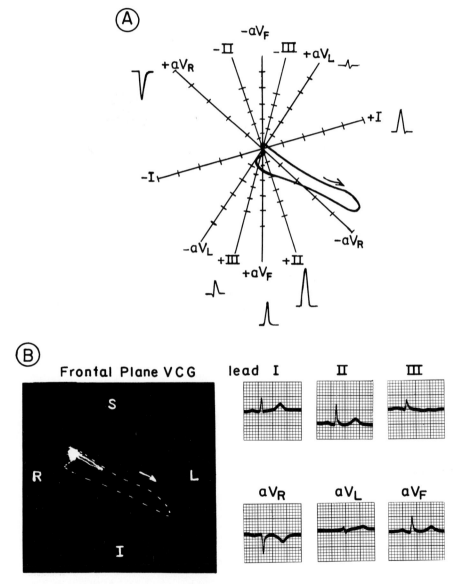

Fig. 4.7. (A) The standard and unipolar limb lead QRS complexes as derived from the frontal plane QRS loop using the improved hexaxial reference system. (B) The frontal plane vectorcardiogram and the standard and unipolar limb leads as actually recorded.

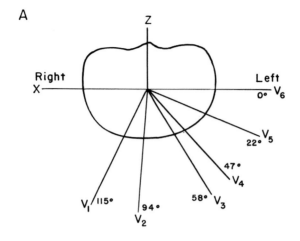

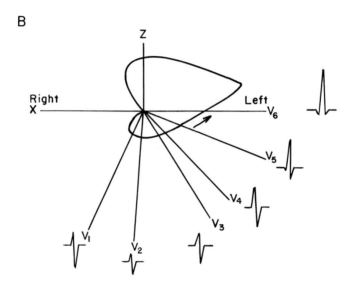

Fig. 4.8. (A) Lead axes corresponding to the precordial leads V_1 through V_6. (B) Derivation of the precordial leads QRS complexes from the transverse plane QRS loop by using the reference system shown in (A).

lead aVF, lead Y. Since the conventional leads are seldom recorded simultaneously in the routine tracing, the vector loop obtained in this fashion is often inaccurate. The configuration and course of the vector loop depend a great deal on the time relationship of the component leads. Valuable information may therefore be lost during the process.

REFERENCES

1. Abildskov JA, Wilkinson RS Jr: The relation of precordial and orthogonal leads. Circulation 27:58, 1963
2. Burger HC, Van Milaan JB: Heart vector and leads. I. Br Heart J 8:157, 1946. II. Ibid 9:154, 1947. III. Ibid 10:229, 1948
3. Helm RA, Fowler NO Jr: A simplified method for determining the angle between two spatial vectors. Am Heart J 45:835, 1953
4. Langner PH Jr: An octaxial reference system derived from a nonequilateral triangle for frontal plane vectorcardiography. Am Heart J 49:696, 1955
5. Pipberger HV: Evaluation of quantitative methods for obtaining mean spatial QRS vectors. Circulation 16:926, 1957
6. Schmitt OH; Cathode-ray presentation of three dimensional data. J Appl Physics 18:819, 1947

5

The Normal Vectorcardiogram

The general configuration of the P, QRS, and T loops has been briefly mentioned and correlated with the normal atrial and ventricular activation processes in Chapter 3. In this chapter the various characteristics of the normal vectorcardiogram recorded with the Frank lead system will be described. The majority of the information is based on a group of 200 normal adults studied by the author. The age of the subjects ranged from 20 to 59 years.

THE PsÊ LOOP

The average normal adult spatial P loop is a small elongated loop requiring great magnification to study its characteristics in detail. The spatial loop is oriented inferiorly, to the left, and either slightly anteriorly or slightly posteriorly. It is often marked by one or more small incisurae or angulations. Because of the atrial repolarization potential, the loop does not close. It ends at a point (O point) superior and slightly posterior and to the right of its origin (E point). Thus the direction of the spatial atrial T vector (**Ta** vector) is usually opposite to the direction of the PsÊ loop itself.

Transverse plane. Among the three planar projections (Fig. 5.1), the transverse plane P loop is usually the smallest in size and presents a variety of configurations. It is oriented to the left with part of it anteriorly and the other part posteriorly located. In the majority of instances it is inscribed in a counterclockwise direction. However, the loop often has a figure-of-eight contour with the proximal part inscribed counterclockwise and the distal part clockwise. The average direction of the planar maximum **P** vector* is —5° with a normal range of —50° to 60°. Its magnitude does not exceed 0.1 mV. The **Ta** vector is oriented to the right and posteriorly and is very small so that the loop often appears to be closed.

---

* Because the P loop is small and may be irregular in configuration, its maximum spatial vector is often difficult to determine. The maximum planar vector instead of the planar projection of the maximum spatial vector is used.

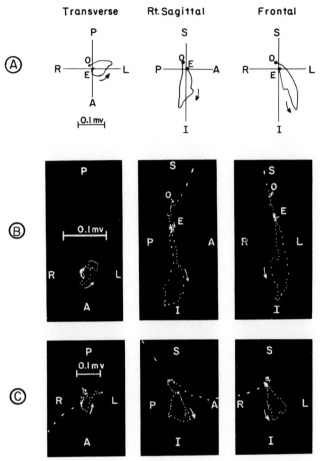

Fig. 5.1. (A) Diagrams of the planar projections of a normal PsÊ loop. (B and C) The planar projections of the PsÊ loops of two normal subjects in which the P loops are "dissected" from the rest of the vectorcardiogram except for a portion of the QRS loop.

Table 5.1

The Direction and Magnitude of the Maximum **P** Vector in Normal Subjects

Plane	Direction (deg)		Magnitude (mV)	
	Mean	95% range*	Mean	95% range*
Transverse	−5	−50—60	0.07	0.04—0.10
Right sagittal	85	50—110	0.12	0.04—0.18
Frontal	65	15—90	0.12	0.06—0.20

    * Throughout the text the 95 percent range given in this and Tables 5.2 and 5.3 will be used as the normal limits.

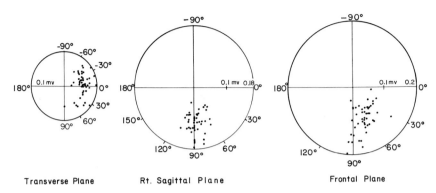

Fig. 5.2. Scattergrams illustrating the magnitude and direction of the maximum **P** vector in 50 normal subjects.

Right sagittal plane. The right sagittal plane P loop is elongated and oval, or occasionally triangular, in shape. The irregularities of its contour, caused by the presence of one or more incisurae, are often well displayed in this projection. The loop is oriented inferiorly; its initial portion is anteriorly located, and its late portion posteriorly located. The loop is thus always inscribed in a clockwise direction. The maximum vector has an average direction of 85° with a normal range of 50° to 110°. The magnitude of the maximum vector is less than 0.2 mV. The **Ta** vector is directed superiorly and posteriorly, opposite to the general direction of the P loop.

Frontal plane. The frontal plane P loop is also somewhat oval in configuration and slightly irregular. It is oriented inferiorly and to the left, and is inscribed in a counterclockwise direction. The average direction of the maximum **P** vector is 65°, and the normal range is between 15° to 90°. The magnitude of the maximum vector does not exceed 0.2 mV. The **Ta** vector is directed superiorly and to the right.

The directions and magnitudes of the maximum **P** vectors in the planar projections in 194 normal subjects are summarized in Table 5.1. Figure 5.2 illustrates the distribution of the vectors in 50 of the individuals in the form of scattergrams.

THE QRSsÊ LOOP

The spatial QRS loop is the largest loop in the vectorcardiogram. Its characteristics have been studied in more detail than those of the P and T loops. The normal QRSsÊ loop has a smooth contour without any notches or irregularities. It forms an almost perfect plane of its own. If the loop is rotated so that its broadside is viewed, it has a configuration resembling that of a "heart."

The great majority of the loop is located in the left inferoposterior octant of the three-dimensional space. The initial deflection (the initial vectors, initial forces, Q loop), which represents mostly the septal and paraseptal activation, is always

NORMAL VECTORCARDIOGRAM

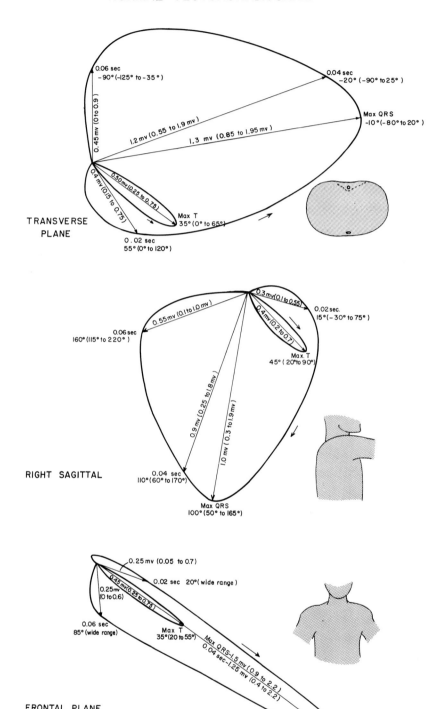

Fig. 5.3. The mean values and 95 percent ranges (in parentheses) of the various measurements of the QRS and T loops obtained from 200 normal adult subjects.

anteriorly directed. It may be oriented to the right or left, either superiorly or inferiorly. However, the anterior, superior, and rightward direction occurs in about 75 percent of the normal subjects. The body of the loop (R loop), representing the dominating left ventricular force or potential, is directed to the left, inferiorly and posteriorly, pointing to the location of the anatomic free wall of the left ventricle. The terminal deflection of the loop (terminal vectors, terminal forces, and S loop) is directed posteriorly, either slightly to the left or to the right, superiorly or inferiorly. These vectors represent the late activation of the posterobasal portion of the ventricles and interventricular septum.

The initial portion of the QRSsÊ loop is inscribed slowly for a very brief period, usually less than 20 mesc. This is followed by a comparatively rapid inscription of the main body of the QRS loop until the terminal portion. Although the slowing of the terminal inscription is quite obvious in most recordings, it seldom exceeds 30 msec in the normal person. The maximum spatial **QRS** vector is directed to the left, inferiorly, and either slightly posteriorly, or less often, slightly anteriorly. It occurs about 38 msec after the beginning of the QRS loop with a normal range of 30 to 48 msec.

Transverse plane QRS loop (Figs. 5.3 and 5.4). In the transverse plane projection the average QRS loop has the shape of a "heart" lying on its side. It is relatively wide with its width more than one-half or one-third of its length. In adults the loop is invariably inscribed in a counterclockwise direction. The initial forces or vectors are usually directed to the right and anteriorly. However, in a small group of persons (less than 15 percent), they are directed anteriorly and to the left. The leftward orientation of the initial vectors in these subjects may be the result of relatively greater contribution of forces from the anterior paraseptal area.* The main

QRS LOOP AREA

NORMAL

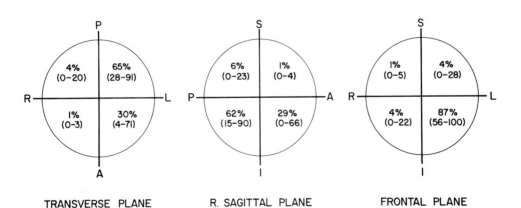

TRANSVERSE PLANE   R. SAGITTAL PLANE   FRONTAL PLANE

Fig. 5.4. The mean value and 95 percent range (in parenthesis) of the percentage of QRS loop area in the various quadrants in 198 normal subjects.

* As it was discussed in Chapter 3, during the initial phase of ventricular activation three areas of the left ventricle are simultaneously depolarized. The forces generated from the anterior and posterior paraseptal regions are essentially opposite to each other and are therefore mostly cancelled. The early QRS forces are mainly represented by those coming from the midseptum. It is conceivable that in some persons there is a greater contribution from the anterior paraseptal area. Its anterior and leftward forces may displace the resultant vectors in that direction.

Table 5.2

Some of the Characteristics of the Normal QRSsÊ Loop

Characteristic	Transverse Plane		Rt. Sagittal Plane		Frontal Plane	
	Mean	95% range	Mean	95% range	Mean	95% range
Max QRS vector						
Direction (deg)	−10	−80—20.0	100	50—165	35	10—65
Magnitude (mV)	1.30	0.85—1.95	1.0	0.3—1.9	1.50	0.9—2.2
0.02 sec vector						
Direction (deg)	55	0—120.0	15	−30—75	20	Widely scattered
Magnitude (mV)	0.40	0.15—0.75	0.30	0.1—0.55	0.25	0.05—0.7
0.04 sec vector						
Direction (deg)	−20	−90—25	110	60—170	35	−10—70
Magnitude (mV)	1.15	0.55—1.9	0.9	0.25—1.8	1.25	0.4—2.2
0.06 sec vector						
Direction (deg)	−90	−125—−35	160	115—220	85	Widely scattered
Magnitude (mV)	0.45	0—0.9	0.55	0.1—1.0	0.25	0—0.6
Time of occurrence						
of max QRS	38	30—48	Same		Same	
vector (msec)						
Direction of						
inscription	Counterclockwise		Clockwise		Clockwise 65%	
					Figure-of-eight 25%	
					Counterclockwise 10%	

body of the loop is directed to the left and slightly posteriorly. The terminal vectors are directed posteriorly and slightly to the right or left, and the loops is usually slowly inscribed just before it returns to its origin.

The maximum **QRS** vector (the projection of the maximum spatial **QRS** vector) is directed to the left with a normal range of −80° to 20°. The magnitude of the maximum vector varies from 0.85 to 1.95 mV with a mean of 1.3mV. The direction and magnitude of the other instantaneous **QRS** vectors are listed in Table 5.2. It is significant that the 0.02-sec instantaneous vector is always directed anteriorly. The values of the 0.04-sec vector are quite similar to those of the maximum vector because the majority of the latter occurs at or about 0.04 sec after the onset of the QRS loop. The 0.06-sec vector is always directed posteriorly with rather marked variation in its magnitude.

The distribution of the QRS loop area in the various quadrants, which serves to indicate whether there is any displacement of the loop, is illustrated in Figure 5.4. The average size of the area in the left posterior quadrant is about 65 percent of the total loop area and is rarely less than 30 percent in the normal adult population. The area in the right posterior quadrant does not normally exceed 20 percent of the total.

Right sagittal plane QRS loop. The QRS loop in the right sagittal projection is generally oval in shape and sometimes has the appearance of a "heart" with its

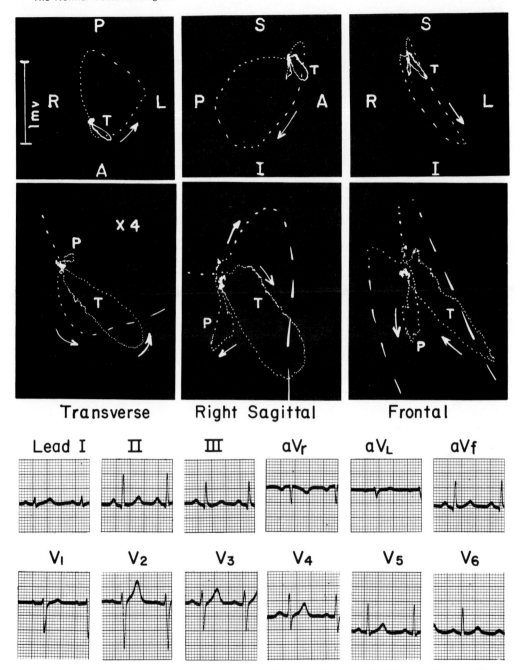

Fig. 5.5. The normal vectorcardiogram and electrocardiogram of a 39-year-old man. Note that the frontal plane QRS loop is relatively vertical and the loop is inscribed clockwise. In this and subsequent vectorcardiograms the loops are interrupted every 2 msec, and the blunt end of the "tear drop" represents the leading end.

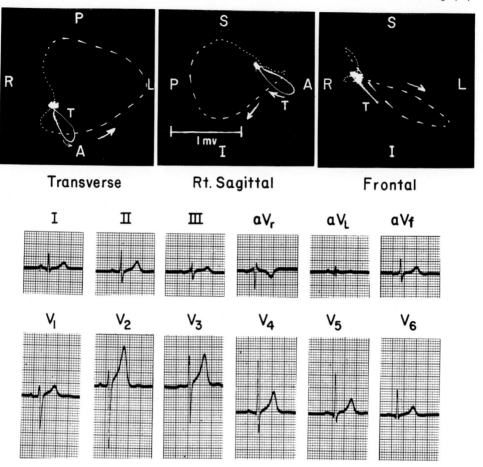

Fig. 5.6. The normal vectorcardiogram and electrocardiogram of a 36-year-old fireman.

correct side up. However, the configuration varies a great deal mostly because of the difference in the length of its vertical component. Thus, some loops appear to be wide, and others appear to be narrow. The loop is practically always inscribed in a clockwise direction. The initial forces are directed anteriorly and usually superiorly, sometimes inferiorly. The main body of the loop is directed inferiorly with most of the efferent limb located anteriorly and most of the afferent limb located posteriorly. The terminal vectors are always directed posteriorly and either superiorly or inferiorly. The terminal slowing of the inscription is also well displayed in this projection. It is particularly in this plane that the projection of the spatial maximum **QRS** vector often fails to present itself as the long axis of the planar loop. The vector representing the planar projection of the maximum spatial vector is usually directed inferiorly and slightly posteriorly. It has a normal range of 50° to 165° with a mean value of 100°. Its magnitude varies from 0.3 to 1.9 mV with an average of about 1 mV. Consistent with the finding in the transverse plane, the 0.02-sec vector is invariably directed anteriorly. The values for the 0.04-sec vector approximate those of the maximum vector. The 0.06-sec vector is oriented posteriorly with extreme variation in its magnitude.

Frontal plane QRS loop.   In contrast to the transverse and right sagittal projections, the frontal plane QRS loop is usually elongated and relatively narrow. This is because the spatial loop is more or less perpendicular to the frontal plane and is thus viewed from its side. The direction of inscription of the loop is variable. In the majority of the subjects (about 65 percent), the loop is inscribed clockwise. A figure-of-eight pattern occurs in about 25 percent and a counterclockwise inscription in 10 percent. The variability of the direction of inscription in the frontal plane can best be appreciated and explained by the use of a wire model. After the direction of inscription is labeled on the spatial loop, the loop is then viewed from its side. It is readily apparent that only a slight degree of rotation of the loop about its longitudinal axis will change the direction of inscription from clockwise to counter-clockwise or vice versa. In general, when the loop is approaching a vertical position,

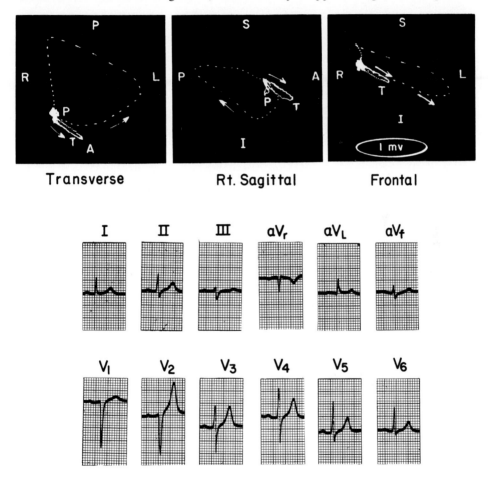

Fig. 5.7.   The normal vectorcardiogram and electrocardiogram of a healthy 52-year-old fireman. In the transverse plane the initial vectors are directed anteriorly and to the left. In the right sagittal plane they are directed anteriorly and inferiorly. The inferior and leftward orientation can also be seen in the frontal plane. The anterior, leftward, and inferior direction of the initial vectors is encountered in a relatively small group of the normal individuals. Note in the frontal plane the QRS loop is inscribed counterclockwise and the T loop clockwise.

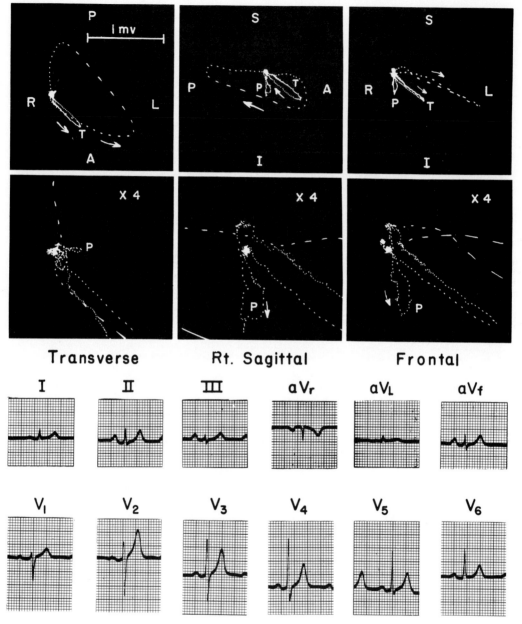

Fig. 5.8. The normal vectorcardiogram and electrocardiogram of a 43-year-old healthy fireman. The transverse plane QRS loop is relatively more anterior in location than it is in the average individual. In the frontal plane the QRS loop is more or less horizontal in orientation. However, the initial QRS loop is inscribed clockwise. Although a horizontally oriented frontal plane QRS loop is usually inscribed counterclockwise, the loop may occasionally be inscribed clockwise in some normal individuals especially if the maximum **QRS** vector is greater than 10°.

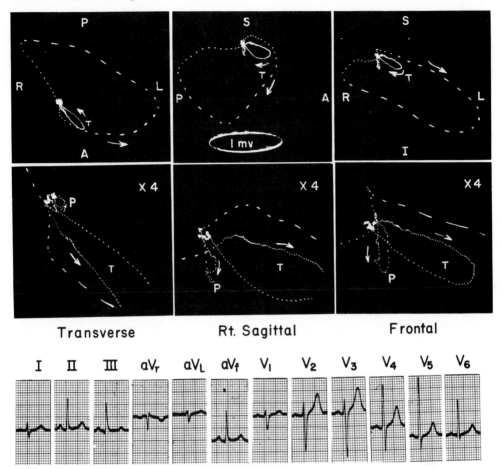

Fig. 5.9. The normal vectorcardiogram and electrocardiogram of a 27-year-old man. Note the relatively large terminal **QRS** vectors as displayed in the transverse plane. Occasionally, in some of the normal individuals, these terminal vectors become very prominent and include the maximum **QRS** vector.

it is inscribed clockwise, and when the loop is horizontal, it is inscribed counterclockwise. It is uncommon to see in the normal subjects a counterclockwise loop when the maximum **QRS** vector is greater than 40° or a clockwise loop when the maximum vector is less than 10°.

The direction of the initial deflection is widely scattered but is usually rightward and superior. The body of the loop is oriented to the left and inferiorly. The direction of the terminal deflection is also widely scattered. The average direction of the maximum **QRS** vector is 35° with a normal range of 10° to 65°. Its magnitude varies from 0.9 to 2.2 mV with a mean value of 1.50 mV. Because the initial and terminal spatial vectors are more or less perpendicular to the frontal plane, the magnitude of their projections is usually very small, and it is in the frontal plane that accurate localization of the various instantaneous vectors is technically most difficult.

As stated previously, most of the QRS loop is in the left inferior quadrant. The area in the left upper, right upper, and right lower quadrants is usually less than 30, 5, and 20 percent of the total, respectively.

Figures 5.5 to 5.9 are examples of normal vectorcardiograms illustrating the various configurations that are seen in the normal subjects.

THE ST VECTOR (FIG. 5.10)

The spatial **ST** vector is very small in normal persons. It is manifested by the failure of the QRS loop to close. It is directed anteriorly, inferiorly, and usually to the left. Thus, in the transverse plane the beginning of the T loop (J point) will appear anterior and to the left of the origin of the QRS loop (O point). In the right sagittal plane the J point is anterior and inferior to the O point and, in the frontal plane it is inferior and usually to the left of the O point. The magnitude of the **ST** vector usually does not exceed 0.1 mV in any of the projections. This is particularly true in older individuals.

THE TsÊ LOOP (FIGS. 5.3, 5.5-5.9)

The normal TsÊ loop is generally elliptical in shape. It is usually elongated and sometimes linear in configuration. It has a smooth contour. The efferent limb is always inscribed slower than the afferent limb. This characteristic corresponds to the more gradual slope of the first half of the normal T wave in the scalar electrocardiogram. The spatial T loop is usually directed to the left, inferiorly and anteriorly.

S – T Vector

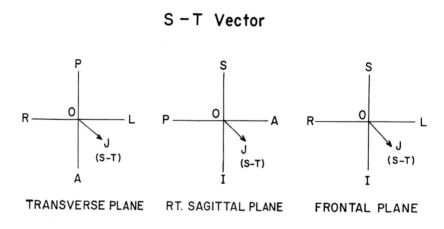

Fig. 5.10. The direction of the normal **ST** vector in the three planar projections. O represents the origin of the QRS loop and J the beginning of the T loop.

Transverse plane. In the transverse plane projection the T loop is typically inscribed in a counterclockwise direction, which is the same as that of the QRS loop in this projection. There are occasional instances in which the loop is linear, and the efferent and afferent limbs superimpose on each other. Only rarely is the loop inscribed clockwise, in which case the loop is always very narrow. The maximum **T** vector is oriented to the left and anteriorly with a normal range of 0° to 65° and a mean value of 35°. Its magnitude varies from 0.25 to 0.75 mV with an average value of 0.50 mV.

Right sagittal plane. In the right sagittal plane projection the direction of inscription of the T loop is also the same as that of the QRS loop in this plane, that is, clockwise. Exceptions in which the T loop is very narrow and inscribed counterclockwise are very rare. The maximum **T** vector is oriented anteriorly and inferiorly. The average direction of the vector is about 45° with a normal range of 20 to 90°. The magnitude of the maximum vector ranges from 0.2 to 0.7 mV with a mean value of 0.4 mV.

Frontal plane. In contrast to the other two planes, the direction of inscription of the frontal plane T loop may be either clockwise or counterclockwise. Furthermore, the direction may occasionally be different from that of the QRS. The maximum **T** vector is oriented inferiorly and to the left with a normal range of 20° to 55° and a mean value of 35°. Its magnitude varies from 0.25 to 0.75 mV with an average of 0.45 mV.

Table 5.3 includes the mean value and the normal range of the direction and magnitude of the maximum **T** vectors in the three planar projections.

THE QRS-T ANGLE

The angle subtended by the maximum spatial **QRS** and **T** vectors is quite variable in normal adult subjects. An angle up to 100° is often found in our series. Draper et al calculated the QRS-T angle using the mean spatial **QRS** and **T** vectors

Table 5.3

The Direction and Magnitude of the Maximum **T** Vector in Normal Subjects (200)

Plane	Direction (deg)		Magnitude (mV)	
	Mean	95% range	Mean	95% range
Transverse	35	0—65	0.5	0.25—0.75
Right sagittal	45	20—90	0.4	0.2 —0.70
Frontal	35	20—55	0.5	0.25—0.75

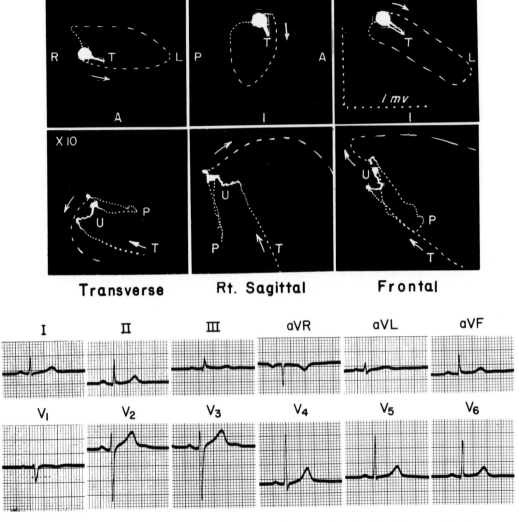

Fig. 5.11. The vectorcardiogram and electrocardiogram of a healthy 27-year-old woman recorded to demonstrate the U loop. In each projection of the vectorcardiogram the U loop is seen in the enlarged picture to begin at the end of the T loop. In recording the U loop a low-frequency filter was used and only the returning portion of the T loop was retained to avoid overlapping of the signal.

and found a wide range of 26° to 134°. These results are distinctly different from those reported by Grant and Estes, who maintained that the spatial angle rarely exceeded 60°. Their values were determined from the mean spatial vectors as derived from the scalar electrocardiograms. Thus the results may not be entirely comparable.

In the planar projections such marked variation in the width of the QRS-T angle is demonstrated in the transverse and sagittal planes. However, in the frontal plane the angle is quite narrow and usually does not exceed 28°.

THE U LOOP (FIG. 5.11)

The normal U loop is difficult to recognize in most of the routine vectorcardiograms. If the area around the null point is greatly magnified, the beginning of the U loop may be identified by the marked slowing of the inscription at the terminal portion of the T loop. The U loop of normal subjects resembles a small, slightly curved club. It is actually a segment or arc rather than a closed loop. It is directed to the left, inferiorly, and mostly anteriorly, and is therefore similar to the direction of the normal T loop. It is inscribed counterclockwise in the transverse plane and clockwise in the right sagittal and frontal planes.

THE EFFECT OF THE CONSTITUTIONAL VARIABLES ON THE VECTORCARDIOGRAM

With advancing age there are significant changes in the QRS and T loops of the adult vectorcardiogram. Pipberger and associates have found that the amplitude of the maximum spatial **QRS** vector decreases at an average rate of 6.5 percent with each decade of the adult life. The planar projections of the maximum vector show similar changes. The direction of the vector shifts anteriorly and superiorly with aging. In normal subjects studied by the author the 97.5 percentile value of the magnitude of the vector for individuals under age 40 is 2.0 mV in the transverse plane and 2.4 mV in the frontal plane; for those age 40 and above, 1.9 and 2.0 mV.

The reduction of the magnitude of the maximum **T** vector with increasing age is even more conspicuous and consistent. According to Pipberger's data the average decrease approaches 10 percent for each decade, but it is somewhat less in the author's series. The maximum **T** vector is oriented more anteriorly in older subjects

Other constitutional variables which may affect the vectorcardiogram include race, sex, and body weight. The black population has higher QRS amplitude than white subjects. Both the **QRS** and **T** vectors are larger in men than they are in women. With increasing body weight the QRS decreases in magnitude and the vector is oriented more superiorly and anteriorly. All of these factors have to be considered in the diagnosis of ventricular hypertrophy when the voltage criteria are used.

REFERENCES

1. Bristow JD: A study of the normal Frank vectorcardiogram. Am Heart J 61:242, 1961
2. Chou TC: Vectorcardiographic lead system and normal vectorcardiogram values: man, in Altman PL, Dittmer DS (eds): Biological Handbooks, Respiration and Circulation. Bethesda, Maryland, Federation of American Societies for Experimental Biology, 1971, pp 294-299
3. Draper HW, Peffer CJ, Stallmann FW, Littmann D, Pipberger HV: The corrected orthogonal electrocardiogram and vectorcardiogram in 510 normal men (Frank lead system). Circulation 30:853, 1964
4. Forkner CE Jr, Hugenholtz PG, Levine HD: The vectorcardiogram in normal young adults. Frank lead system. Am Heart J 62:237, 1961
5. Grant RP, Estes EH Jr: Spatial Vector Electrocardiography. Philadelphia, Blakiston, 1951

6. McCall BW, Wallace AG, Estes EH Jr: Characteristics of the normal vectorcardiogram recorded with the Frank lead system. Am J Cardiol 10:514, 1962
7. Pipberger HV, Goldman MJ, Littmann D, Murphy GP, Cosma J, Synder JR: Correlations of the orthogonal electrocardiogram and vectorcardiogram with constitutional variables in 518 normal men. Circulation 35:536, 1967
8. Sano T, Tsuchihashi H, Takigawa S, Shimamoto T; U vector loop or arc in normal subjects and in those with left ventricular hypertrophy. Am Heart J 61:802, 1961
9. Sotobata I, Richman H, Simonson E: Sex differences in the vectorcardiogram. Circulation 37:438, 1968

6

Left Ventricular Hypertrophy

In left ventricular hypertrophy the increase in the muscle mass of the left ventricle exaggerates the normal preponderance of the left ventricular potential. Consequently, the vector representing the resultant of the left and right ventricular potentials has a larger magnitude and is rotated further toward the direction of the left ventricular force (Fig. 6.1). Indeed, an abnormally large QRS loop oriented to the left is the most characteristic vectorcardiographic finding in left ventricular hypertrophy. The following description is based mainly on the changes observed in patients with hypertensive cardiovascular and aortic valvular diseases.

QRSsÊ LOOP

The spatial QRS loop in left ventricular hypertrophy has a smooth contour and is abnormally large in magnitude. In the majority of instances the loop is oval and elongated in configuration. There is a tendency for the initial vectors to be displaced from the normal rightward, anterior and superior orientation to that of a leftward, anterior and inferior direction. The body of the QRSsÊ loop is located in the left, posterior, and usually inferior octant of three-dimensional space. The terminal deflection is directed posteriorly and mostly to the left, either superiorly or inferiorly. The duration of the QRS loop is often slightly prolonged. However, in the uncomplicated cases, there is no evidence of a conduction delay as indicated by the speed of inscription. The maximum spatial **QRS** vector is directed to the left, posteriorly and usually inferiorly. Its time of occurrence after the beginning of the QRS loop is sometimes prolonged, especially when the hypertrophy is marked.

Planar Projections of the QRSsÊ Loop (Figs. 6.2-6.9)

Transverse plane QRS loop. The QRS loop in the transverse plane is usually elongated and narrower than normal. Its magnitude is abnormally increased. In the majority of instances, the direction of inscription remains normal, that is, counterclockwise. However, frequently the loop presents a figure-of-eight pattern, especially

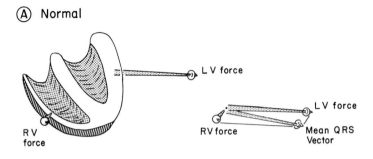

(A) Normal

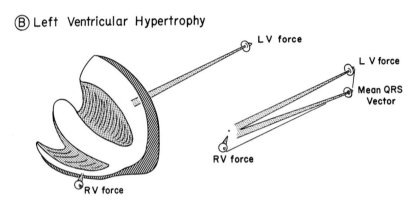

(B) Left Ventricular Hypertrophy

Fig. 6.1. Vector representation of the left and right ventricular potentials and their resultant forces. (A) Normal heart, (B) Left ventricular hypertrophy.

in those cases in which the hypertrophy is severe. When the loop has a figure-of-eight configuration, the proximal portion is always inscribed counterclockwise and the distal portion clockwise. The relative sizes of the proximal and distal portions vary. Rarely, a clockwise loop is inscribed to mimic anterolateral myocardial infarction.

The normal initial anterior and rightward forces are often reduced or replaced by vectors directed anteriorly and to the left. In 100 patients with left ventricular hypertrophy caused either by hypertension or by aortic valvular disease, studied by one of the authors (Chou), a leftward and anterior initial deflection was observed in 60 percent. A similar initial deflection was seen in only 13 percent of the normal subjects. As a result of the leftward displacement, the initial deflection frequently becomes continuous with the efferent limb of the body of the QRS loop so that a distinct turning point is no longer present. In rare instances the initial deflection may be directed posteriorly in the absence of myocardial infarction. The body of the QRS loop is located in the left and posterior quadrant and occupies a more posterior position than that of the normal loop. The terminal deflection is usually also directed to the left and posteriorly, and is often continuous with the afferent limb of the body without any change in the direction before the loop returns toward its origin. The

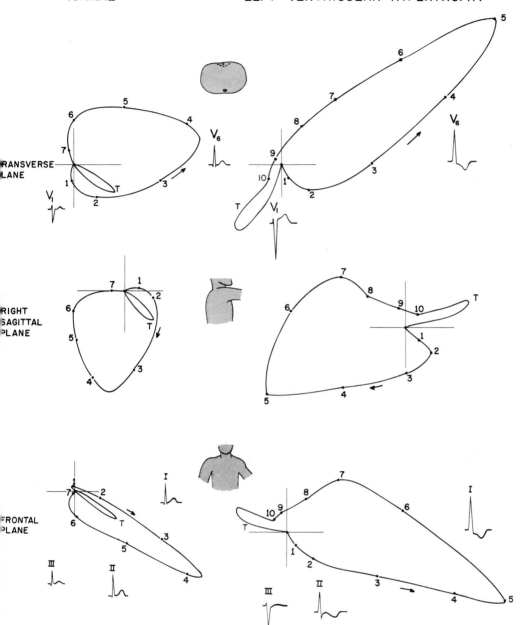

Fig. 6.2. Schematic diagrams of the vectorcardiogram in left ventricular hypertrophy as compared with that of the normal. The numerals indicate the time in hundredths of a second after the beginning of the QRS loop. The representative scalar lead QRS-T complexes are given. The P loops are not shown.

73

duration of the QRS loop is sometimes slightly prolonged, but there is no evidence of abnormal slowing of the speed of inscription to indicate a conduction delay.

The maximum **QRS** vector is directed to the left and is displaced further posteriorly than that of the normal. Its magnitude exceeds the normal upper limit which is 2.0 mV for subjects under 40 years of age and 1.9 mV for those age 40 or older. This increase in the magnitude of the maximum **QRS** vector is one of the most consistent vectorcardiographic findings in left ventricular hypertrophy. The time of occurrence of the maximum **QRS** vector is sometimes delayed (equal to or exceeding 0.05 sec), especially when the hypertrophy is severe.

Figure 6.3 illustrates a convenient way to visualize the changes of the transverse plane QRS loop in left ventricular hypertrophy. The application of an additional pulling force on the early, mid, and late portions of a normal transverse QRS loop from the left and posterior direction results in the elongation and increase in the magnitude of the loop in that direction. The initial and terminal deflections will also be displaced in the manner described in the preceding paragraphs.

The reduction of the initial right anterior forces can be seen in the scalar electrocardiogram as a decrease in the size of the Q wave in leads V_5 and V_6. The leftward displacement of the initial vectors also explains the decrease of the R wave in the right precordial leads. The increase in the maximum **QRS** vector in the leftward direction is reflected in leads V_5 and V_6 as a tall R wave, and the posterior displacement of the vector is manifested in the right precordial leads as a deep S wave. If the QRS loop has a figure-of-eight pattern, notching of the R or S wave may appear in the midprecordial leads. The delay in the time of occurrence of the maximum **QRS** vector corresponds to the delay in the onset of the intrinsicoid deflection in the left precordial leads. The leftward displacement of the terminal deflection explains the infrequent appearance of an S wave in the left precordial leads in patients with left ventricular hypertrophy.

Sagittal plane QRS loop.   In the right sagittal plane the initial **QRS** vectors in most of the normal individuals are directed anteriorly and superiorly. In left ventricular hypertrophy there is a displacement of the initial vectors downward, even though they remain anteriorly oriented. The loop is usually inscribed clockwise. Occasionally, it presents a figure-of-eight pattern with the proximal portion inscribed clockwise. The majority of the QRS loop occupies a position in the inferior and posterior quadrant. The terminal vectors are displaced superiorly. The maximum **QRS** vector is increased in magnitude and exceeds the normal upper limit of 2.0 mV.

Frontal plane QRS loop.   In the frontal plane the initial **QRS** vectors are usually directed toward the left and inferiorly. Only a relatively small percentage of cases of left ventricular hypertrophy retains the usual rightward and superior direction of the normal subject. The body of the loop becomes more horizontal or even slightly superior in position, and the afferent limb is quite consistently displaced superiorly. As a result the QRS loop is frequently inscribed in a counterclockwise direction and is often wider than normal. Marked superior displacement of the QRS loop, however, is usually caused by the coexistence of left anterior fascicular block. There is a significant increase in the magnitude of the maximum **QRS** vector (exceeding 2.4 mV in subjects under 40 years of age and 2.0 mV age 40 or older) and occasionally a delay in its time of occurrence. The terminal deflection is directed

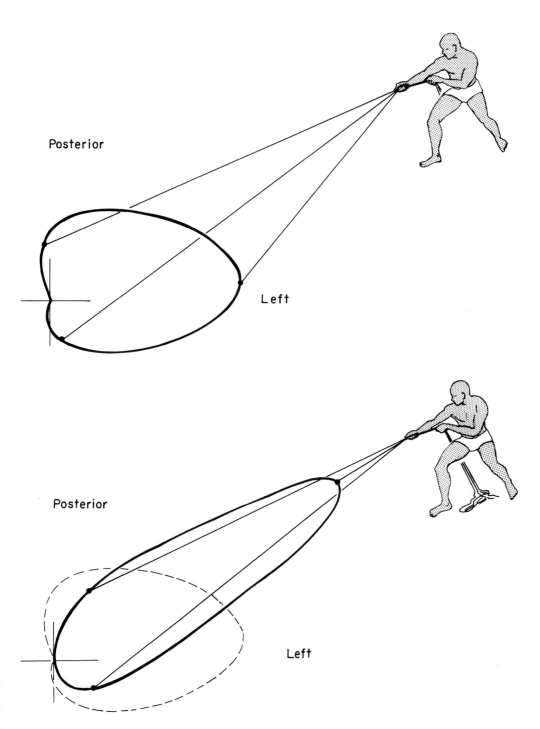

Fig. 6.3. A convenient way to visualize the effect of left ventricular hypertrophy on the normal transverse plane QRS loop. The added left ventricular force pulls the loop to a more posterior and leftward direction with an increase in its magnitude. The initial and terminal deflections, as well as the body of the loop, may be affected.

TRANSVERSE PLANE   RIGHT SAGITTAL PLANE   FRONTAL PLANE

A

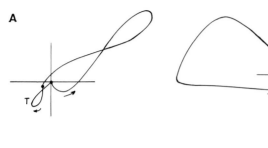
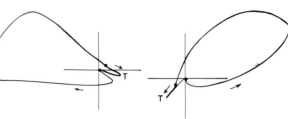

B

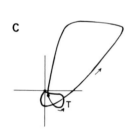
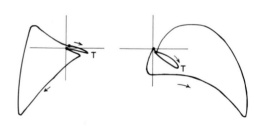

C

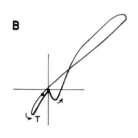
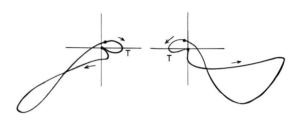

D

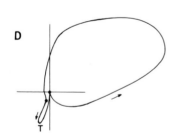
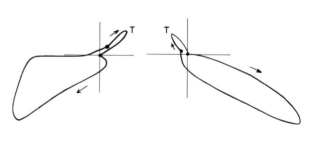

Fig. 6.4. Schematic diagrams of the various configurations of the QRS and T loops seen in patients with left ventricular hypertrophy. In (A) the marked superior displacement of the QRS loop suggests the coexistence of left anterior fascicular block.

usually to the left and superiorly and is often continuous with the afferent limb of the body without any distinct turning point.

The changes in the frontal plane QRS loop can readily be correlated with those observed in the limb leads of the scalar electrocardiogram. The leftward and inferior direction of the initial deflection explains the diminution or absence of the Q wave in leads I and aVL. The increase in the magnitude of the maximum **QRS** vector with its horizontal orientation explains the high voltage of the R wave in these leads. The superior displacement of the afferent limb of the body and of the terminal deflection of the loop is seen in leads II, III, and aVF as a deeper S wave. When the loop remains relatively vertical, a tall R wave instead of a deep S wave is seen in the inferior leads.

ST VECTOR AND THE TsÊ LOOP

In left ventricular hypertrophy the QRSsÊ loop terminates usually at a point (J point) to the right, anterior, and superior to its point of origin. Thus, the direction of the spatial **ST** vector is opposite to that of the QRSsÊ loop itself. The magnitude of the **ST** vector is often increased. In the planar projections the **ST** vector is directed to the right and anteriorly in the transverse plane, anteriorly and superiorly in the right sagittal plane, and to the right and superiorly in the frontal plane.

The TsÊ loop is usually elongated but may be abnormally wide. When the **ST** vector is large, the loop remains widely opened. There is a tendency for the TsÊ loop to be displaced anteriorly, rightward and superiorly; in a fully developed case the direction of the TsÊ loop is opposite to that of the QRSsÊ loop and is parallel to the axis of the **ST** vector. The initial portion of the TsÊ loop is slowly inscribed as in the normal individual, and the magnitude of the T loop (or its maximum vector) can be normal, reduced, or increased. In the transverse plane projection the typical left ventricular hypertrophy has a T loop oriented to the right and anteriorly. It is directed anteriorly and superiorly in the right sagittal plane and to the right and superiorly in the frontal plane. The direction of inscription of the T loop may be either clockwise or counterclockwise in each of the planar projections. The angle subtended by the maximum **QRS** and **T** vectors in all three planes often approaches 180°.

The divergent maximum **QRS** and **ST-T** vectors are represented in the scalar leads as QRS and ST-T waves of opposite polarities. The rightward and anterior direction of the **ST** and **T** vectors, as seen in the transverse plane, results in an elevation of the ST segment with an upright T wave in the right precordial leads since the vectors are pointing to the positive side of the lead of derivation of the right precordial leads. The ST segment is depressed and the T wave is inverted in the left precordial leads because the vectors are pointing to the negative side of the lead axis of these leads. Similar relationship exists in the limb leads, where ST-segment depression and T-wave inversion are usually seen in the leads with an upright R wave and vice versa.

Figures 6.5 to 6.8 illustrate the various vectorcardiographic features and their electrocardiographic counterparts recorded in patients with definite clinical evidence of left ventricular hypertrophy.

T. A. 421937

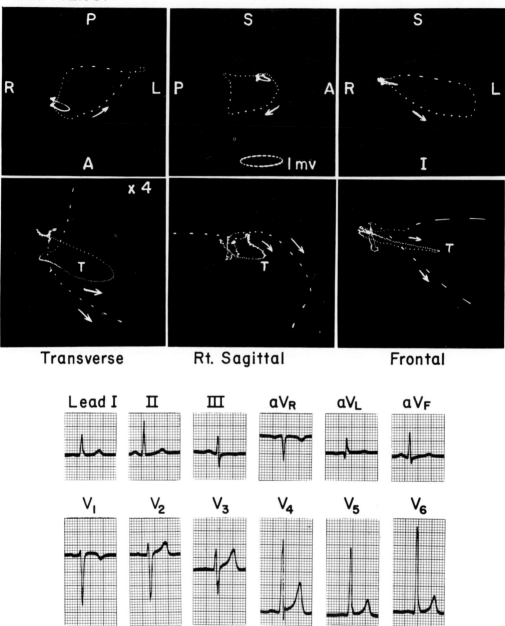

Transverse   Rt. Sagittal   Frontal

Fig. 6.5. Left ventricular hypertrophy. The vectorcardiogram and electrocardiogram were recorded from a 42-year-old man with hypertensive cardiovascular disease. The magnitude of the QRSsÊ loop is abnormally large and the maximum **QRS** vector exceeds 2.0 mV in both the transverse and frontal planes. There is a twisting of the distal portion of the QRS loop in the transverse plane projection. In the same projection the **ST** vector is displaced to the right and anteriorly. However, the TsÊ loop is normal in its orientation, magnitude, and direction of inscription. The vector loops are interrupted every 2 msec.

S.M. 376171

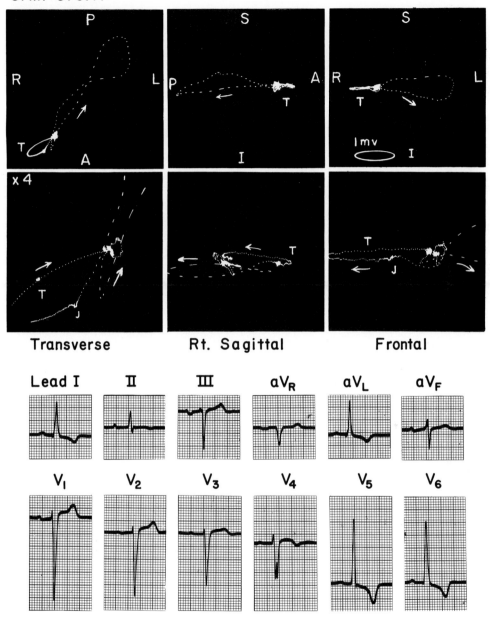

Transverse **Rt. Sagittal** **Frontal**

Fig. 6.6. Left ventricular hypertrophy. The vectorcardiogram and electrocardiogram were recorded from a 47-year-old woman with hypertensive cardiovascular disease. The QRSs loop is large and is oriented posteriorly and to the left. Note the figure-of-eight configuration of the QRS loop in the transverse plane. The duration of the QRS loop is prolonged, and there is a delay in the time of occurrence of the maximum **QRS** vector. The **ST** vector is abnormally large. Both the **ST** vector and the TsÊ loop are discordant to the QRSsÊ loop (dash interval 2 msec).

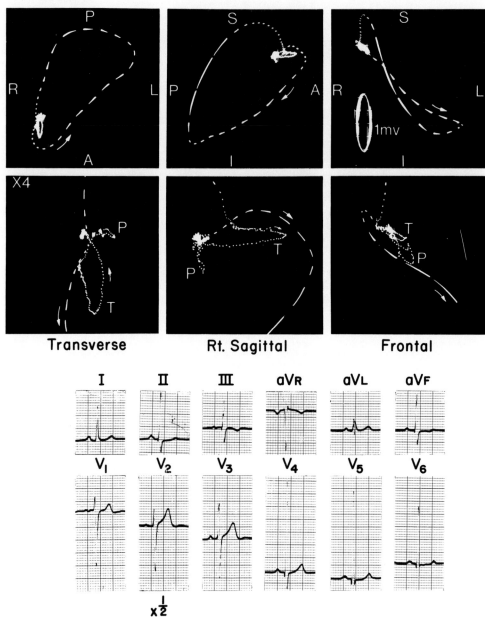

Fig. 6.7. Left ventricular hypertrophy. The vectorcardiogram and electrocardiogram were recorded from a 17-year-old boy with moderately severe aortic insufficiency proved by aortography. The magnitude of the maximum **QRS** vector in the transverse plane is greater than 2.0 mV. The direction of the T loop in this projection exceeds 70°. There is also a superior displacement of the T loop which is best seen in the sagittal plane. Note in the transverse plane the distal QRS loop area is larger than the proximal area (dash interval 2 msec).

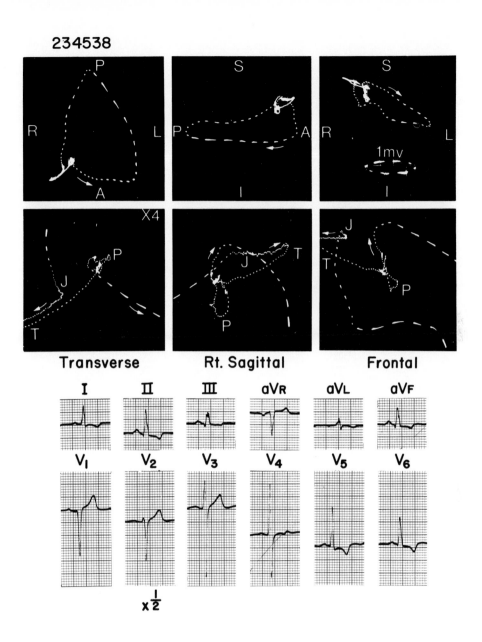

Fig. 6.8. Left ventricular hypertrophy. The vectorcardiogram and electrocardiogram were recorded from a 24-year-old man with severe calcific aortic stenosis. The pressure gradient across the aortic valve was 122 mm Hg. The magnitude of the maximum **QRS** vector is within normal limits in all planes. There is a posterior displacement of the maximum **QRS** vector and the maximum posterior force measures 1.75 mV. The **ST** vector and T loop are displaced rightward and superiorly (dash interval 2 msec).

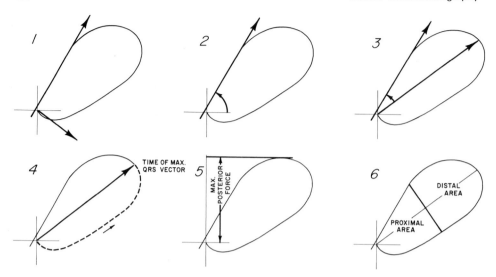

Fig. 6.9. Diagrams of the transverse plane QRS loop illustrating some additional measurements which are useful in the diagnosis of left ventricular hypertrophy (see text, criteria 1 to 6).

During routine interpretation of the vectorcardiogram the diagnosis of left ventricular hypertrophy is usually based on the increased magnitude of the maximum **QRS** vector in one or more planar projections. However, a significant number of patients with anatomical left ventricular hypertrophy do not display abnormally large QRS voltage. The recognition of other changes in the QRS loop, as described previously, may often lead to the correct diagnosis. The following criteria (Fig. 6.9) based on the transverse plane QRS loop may be applied provided the magnitude of the maximum **QRS** vector to the left is greater than 1.3 mV (normal mean):

1. Both the initial and terminal deflections are directed leftward. The direction of the initial deflection is determined by a line joining the beginning of the QRS to the midpoint of the initial deflection. The direction of the terminal deflection is determined by a line joining the end of the QRS (J point) to the midpoint of the terminal deflection.
2. The direction of the terminal deflection is anterior to −65°.
3. The angle between the maximum **QRS** vector and terminal deflection is less than 35°.
4. The time of inscription of the maximum **QRS** vector is later than 0.0475 sec.
5. The maximum leftward posterior force is greater than 1.2 mV.
6. The distal loop area is larger than the proximal loop area. These areas are defined by a perpendicular line bisecting the maximum **QRS** vector.
7. The direction of the **ST** vector is to the right of 120° or the direction of the maximum **T** vector is to the right of 70°.

When two or more of these findings are present, anatomical left ventricular hypertrophy usually exists. These criteria are also useful to confirm the diagnosis of left ventricular hypertrophy based on the voltage criteria, especially in the young subjects.

Although the *pathophysiology* responsible for the vectorcardiographic and electrocardiographic changes in left ventricular hypertrophy appears to be quite simple, its details have not been well elucidated. The explanation for the reduction of the initial rightward and superior forces remains a controversial subject. In left ventricular hypertrophy there is hypertrophy of the interventricular septum so that one would expect the septal vectors (i.e., the initial rightward, anterior, and superior vectors) to increase in their magnitude. However, in the adult patients the opposite is usually true and has been explained in the following ways:

1. The right septal surface is facing downward instead of upward because of either a counterclockwise rotation of the heart along its longitudinal axis or an increase in the rightward convexity of the septum. The left-to-right septal activation would thus result in a vector which is directed inferiorly instead of superiorly.

2. There is a complete or partial disappearance of left septal forces caused by myocardial fibrosis or infarction. It has been postulated that as the subaortic portion of the interventricular septum hypertrophies and bulges into the left ventricular outflow tract, it is subjected to unusual trauma. As a result of this trauma, local endocardial fibrosis occurs. Since the origin of the left bundle branch is located in this subaortic region, it may become involved in the fibrotic lesions with resultant incomplete left bundle branch block, which further decreases the early left-to-right septal forces.

3. It has been suggested that the electrical activity of the hypertrophied free wall of the left ventricle can manifest itself from the beginning to the end of the ventricular depolarization. It is possible that by these predominant forces the initial septal forces are "pulled" to the left and backward and incorporated into the main body of the QRS loop.

The increase in the magnitude of the QRS loop and its posterior displacement can readily be related to the increased muscular mass of the left ventricle, although the basic mechanism responsible for the high electrical potential in hypertrophy is not entirely clear. The superior displacement of the terminal forces has been attributed by Grant to the hypertrophy, elongation and bowing superiorly of the basal portion of the left ventricular free wall. Marked superior displacement of the late **QRS** vectors, however, occurs only when there is co-existing left anterior hemiblock. The prolongation of the QRS interval and the delay in the occurrence of the maximum **QRS** vector may be related to the increase in the thickness of the hypertrophied ventricle, since the distance the activation wave must travel to reach the epicardium is increased. In some instances a localized conduction disturbance may also contribute to the prolongation of the QRS interval. Indeed, the figure-of-eight configuration of the QRS loop in patients with rather severe left ventricular hypertrophy is probably a manifestation of incomplete left bundle branch block.

Because of the increased thickness of the hypertrophied wall and a delay for the activation process to reach the epicardial layers, repolarization begins in the endocardium before the depolarization process has been completed. The spread of the repolarization process is therefore also from the endocardial to the epicardial surface and is opposite to the normal process. The resultant forces or vectors (**T** vectors) are thus directed away from the **QRS** vectors. Since the repolarization process begins before the completion of the depolarization process, it causes a deviation of the terminal portions of the QRS loop, and the J point is displaced in the direction of the **T** vector and is represented by the abnormal **ST** vector.

REFERENCES

1. Abbott-Smith CW, Chou TC: Vectorcardiographic criteria for the diagnosis of left ventricular hypertrophy. Am Heart J 79:361, 1970
2. Bell H, Pugh D, Dunn M: Vectorcardiographic evolution of left ventricular hypertrophy. Br Heart J 30:70, 1968
3. Bristow JD, Porter GA, Griswold HE: Observations with the Frank system of vectorcardiography in left ventricular hypertrophy. Am Heart J 62:621, 1961
4. Cabrera E, Gaxiola A: A critical reevaluation of systolic and diastolic overloading patterns. Prog Cardiovasc Dis 2:219, 1959
5. Cabrera E, Gaxiola A: Diagnostic contribution of the vectorcardiogram in hemodynamic overloading of the heart. Am Heart J 60:296, 1960
6. Castellanos A, Hernandez FA, Lemberg L, Castellanos A Jr: The vectorcardiographic criteria of hemodynamical overloadings in congenital heart disease. Cardiologia 44:392, 1964
7. Estes EH Jr: Left ventricular hypertrophy in acquired heart disease: A comparison of the vectorcardiogram in aortic stenosis and aortic insufficiency. Proc Long Island Jewish Hosp Symp Vectorcardiography. Amsterdam, North Holland, 1965, p 157
8. Grant RP: Relation between anatomical axis of the heart and the electrocardiogram. Circulation 7:890, 1953
9. Hugenholtz PG, Gamboa R: Effect of chronically increased ventricular pressure on electrical forces of the heart. A correlation between hemodynamic and vectorcardiographic data (Frank system) in 90 patients with aortic or pulmonic stenosis. Circulation 30:511, 1964
10. Romhilt DW, Greenfield JC Jr, Estes EH Jr: Vectorcardiographic diagnosis of left ventricular hypertrophy. Circulation 37:15, 1968
11. Toole JG, von der Groeben J, Spivack AP: The calculated temperospatial heart vector in proved isolated left ventricular overwork. Am Heart J 63:537, 1962
12. Varriale P, Alfenito JC, Kennedy RJ: The vectorcardiogram of left ventricular hypertrophy. Analysis and criteria (Frank lead system). Circulation 33:569, 1966
13. Wallace AG, McCall BW, Estes EH Jr: The vectorcardiogram in left ventricular hypertrophy. A study using the Frank lead system. Am Heart J 63:466, 1962
14. Yano K, Pipberger HV: Correlations between radiologic heart size and orthogonal electrocardiograms in patients with left ventricular overload. Am Heart J 67:44, 1964

7

Right Ventricular Hypertrophy

In right ventricular hypertrophy the increase in the muscle mass of the right ventricle is accompanied by an increase in the right ventricular electrical potential. The right ventricular forces which are normally masked by the dominant left ventricular potential may now become evident. The resultant forces will be modified depending on the degree of right ventricular hypertrophy, the extent of the deviation of the resultant forces from those of normal varies (Fig. 7.1). When the right ventricular hypertrophy is severe, the right ventricular potential may even become the dominant force and the resultant vector is oriented toward the direction of the anatomic right ventricle, that is, to the right, anteriorly, either inferiorly or superiorly. The vectorcardiogram representing right ventricular hypertrophy shows a much greater variation in its configuration and orientation than it does in left ventricular hypertrophy. The types of changes depend not only on the severity of the hypertrophy but also, to a certain degree, on the etiology of the heart disease and type of hemodynamic alteration (pressure overload or volume overload). For the convenience of description three types of right ventricular hypertrophy based on certain characteristics of the QRSsÊ loop will be presented. Types A and B right ventricular hypertrophy include those in which the QRSsÊ loop is displaced anteriorly, and in type C, it is displaced posteriorly.

TYPE A RIGHT VENTRICULAR HYPERTROPHY (Figs. 7.2 - 7.8)

Type A is generally considered the most typical type of right ventricular hypertrophy. It is seen most commonly in patients with congenital heart disease, such as pulmonic stenosis, tetralogy of Fallot, and Eisenmenger syndrome, but it is also encountered in advanced cases of chronic cor pulmonale and mitral stenosis.

QRSsÊ Loop

The spatial QRS loop in type A right ventricular hypertrophy is displaced anteriorly and to the right so that an abnormally large portion of the loop is located

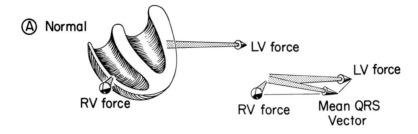

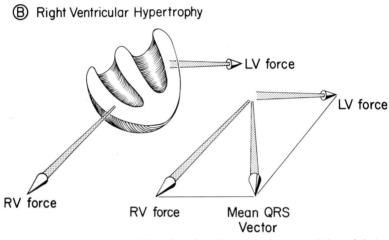

Fig. 7.1. Vector representation of the left and right ventricular potentials and their resultant forces. (A) Normal heart, (B) Heart with rather severe right ventricular hypertrophy.

in the right, anterior, and usually inferior octant. The loop has a smooth contour and its magnitude may or may not exceed that of normal. It is usually rather wide and oval in shape. The duration of the QRS loop may be slightly prolonged but is often within the normal range. The maximum spatial **QRS** vector is displaced anteriorly. In some cases it retains its leftward and inferior orientation, but it is accompanied by abnormally large rightward forces in the later part of the QRS loop. In other instances the maximum **QRS** vector is directed rightward, anteriorly, and inferiorly. It is also not unusual to see prominent superiorly directed forces in the late portion of the QRS loop.

Planar Projections of the QRSsÊ Loop

Transverse plane QRS loop. The configuration of the QRS loop in the transverse plane varies considerably. It may be wide and oval in shape or quite narrow if the spatial loop is vertical. The loop size may or may not be enlarged. Typically, the majority of the loop is located anteriorly and to the right. The direction of inscription is *clockwise*, which has been considered one of the most characteristic vectorcardiographic signs of right ventricular hypertrophy. In some instances the loop presents a figure-of-eight pattern, and the initial portion of the loop is inscribed counterclockwise and the later portion, clockwise.

The initial deflection may retain its normal anterior and rightward direction. However, its amplitude is often reduced, or the vectors are displaced to the left, and in some cases they may even be directed leftward and posteriorly. The efferent limb of the body of the QRS loop is inscribed leftward, either slightly anteriorly or posteriorly. The leftward vectors are usually relatively small. After it reaches its maximum leftward location, the loop begins to turn more anteriorly and toward the right. The magnitude of the right anterior forces may or may not exceed that of the leftward forces. The terminal deflection is directed to the right, either anteriorly or posteriorly. In contrast to right bundle branch block, the uncomplicated case of right

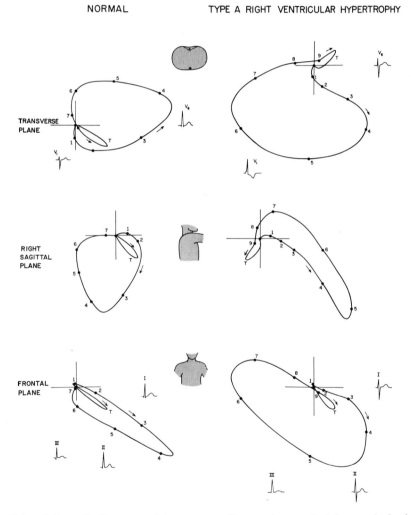

Fig. 7.2. Schematic diagrams of the vectorcardiogram in type A right ventricular hypertrophy as compared with that of the normal. The numerals indicate the time in hundredths of a second after the beginning of the QRS loop. The representative conventional scalar lead QRS-T complexes are given. The P loops are not shown.

TYPE A   RIGHT   VENTRICULAR   HYPERTROPHY

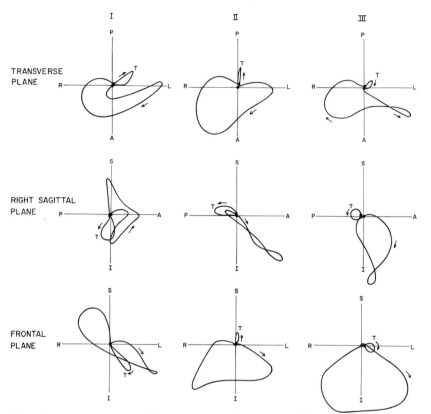

Fig. 7.3. Schematic diagrams of the various configurations of the QRS and T loops seen in patients with vectorcardiographic type A right ventricular hypertrophy.

ventricular hypertrophy does not show an abnormal prolongation of the terminal slow inscription. The total duration of the QRS loop may be within normal limits or slightly prolonged.

The planar projection of the maximum spatial **QRS** vector may be directed either to the left or to the right, but is usually located anteriorly. If the leftward orientation is maintained, there are abnormally large right, anterior vectors during the later part of the QRS interval.

To correlate with the conventional electrocardiogram, the overall anterior and rightward direction of the QRS loop is responsible for the large upright deflections (R or R') in the right precordial leads. Depending on the orientation of the initial deflection and efferent limb, the QRS complex in lead V_1 may assume the pattern of a tall R wave with or without slurring or notching of its ascending portion, an RSR' or a qR pattern. If the initial deflection is oriented anteriorly and is on the positive side of the lead axis of V_1 (i.e., anterior to 25°), an initial r wave will be recorded which will continue as a part of a tall R wave if the succeeding leftward inscription of the loop becomes increasingly anterior. However, slurring or notching of the R wave will result if its anterior movement is slowed down or the direction is temporarily

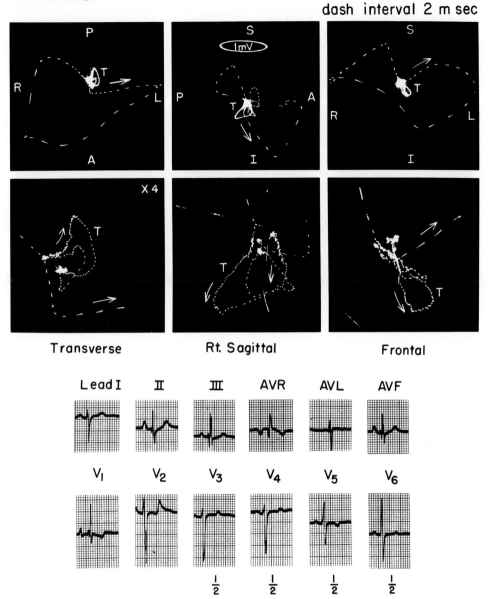

Fig. 7.4. Type A right ventricular hypertrophy. The vectorcardiogram and electrocardiogram were recorded from a 14-year-old boy with tetralogy of Fallot. In the transverse plane the QRS loop is displaced anteriorly and to the right and the loop is inscribed clockwise. The T loop is directed to the left and posteriorly and is inscribed clockwise. In the sagittal plane the QRS loop appears to be quite tortuous with the major portion of the loop located anteriorly and inferiorly and inscribed counterclockwise. The T loop is posterior and inferior and is inscribed counterclockwise. In the frontal plane an abnormally large portion of the QRS loop is located to the right and superiorly, and the loop is inscribed clockwise.

J. A.

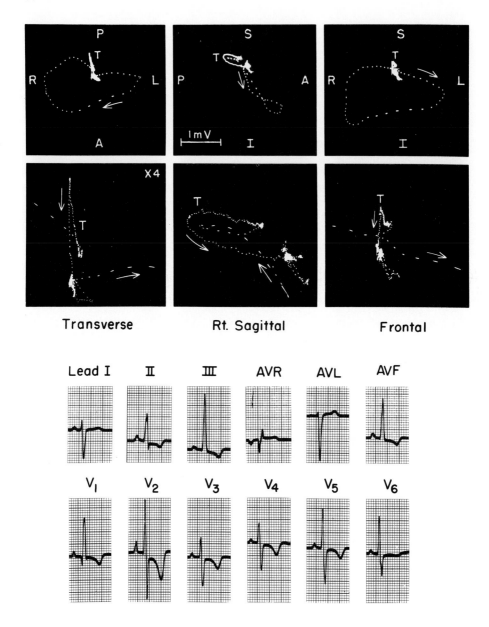

Fig. 7.5. Type A right ventricular hypertrophy. The vectorcardiogram and electrocardiogram were recorded from a 21-year-old woman with multiple pulmonary branch stenosis. The diagnostic vectorcardiographic findings include a clockwise transverse plane QRS loop which is displaced anteriorly and to the right, a wide clockwise frontal plane QRS loop with its major portion located on the right. Note the leftward and posterior displacement of the initial deflection, which is best seen in the transverse plane and is manifested in lead V_1 of the electrocardiogram as a Q wave. The TsÊ loop is oriented posteriorly, superiorly, and rather atypically slightly to the right.

reversed. If part of the loop reaches the negative side of the lead axis of V_1, an S wave will be recorded, and an RSR′ pattern will be seen after the loop completes its later anterior and rightward course. A qR pattern is formed if the initial deflection and part of the efferent limb are located on the negative side of the lead axis. Since the peak of the R or R′ wave usually represents the projection of an anterior and rightward vector of the afferent limb of the QRS loop, it thus appears in the later part of the QRS interval and results in a delay of the onset of the "intrinsicoid deflection" in V_1. In the left precordial leads (V_5 and V_6), the decrease in the leftward forces results in a smaller R wave, and the increase in the late rightward forces, a larger S wave. An initial small Q will be seen in these leads only when the initial deflection is oriented to the right.

Sagittal plane QRS loop. In the right sagittal plane the major portion of the QRS loop is located anteriorly and inferiorly. With or without an initial small upward deflection, the early portion of the loop is directed inferiorly either slightly anteriorly or posteriorly. The loop then turns more anteriorly inscribing a *counterclockwise* loop. The later portion of the loop is usually located superiorly and may occasionally be quite large. A figure-of-eight pattern is often seen, and sometimes the loop may cross itself more than once before it returns to its origin.

Frontal plane QRS loop. In the frontal plane most of the QRS loop is located inferiorly with the exception of the terminal portion which may be displaced superiorly. Unlike the rather narrow normal frontal plane QRS loop, the loop in right ventricular hypertrophy is usually wide. Its magnitude may or may not be abnormally increased. With few exceptions the loop is inscribed *clockwise*.

With or without an initial upward deflection, the loop is inscribed inferiorly and to the left. The leftward vectors are usually relatively small, and after the efferent limb reaches its maximal leftward location the afferent limb swings quickly to the right giving rise to an abnormally large rightward bulge of the loop. The abnormally large rightward vectors may or may not be larger than the leftward forces. The terminal deflection is directed to the right, either inferiorly or superiorly.

The decrease in the leftward forces and the increase in the rightward forces result in a small R and a large S wave in lead I of the scalar electrocardiogram. The inferior orientation of the loop gives a prominent R wave in the inferior leads. In some instances, when the terminal superior and rightward vectors are very prominent, leads II, III, and aVF will register an RS or rS complex. These large terminal right superior forces are the counterpart of the $S_1S_2S_3$ pattern in the conventional electrocardiogram.

The basic mechanism responsible for the QRS changes in this type of right ventricular hypertrophy can be related mainly to the dominant electrical potential from the hypertrophied free wall of the right ventricle. In certain congenital heart diseases the underdevelopment of the left ventricle may further contribute to the changes. The difference in the configuration of the QRS loop can be attributed to the variation in the degree of right ventricular preponderance and its time of onset during the ventricular depolarization process. The characteristic clockwise rotation of the QRS loop in the transverse plane is chiefly attributed to the major effect of right ventricular dominance being manifested during the mid and late periods of the ventricular activation, and the afferent limb becomes anterior and to the right of the

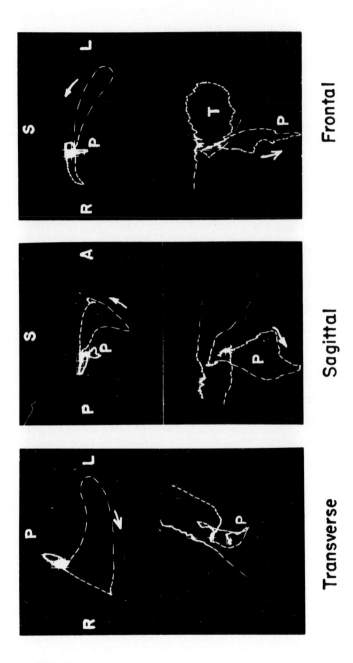

Frontal

Sagittal

Transverse

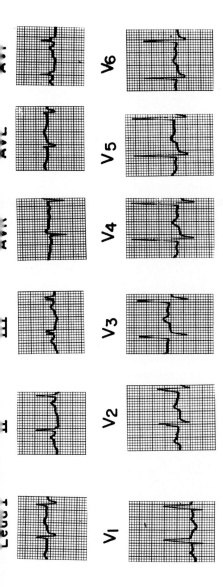

Fig. 7.6. Type A right ventricular hypertrophy. The patient is a 48-year-old woman with mitral stenosis. The changes of the QRS and T loops in the transverse and sagittal planes are quite typical of right ventricular hypertrophy. The QRS loop in the frontal plane is, however, inscribed counterclockwise, which suggests the possibility of left ventricular disease. In this illustration the loops are interrupted every 2.5 instead of 2 msec.

93

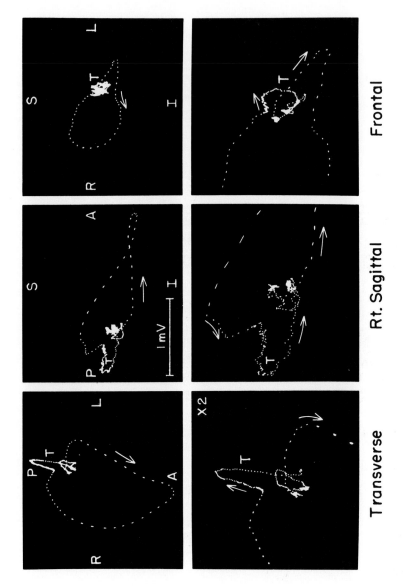

R.J. 292611

Transverse   Rt. Sagittal   Frontal

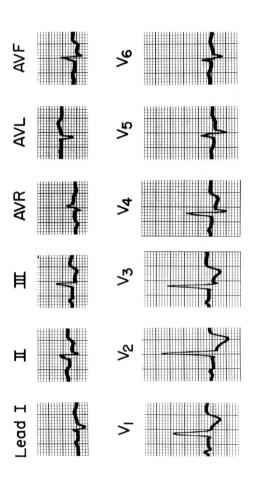

Fig. 7.7. Type A right ventricular hypertrophy. The patient has severe chronic lung disease with advanced cor pulmonale and right-sided heart failure. Both the vectorcardiogram and electrocardiogram are diagnostic of right ventricular hypertrophy.

D.V. 3l7376   dash interval 2 msec

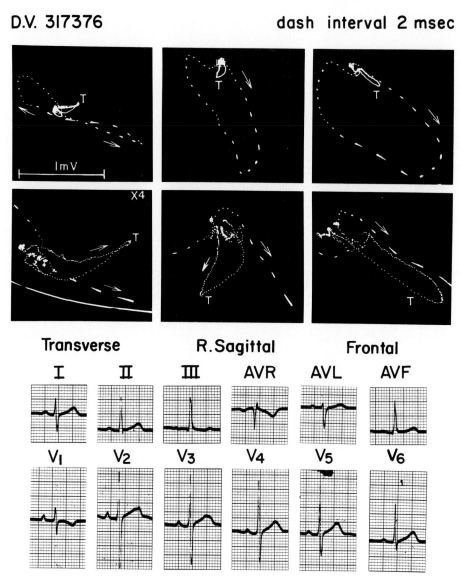

Fig. 7.8. Type A right ventricular hypertrophy. The patient is a 19-year-old girl with proved secundum type of atrial septal defect. The QRSsÊ loop is displaced anteriorly and rightward. In the transverse plane the QRS loop has a figure-of-eight pattern. In the frontal plane it is inscribed clockwise. The T loop is also abnormal with a reversal of the direction of its inscription in the transverse and sagittal projections. Although the vectorcardiographic changes are diagnostic of right ventricular hypertrophy, the electrocardiographic findings are equivocal for a 19-year-old patient.

efferent limb. However, if the right ventricular preponderance occurs mostly during the later phase, a figure-of-eight loop is inscribed. It is quite possible that the latter configuration is associated with more selective hypertrophy of the basal portion of the right ventricle, including the crista supraventricularis which is normally the last region of the right ventricle to be depolarized. It is of interest that a significant relationship has also been demonstrated between the magnitude of the maximum rightward forces and the right ventricular peak pressure as in the cases of pulmonic stenosis (Hugenholtz and Gamboa).

There is no general agreement as to the genesis of the leftward initial deflection or the q wave in lead V_1 in many patients with right ventricular hypertrophy. Some have attributed the change to a reversal of the direction of the septal activation, the septum being activated from right to left instead of left to right. The right septal potential may be greater than the left septal potential with the resultant forces being directed from right to left. Others believe that the clockwise rotation of a vertical heart around its longitudinal axis is responsible for the leftward orientation of the initial QRS vectors.

ST Vector and TsÊ Loop

The magnitude of the **ST** vector in right ventricular hypertrophy is generally small and often difficult to identify. In fact, it is only in type A right ventricular hypertrophy that the vector occasionally becomes abnormally large. The latter condition is usually associated with very large anterior and rightward **QRS** vectors. Even then the magnitude seldom approaches that seen in left ventricular hypertrophy. However, the vector is displaced posteriorly, to the left, either inferiorly or superiorly, instead of the normal anterior, leftward and inferior orientation. Thus, in the transverse plane projection the vector points posteriorly and to the left; in the sagittal plane, posteriorly, inferiorly or superiorly; and in the frontal plane, mostly leftward, either inferiorly or superiorly.

The spatial T loop is either abnormally small or at the lower limits of normal in its magnitude. The configuration of the loop is mostly oval, sometimes quite wide. In many cases the loop is asymmetrical with the efferent limb shorter than the afferent limb and appears as a straight line. However, the normal slow inscription of the efferent limb remains. The loop is oriented posteriorly (occasionally anteriorly), to the left and inferiorly. Its direction is similar to that of the **ST** vector. It is quite characteristic of this type of right ventricular hypertrophy that the general direction of the spatial T loop, as well as the **ST** vector, is discordant to the terminal vectors of the QRS loop. In the transverse plane projection the T loop is directed to the left, usually posteriorly and occasionally anteriorly. In the majority of instances the loop is inscribed clockwise. In the right sagittal plane the loop is directed inferiorly and posteriorly even though an occasional anterior loop is also seen. The loop is usually inscribed counterclockwise. The reversal of the direction of inscription from that of the normal in these two planes is a useful feature, since the general orientation of the T vectors may sometimes be normal (leftward, anterior, and inferior), and no apparent abnormality is seen in the T wave of the scalar electrocardiogram. In the frontal plane the loop is directed inferiorly and leftward. With few exceptions it is inscribed clockwise.

In the conventional electrocardiogram the small posterior and leftward **ST** vector (as seen in the transverse plane) is recorded as a slightly depressed J junction and ST segment in the right precordial leads and an isoelectric or slightly elevated ST segment in the left precordial leads. In the occasional patient in whom the **ST** vector is abnormally large, the ST segment depression in the right precordial leads will be more prominent and is frequently associated with a tall R wave. The ST segment in lead I is usually isoelectric or elevated because of the leftward orientation of the vector. It may be depressed or elevated in the inferior leads owing to the variable superior or inferior direction of the **ST** vector in the frontal plane.

The leftward and posterior orientation of the T loop is responsible for the presence or increase in the T wave negativity in the right precordial leads. As the T loop rotates from a position of approximately 25° backward in a counterclockwise direction, additional right and midprecordial leads will show T wave inversion (i.e., lead V_1 through V_4). The left precordial leads usually record an upright T wave owing to the leftward orientation of the **T** vector loop. In general, since the **ST** vector and T loop are approximately 180° away from the late **QRS** vectors, ST segment depression and an inverted T wave will be seen in leads which display a tall, upright R wave, and ST segment elevation, and an upright T wave will be seen in leads which display a deep terminal negative deflection (S wave).

The probable pathophysiology responsible for the alterations of the **ST** and **T** vectors is similar to that for left ventricular hypertrophy. The initiation of the repolarization of the endocardial layer of the hypertrophied right ventricle before depolarization has been completed results in the displacement of the J junction and, consequently, the ST segment. Since there is an accentuation of the repolarization potential from the right ventricle, the resultant **T** vector will adopt a direction similar to that originating from the right ventricle instead of the left ventricle. The endocardium to epicardium spread of the repolarization process in the right ventricle results in **ST** and **T** vectors which are leftward, posterior and inferior or superior.

TYPE B RIGHT VENTRICULAR HYPERTROPHY (Fig. 7.9 and 7.10)

QRSsÊ Loop

In type B right ventricular hypertrophy pattern, the QRSsÊ loop is also displaced anteriorly. In contrast to type A, the spatial relationship among the successive instantaneous vectors is relatively undisturbed. In other words, the entire spatial loop is displaced forward, but the rotation of the loop itself remains unchanged.

Transverse plane.   The major portion of the QRS loop is located anteriorly in the transverse plane projection, and the loop is inscribed counterclockwise. Since the transverse plane QRS loop in the normal individual often has more than 50 percent of its area located anteriorly, a loop cannot be considered as abnormally anterior unless over 70 percent of the loop is so located.

Sagittal plane.   In the right sagittal plane projection the anterior displacement of the QRS loop can also be seen, and the loop is usually oriented inferiorly. The direction of inscription is clockwise as it is in the normal individuals.

Frontal plane.   In the frontal plane projection, the loop remains relatively narrow in most of the cases. Occasionally, however, the loop is abnormally wide owing to a late, large, rightward component. The direction of inscription is clockwise in the great majority.

In the conventional electrocardiogram the abnormal findings are usually limited to a large R wave (5 mm or more) in lead V_1 with an R/S ratio greater than one and sometimes a significant S wave in leads I, V_5, and V_6. Anatomically, the right ventricular hypertrophy associated with this pattern is usually moderate.

ST Vector and TsÊ Loop

The magnitude of **ST** vector in type B right ventricular hypertrophy is usually within normal limits. However, the vector is oriented posteriorly, to the right, and superiorly. The direction is thus approximately opposite to that of the QRS loop. The magnitude of the spatial T loop is either small or normal. It is often wide and becomes almost circular in appearance. The loop is oriented to the left, inferiorly, and anteriorly or slightly posteriorly. Although its orientation may be similar to that of the normal T loop, its direction of inscription is frequently reversed, being

TYPE B RIGHT VENTRICULAR HYPERTROPHY

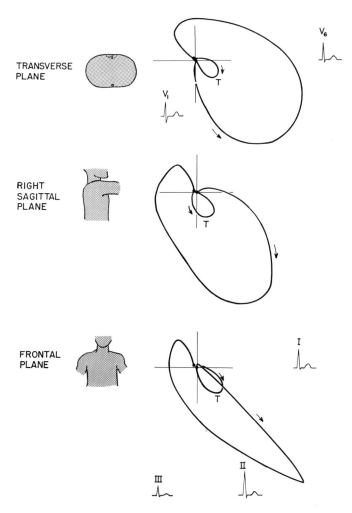

Fig. 7.9. Schematic diagrams of QRS and T loops in type B right ventricular hypertrophy and the representative scalar lead QRS-T complexes.

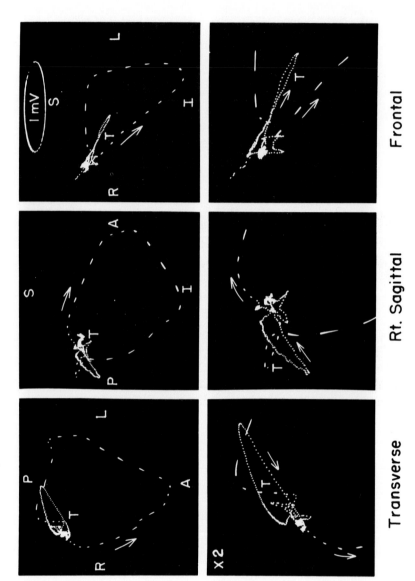

J.H. 436262

Frontal

Rt. Sagittal

Transverse

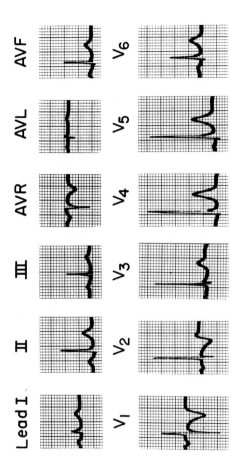

Fig. 7.10. Type B right ventricular hypertrophy. The patient is a 56-year-old man with rheumatic heart disease and severe mitral stenosis and pulmonary hypertension. In the vectorcardiogram the QRS loop is displaced anteriorly as can be seen in the transverse and right sagittal planes. The direction of inscription, however, remains counterclockwise in the transverse plane and clockwise in the right sagittal plane. In the transverse plane the T loop is directed to the left and posteriorly, and the loop is inscribed clockwise. In the right sagittal plane the T loop points posteriorly and inferiorly and is inscribed counterclockwise. In the frontal plane the QRS loop is inscribed counterclockwise, which is atypical. The T loop is normal in its orientation.

TYPE C   RIGHT VENTRICULAR HYPERTROPHY

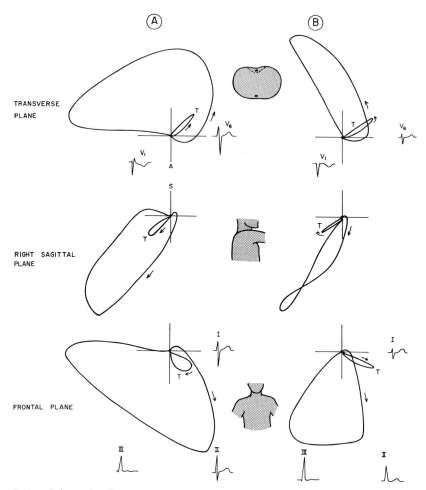

Fig. 7.11. Schematic diagrams of the QRS and T loops in type C right ventricular hypertrophy. In (A) the increase of the rightward forces is more marked than that of (B) so that the larger part of the QRS loop area is located to the right as seen in the transverse and frontal planes. There is also a tendency of the terminal deflection of the QRS loop to be displaced more anteriorly in (A) as demonstrated in the transverse plane projection. A late positive deflection (r′) is thus seen in lead V_1 of the conventional electrocardiogram.

clockwise in the transverse plane and counterclockwise in the right sagittal plane. The loop is usually inscribed clockwise in the frontal plane.

In the scalar electrocardiogram the ST segment and the T wave usually appear to be quite normal except for the occasional slight ST depression in the precordial leads and the inferior limb leads owing to the abnormal posterior, rightward and superior orientation of the **ST** vector. The relatively minor changes in the **ST** and **T** vectors are probably also related to the lesser degree of right ventricular hypertrophy in this type of pattern.

TYPE C RIGHT VENTRICULAR HYPERTROPHY (Figs. 7.11–7.13)

The main feature of type C right ventricular hypertrophy is the posterior orientation of the QRS loop. It is seen most commonly in patients with chronic cor pulmonale but also in patients with mitral stenosis and occasionally congenital heart disease such as atrial septal defect.

QRSsÊ Loop

The spatial QRS loop in this type of right ventricular hypertrophy is displaced posteriorly and to the right. It may be oriented either inferiorly or superiorly. The magnitude of the loop is often within the normal range. The duration of the QRS loop may or may not be slightly prolonged. There is no evidence of an abnormal terminal conduction delay. The maximum spatial **QRS** vector is directed posteriorly and to the right, most often inferiorly, but occasionally superiorly.

Planar Projections of the QRSsÊ Loop

Transverse plane QRS loop. The configuration of the QRS loop in this projection may either be wide or narrow; the latter is seen mostly in patients with chronic cor pulmonale. The great majority of the loop area is located posteriorly. The extent of the rightward deviation varies, but the area in the right posterior quadrant is larger than 20 percent of the total QRS area (upper normal limit) in this plane. The loop is inscribed *counterclockwise.* In certain instances there is a figure-of-eight pattern with the distal portion inscribed clockwise.

The initial deflection inscribes mostly anteriorly and to the left. After a limited leftward course, the efferent limb of the QRS loop inscribes rapidly in a posterior and rightward direction. When the loop is narrow, the afferent limb returns toward the origin of the loop and becomes continuous with the terminal deflection without a distinct change in its direction. In other cases the later portion of the QRS loop may bulge more to the right or forward and present itself in the right anterior quadrant. The planar projection of the maximum spatial **QRS** vector is usually directed posteriorly and to the right.

The posterior displacement of the major portion of the QRS loop is responsible for the leftward displacement of the transitional zone in the precordial leads of the scalar electrocardiogram. Most of the loop is now projected on the negative side of the lead axes of the right and mid precordial leads, and the initial positivity is small and increases slowly from lead V_1 through V_6. Depending on whether the initial deflection is anterior or posterior to 25°, lead V_1 may display an rS or a QS deflection. When the late **QRS** vectors are directed rightward and anteriorly, a secondary wave (R′) will be seen in lead V_1. In the left precordial leads the reduction of the normal leftward forces and the increase of the late rightward forces are manifested as smaller R and deeper S waves.

Sagittal plane QRS loop. In the right sagittal plane the QRS loop is located mostly in the posterior-inferior quadrant. Occasionally, a significant late por-

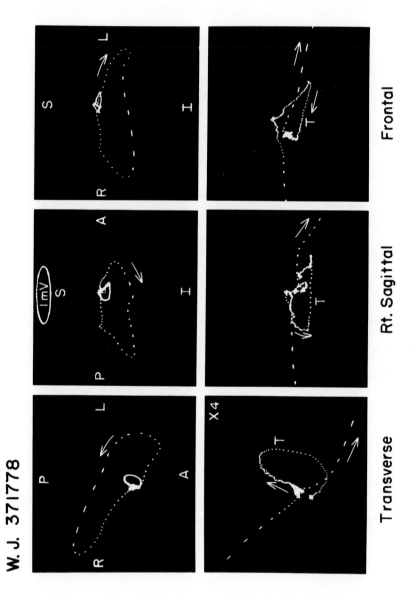

W.J. 371778

Transverse   Rt. Sagittal   Frontal

104

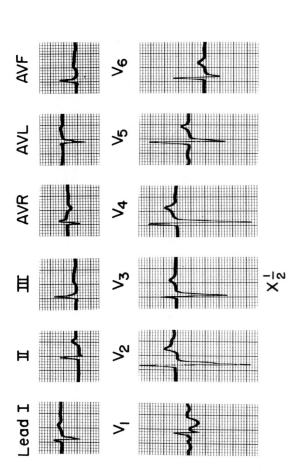

Fig. 7.12. Type C right ventricular hypertrophy. The vectorcardiogram and electrocardiogram were recorded from a 46-year-old man with rheumatic heart disease, mitral stenosis and functional tricuspid regurgitation. The P loop and P wave cannot be identified because of atrial fibrillation. In the vectorcardiogram the transverse plane projection reveals a QRS loop which is displaced to the right and posteriorly. The direction of inscription is counterclockwise. The T loop is oriented to the left and posteriorly and is inscribed clockwise. In the right sagittal plane the QRS loop is not remarkable, but the T loop is inscribed counterclockwise. In the frontal plane over half of the QRS loop area is located on the right side. The loop is inscribed clockwise.

tion of the loop is located superiorly. There is considerable variation of the direction of the initial deflection although the superior and anterior direction is the most common. The loop may be inscribed either clockwise or occasionally counterclockwise, and a figure-of-eight pattern is also seen.

Frontal plane QRS loop. In the frontal plane projection the QRS loop is inferior and more or less vertical in position. The loop may be narrow or wide. The magnitude may or may not be abnormally increased. The majority shows a clockwise inscription.

The initial deflection is usually inscribed to the left and superiorly but occasionally inferiorly. The course of the efferent limb is downward, at first slightly toward the left and then gradually toward the right; its leftward component is much smaller than that of the normal. The afferent limb extends abnormally to the right. The terminal deflection may be directed inferiorly or superiorly. Frequently, a considerable portion of the terminal QRS loop is located in the right upper quadrant.

The vertical position of the QRS loop with the decrease of the leftward forces and increase of rightward forces results in an rs or rS complex in lead I of the conventional electrocardiogram. An rS complex is associated with a wider loop with a larger terminal rightward component and usually a more severe degree of right ventricular hypertrophy. In the inferior leads (leads II, III, and aVF) a qR pattern is most frequently seen because of the superior direction of the initial vectors and inferior direction of the main body of the loop. It is also common to see an rS complex in these leads owing to a large, superiorly located terminal portion of the QRS loop.

The genesis of type C right ventricular hypertrophy is probably dependent upon more than one factor. In patients with chronic cor pulmonale, in whom this type of QRS loop is most frequently seen, both the hypertrophy and the change in the position of the heart are probably responsible. There is usually a lowering of the diaphragm accompanied by a vertical heart with clockwise rotation along its longitudinal axis. The left ventricular free wall is now facing more posteriorly. The vectoral sum of the left ventricular forces and the increased right ventricular forces will result in a mean **QRS** vector which is directed posteriorly and to the right (Fig. 7.13A). Schepers has demonstrated pathologically that in the early stage the hypertrophy of the right ventricle in chronic cor pulmonale involves chiefly the region of the outflow tract. A study at the authors' institution (Bove and Scott) also revealed that the basal portion of the right ventricle is hypertrophied to a greater degree than the apical portion in the more advanced cases. As the vectors representing the activation of this portion of the right ventricle are directed to the right, superiorly, and posteriorly, and the vectors of the basal portion of the left ventricle are directed to the left, posteriorly, and inferiorly, the resultant forces will thus be oriented to the right, posteriorly, and usually superiorly (Fig. 7.13B). It is probably true that this type of QRS loop is associated with a lesser degree of right ventricular hypertrophy than that represented by the type A loop. Many of the more severe cases of chronic cor pulmonale eventually develop an anterior QRS loop with clockwise inscription of the loop in the transverse plane projection. A similar mechanism is probably also responsible for the large posterior and rightward terminal vectors seen in many cases of atrial septal defect.

As will be discussed in a later chapter, the QRS loop in type C right ventricular hypertrophy closely resembles that of left posterior hemiblock. Other clinical information is often needed before a definite diagnosis can be reached.

ST Vector and TsÊ Loop

The magnitude and direction of the **ST** vector in type C right ventricular hypertrophy are usually normal. The spatial T loop is usually normal in its magnitude and has an elongated and elliptical configuration. It is oriented to the left,

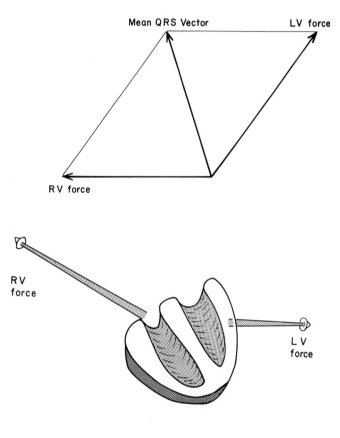

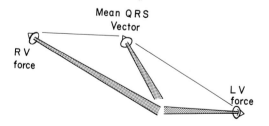

Fig. 7.13. (A) and (B). Possible explanations for the posterior and rightward orientation of the QRS loop in type C right ventricular hypertrophy (see text). In (A) the vectors are viewed in the transverse plane projection.

inferiorly, and posteriorly, although occasionally an anterior loop is seen. The normal slow inscription of the efferent limb is retained. In the transverse plane the loop is directed to the left and posteriorly (occasionally anteriorly). It is usually inscribed counterclockwise. In the right sagittal plane it is directed inferiorly and posteriorly (occasionally anteriorly) and is inscribed clockwise. In the frontal plane it is directed inferiorly and to the left and is inscribed clockwise.

The ST segment in the scalar electrocardiogram is usually within normal limits owing to the normal orientation and magnitude of the ST vector. The posterior orientation of the T loop is manifested in the right precordial leads as inverted T waves, and its leftward orientation results in upright T waves in the left precordial leads and standard lead I. The T waves in the standard leads II, III, and aVF are usually upright due to the inferior direction of the T loop.

Summary of transverse plane QRS loop configurations.   A convenient way to summarize and visualize the mechanism of production of the various configurations of the transverse plane QRS loop in the three types of right ventricular hypertrophy is given in Figure 7.14. The different segments of a normal QRS loop may be "pulled" by the increased right ventricular forces in either the right anterior or the right posterior direction as depicted in Figure 7.14.A. Depending on the portion that is involved and the direction of the displacement, various forms of the loop may be seen and are illustrated in Figure 7.14B. In all the diagrams in (B), the segments of the loop which are most affected are drawn in a heavy line. Diagrams (a) to (d) are representative of the type A right ventricular hypertrophy. In (a) the afferent limb and the terminal deflection are displaced anteriorly and to the right because of the increased right anterior force. The loop presents a figure-of-eight pattern. Lead V_1 of the conventional electrocardiogram displays an rSr' complex with the r' representing the displaced late portion of the QRS loop. If the afferent limb and the terminal deflection are "pulled" further in the right anterior direction, they may become anterior to the efferent limb and an essentially clockwise loop will be inscribed as is demonstrated in diagrams (b) and (c). A part of the efferent limb may now also be involved. As the extent of the displacement increases, a greater portion of the QRS loop will be located on the positive side of the lead axis of V_1 and a smaller portion, on the negative side. Consequently, the S wave in V_1 gradually decreases and the R' increases in amplitude, and an rsR' or a notched R is recorded. In (d) there is also involvement of the initial deflection, which is displaced posteriorly and to the left because of the increase of the right septal force (not represented in diagram A). A qR complex is displayed in lead V_1 as the initial deflection is now written on the negative side of the lead axis of V_1.

If the right anterior "pulling" force is now applied equally on both the efferent and afferent limbs of the QRS loop, the loop will be oriented more anteriorly and less leftward (diagram e). The spatial relationship between the efferent and the afferent limbs is unchanged. The loop is inscribed in the normal counterclockwise direction and represents the pattern seen in type B right ventricular hypertrophy. An Rs complex is recorded in lead V_1.

In contrast to the changes that have just been described, all of which may be explained on the basis of increased right anterior force, the alteration of the QRS loop illustrated in diagram (f) is the result of increased right *posterior* force. The

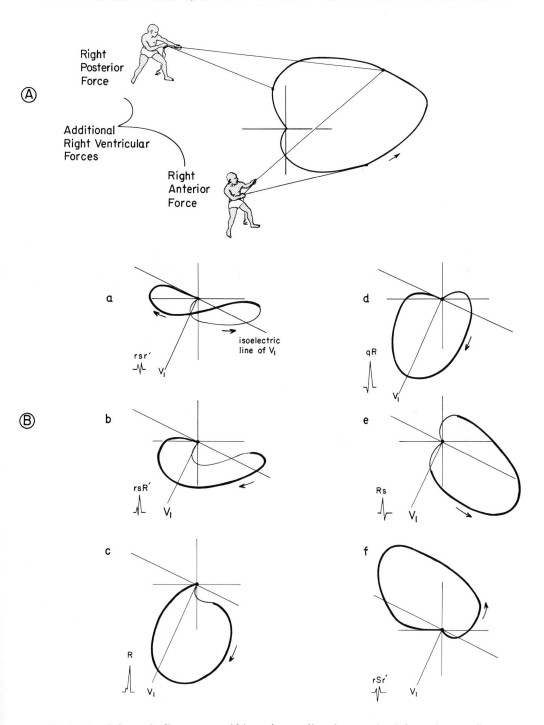

Fig. 7.14. Schematic diagrams to aid in understanding the genesis of the various configurations of the transverse plane QRS loop in right ventricular hypertrophy.

QRS LOOP AREA
RIGHT VENTRICULAR HYPERTROPHY

TRANSVERSE PLANE

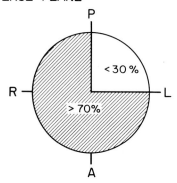
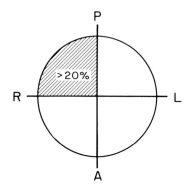

FRONTAL PLANE

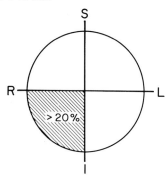

Fig. 7.15. Diagrams illustrating some quantitative criteria for the diagnosis of right ventricular hypertrophy. The numbers indicate the percentage of loop area located in the corresponding quadrant or quadrants.

entire loop is more or less equally affected and "pulled" in that direction. The direction of inscription of the loop remains counterclockwise. This is the pattern seen in type C right ventricular hypertrophy. Since the small initial and terminal deflections are now on the positive side, and the major portion of the loop is on the negative side of the lead axis of V_1, an rSr′ complex is recorded in this lead.

Based on the rightward, anterior, or posterior displacement of the QRS loop area, a group of simple quantitative criteria have been used by the author for the diagnosis of right ventricular hypertrophy in the absence of conduction defect (Fig. 7.15). They are applicable for all three types of right ventricular hypertrophy.

A. In the transverse plane:
1. The QRS loop area in the left posterior quadrant is less than 30 percent of the total (or the anterior and rightward area is greater than 70 percent of the total)

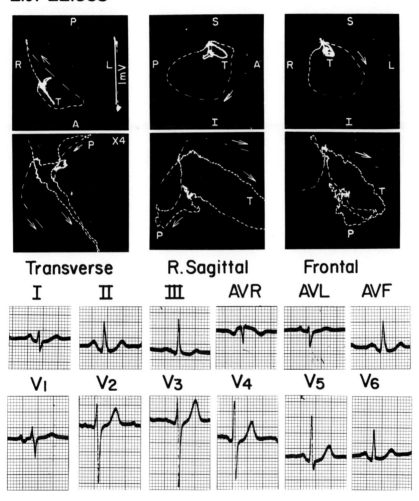

Fig. 7.16. Right ventricular hypertrophy. The tracings were obtained from a 33-year-old man with mitral stenosis. In the vectorcardiogram the QRS loop area in the left posterior quadrant of the transverse plane is less than 30 percent of the total. The area in the right inferior quadrant of the frontal plane is greater than 20 percent of the total. The electrocardiogram does not reveal definite evidence of right ventricular hypertrophy.

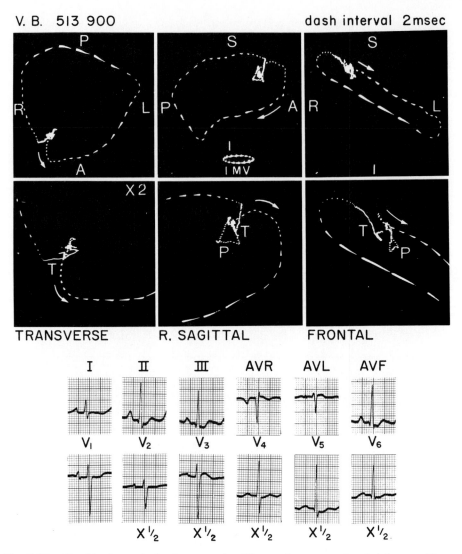

Fig. 7.17. Combined ventricular hypertrophy. The tracings were recorded from a 45-year-old woman with idiopathic cardiomyopathy. Autopsy revealed combined ventricular hypertrophy. The vectorcardiogram meets the voltage criteria for left ventricular hypertrophy. In the transverse plane the QRS loop area in the right posterior quadrant is slightly greater than 20 percent of the total suggesting coexisting right ventricular hypertrophy.

    2.   The loop area in the right posterior quadrant is greater than 20 percent of
        the total

B.   In the frontal plane:

    1.   The area in the right inferior quadrant is greater than 20 percent of the
        total

Right ventricular hypertrophy is considered to be present if one or more of the three criteria are met. These criteria are derived from the planimetry studies of 198 normal subjects (Chapter 5) and have been tested in 100 proved cases of right ventricular hypertrophy with high degree of sensitivity. An example is illustrated in Figure 7.16. As true posterior myocardial infarction may also result in a reduction of the loop area in the left posterior quadrant and left posterior hemiblock in an increase of the right side area, these possibilities should be considered before the diagnosis is made.

COMBINED VENTRICULAR HYPERTROPHY (Fig. 7.17)

In combined ventricular hypertrophy the increased electric potentials from the left and right ventricles may counterbalance each other and their effect is not detectable in the vectorcardiogram. When the degree of hypertrophy is more marked in one ventricle than the other, the resultant forces may adapt the characteristics of those of the preponderant ventricle, and the vectorcardiogram reveals hypertrophy of that ventricle alone. In most instances, because of the normal preponderance of the left ventricle, a proportional increase of the muscle mass of both ventricles usually results in changes suggestive of left ventricular hypertrophy only. However, in some cases the vectorcardiographic signs of either left or right ventricular hypertrophy are so modified that coexisting hypertrophy of the other ventricle may be suspected.

There are only a few reports concerning the vectorcardiographic findings of combined ventricular hypertrophy. In an analysis of 60 patients with acquired heart disease and hemodynamic or anatomic evidence of combined ventricular hypertrophy in the author's institution, we have found the following signs helpful. However, they are disappointingly insensitive. The majority of cases displayed only evidence of either left or right ventricular hypertrophy alone or nonspecific changes.

1. The presence of large anterior forces in the QRS loop with the maximum anterior voltage greater than 0.6 mV when the loop is otherwise typical of left ventricular hypertrophy.
2. The presence of large right posterior forces with the loop area in the right posterior quadrant greater than 20 percent of the total when the vectorcardiogram is otherwise typical of left ventricular hypertrophy.
3. The QRS loop is anteriorly oriented and is inscribed either clockwise or counterclockwise in the transverse plane to suggest right ventricular hypertrophy. However, the loop is inscribed counterclockwise in the frontal plane.

REFERENCES

1. Bove KE, Scott RC: The anatomy of chronic cor pulmonale secondary to intrinsic lung disease. Prog Cardiovasc Dis 9:227, 1966
2. Brown IK: Electrocardiography and vectorcardiography in right ventricular hypertrophy from chronic bronchitis. Br Heart J 30:470, 1968
3. Cabrera E, Gaxiola A: Diagnostic contribution of the vectorcardiogram in hemodynamic overloading of the heart. Am Heart J 60:296, 1960
4. Castellanos A, Hernandez FA, Lemberg L, Castellanos A Jr: The vectorcardiographic

criteria of hemodynamical overloadings in congenital heart disease. Cardiologia 44:392, 1964

5. Chou TC, Masangkay MP, Young R, Conway GP, Helm RA: Simple quantitative vectorcardiographic criteria for the diagnosis of right ventricular hypertrophy. Circulation 48:1262, 1973

6. Cueto J, Toshima H, Armijo G, Tuna N, Lillehei CW: Vectorcardiographic studies in acquired valvular disease with reference to the diagnosis of right ventricular hypertrophy. Circulation 33:588, 1966

7. Dack S: The electrocardiogram and vectorcardiogram in ventricular septal defect. Am J Cardiol 5:199, 1960

8. Fowler NO, Helm RA: The spatial QRS loop in right ventricular hypertrophy with special reference to the initial component. Circulation 7:573, 1953

9. Gamboa R, Hugenholtz PG, Nadas AS: Corrected (Frank), uncorrected (Cube), and standard electrocardiographic lead systems in recording augmented right ventricular forces in right ventricular hypertension. Br Heart J 28:62, 1966

10. Hugenholtz PG, Gamboa R: Effect of chronically increased ventricular pressure on electrical forces of the heart. A correlation between hemodynamic and vectorcardiographic data (Frank system) in 90 patients with aortic or pulmonic stenosis. Circulation 30:511, 1964

11. Khoury GH, DuShane JW, Ongley PA: The preoperative and postoperative vectorcardiogram in tetralogy of Fallot. Circulation 31:85, 1965

12. Kovats-Hopff L, Wyss OAM: Vectorcardiographic signs of biventricular hypertrophy. Cardiologia 48:269, 1966

13. Lal S, Fletcher E, Binnion P: Frank vectorcardiogram correlated with haemodynamic measurements. Quantitative analysis. Br Heart J 31:15, 1969

14. Lasser RP, Borun ER, Grishman A: Spatial vectorcardiography: right ventricular hypertrophy as seen in congenital heart disease. VII. Am Heart J 42:370, 1951

15. Mathur VS, Levine HD: Vectorcardiographic differentiation between right ventricular hypertrophy and posterobasal myocardial infarction. Circulation 42:883, 1970

16. McCaughan D, Koroxenidis GT, Hopff LG, Williams C: New vectorcardiographic criteria for the diagnosis of acquired right ventricular hypertrophy: Comparison with standard electrocardiographic criteria. (P). Circulation 28:766, 1963

17. Richman JL, Wolff L: The spatial vectorcardiogram in congenital heart disease and right ventricular hypertrophy. Am Heart J 50:85, 1955

18. Schepers GWH: The pathology of cor pulmonale. Trans Am Coll Cardiol 7:48, 1957

19. Taymor RC, Hoffman I, Henry E: The Frank vectorcardiogram in mitral stenosis. A study of 29 cases. Circulation 30:865, 1964

20. Varriale P, Kennedy RJ, Alfenito JC: Vectorcardiogram of combined ventricular hypertrophy: Posterior counterclockwise loop (Frank System). Br Heart J 31:457, 1969

21. Walsh TJ, Roman GT Jr, Massie E: The vectorcardiographic QRSsÊ-loop findings in chronic cor pulmonale. Am Heart J 60:592, 1960

8

Left Bundle Branch Block

SEQUENCE OF VENTRICULAR ACTIVATION IN LEFT BUNDLE BRANCH BLOCK

It will be recalled that the bundle of His bifurcates at the lower edge of the membraneous interventricular septum into the left and right bundle branches. The two bundle branches descend subendocardially on each side of the muscular interventricular septum. The left bundle branch divides into an anterior and a posterior division soon after its origin to supply fibers to the left septal mass and the free wall of the left ventricle. The right bundle branch descends as a single cord until it reaches the base of the anterior papillary muscle of the right ventricle, where it arborizes and supplies fibers to the right septum and the free wall of the right ventricle. In the presence of a normal conduction system the ventricular activation begins at the left midseptal and paraseptal regions and the impulse spreads in an essentially rightward direction. Shortly afterwards the activation also begins at the lower right septal surface and the impulse spreads leftward. Therefore, the depolarization of the ventricular septum involves a double envelopment process. However, the net effect of the septal activation is from left to right owing to the slightly earlier initiation and a much larger area of involvement of the left septum. Activation of the free wall of the ventricles soon proceeds in an endocardium-to-epicardium direction. As has been stated previously, the electrical potential manifested is mainly that of the left ventricle.

When the conduction through the main left bundle branch is interrupted, or if there is simultaneous block of the two divisions, the earliest ventricular excitation occurs in the tissue supplied by the right bundle, that is, the right septal and ventricular myocardium (Fig. 8.1). The wave of excitation then spreads transseptally from right to left. Since the septal depolarization now depends solely on the impulse coming from the right side instead of both sides, the process requires a much longer duration for its completion. Rodriquez and Sodi-Pallares maintain that the boundary between the right and left septal mass serves as an electrical "barrier" which causes considerable delay in the advancement of the impulse across the septum. Becker and associates have failed to demonstrate such a "barrier," and their experiments

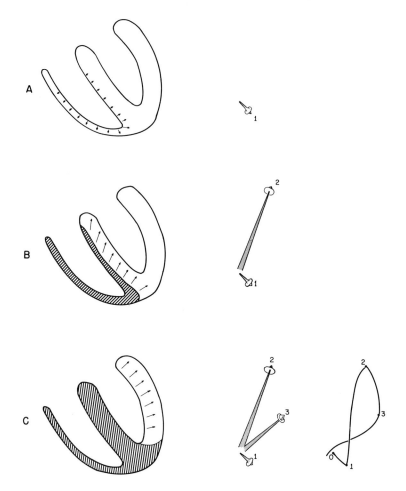

Fig. 8.1. See text. The vectors and resultant loop are viewed in their transverse plane presentation.

indicated that the wave front advanced throughout the septum at a uniform speed. Nevertheless, it is generally agreed that the alteration of the septal activation in complete left bundle branch block is responsible for most of the prolongation of the QRS duration.

There is also some difference of opinion in regard to the sequence of activation of the free wall of the left ventricle in left bundle branch block. Some believe that although there is a delay of the arrival of the excitation impulse, the free wall of the left ventricle is depolarized in a normal fashion once the process is begun. The direction is thus from the endocardium to epicardium. Others have found that there is also alteration in the pattern of depolarization in the free wall. According to Kennamer and Prinzmetal, the impulse enters the mural myocardium without passing through the Purkinje system. Becker and associates have demonstrated that while the septal depolarization is still going on, there is activation of the anterior and posterior epicardium adjoining the septum, and the spread of the impulse in these areas is from the epicardium to endocardium. This spread is by means of muscle conduction. The remaining left lateral myocardium is excited through the Purkinje network.

If the ventricular activation process in left bundle branch block (or simultaneous block of its two divisions) is arbitrarily simplified and divided into three phases, they may be represented by three vectors (Fig. 8.1). During the initial phase the right septum and the free wall of the right ventricle, which are supplied by the intact right bundle branch, are depolarized. As the activation wave front bordering the right ventricular cavity assumes the configuration of a cone, the resultant force will thus be directed toward the apex of the right ventricle. The mean vector representing the initial phase (vector 1) is therefore directed anteriorly, to the left and inferiorly. During the second phase the left septal mass and its adjacent myocardium of the free wall of the left ventricle are depolarized. The direction of the spread is from right to left. Since anatomically the left septal surface is oriented to the left, inferiorly and posteriorly, a right to left septal activation will result in a vector pointing in the same direction (vector 2). During the last phase the lateral wall of the left ventricle is activated from the endocardium to the epicardium. The vector (vector 3) representing the wave front is directed to the left, posteriorly, either superiorly or inferiorly, but is more superior than vector 2.

It is to be emphasized that the foregoing description of the sequence of activation in left bundle branch block is based on observations from dog experiments. The application of these findings to human hearts may or may not be entirely acceptable. However, the vectorcardiogram deducted from the above outlined sequence does correlate quite well with that observed in clinical left bundle branch block. Furthermore, since the great majority of patients manifesting left bundle branch block have other associated abnormalities, it is expected that the pattern of left bundle branch block will often be modified and be different from a surgically induced left bundle branch block in animals.

VECTORCARDIOGRAPHIC FINDINGS IN LEFT BUNDLE BRANCH BLOCK

QRSsÊ Loop

The spatial QRS loop in left bundle branch block is elongated and narrow. In the majority of instances its magnitude exceeds the normal limit. Practically the entire loop is located posteriorly and to the left, either superiorly or inferiorly. In the uncomplicated case a small initial deflection is inscribed to the left, mostly anteriorly and inferiorly. The efferent limb of the body of the loop turns rather sharply in the posterior direction although its inferior and slightly leftward orientation persists. The afferent limb is invariably more superior and to the left than the efferent limb. The terminal deflection usually cannot clearly be separated from the afferent limb as it is inscribed in the same direction. Its end point (J) is to the right, anterior, either superior or inferior to the origin of the loop. The duration of the QRS loop is prolonged to 0.12 sec or more. One of the diagnostic features is the presence of conduction delay involving the mid and late portions of the loop. The maximum spatial **QRS** vector is oriented to the left, posteriorly and either inferiorly or superiorly. Its time of occurrence after the beginning of the QRS loop is characteristically delayed.

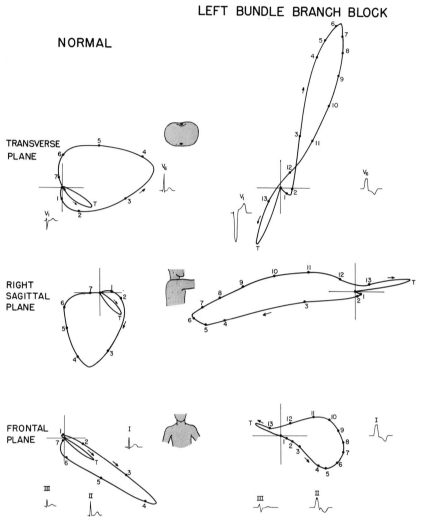

Fig. 8.2. Schematic diagrams of the vectorcardiogram in left bundle branch block as compared with that of the normal person. The numerals indicate the time in hundredths of a second after the beginning of the QRS loop. The representative scalar lead QRS-T complexes are illustrated.

Planar Projections of the QRSsÊ Loop and Correlation with the Conventional Electrocardiogram (Figs. 8.2–8.5, 8.7)

Transverse plane QRS loop.   In the transverse plane projection the QRS loop is usually longer and narrower than normal. Characteristically, with the exception of a small initial portion, the majority of the loop is inscribed clockwise. Frequently, the loop has a figure-of-eight pattern or it may have a double twist. Otherwise, the contour of the loop is relatively smooth.

In the uncomplicated case of left bundle branch block the initial deflection is invariably directed leftward and is usually anterior. In our experience a leftward and

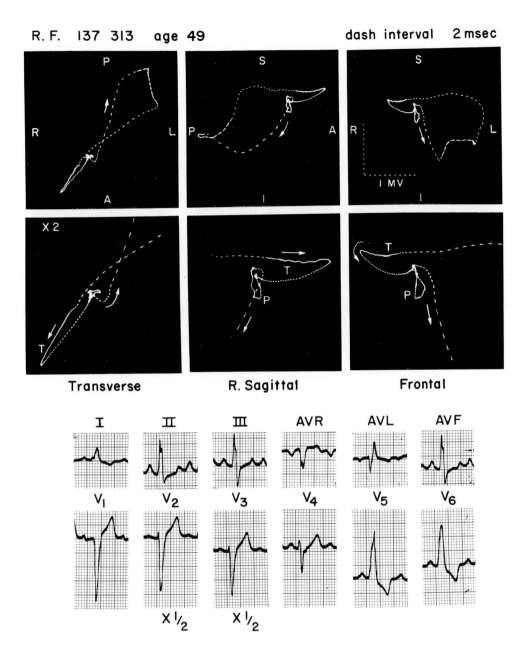

Fig. 8.3. Complete left bundle branch block. The vectorcardiogram and electrocardiogram were recorded from a 49-year-old woman with idiopathic cardiomyopathy and congestive heart failure. The magnitude of the QRSsÊ and T loops is increased. The spatial QRS loop is directed leftward, posteriorly, and inferiorly. Its duration is prolonged to 0.12 sec. There is a slow inscription of the midportion of the QRS loop. In the transverse plane the initial deflection is directed anteriorly and leftward. The QRS loop is inscribed in a figure-of-eight pattern with its major portion inscribed clockwise. The loop is inscribed counterclockwise in the frontal plane. The **ST** vector and T loop are discordant to the QRS loop in all of the projections.

119

G. D. 435401

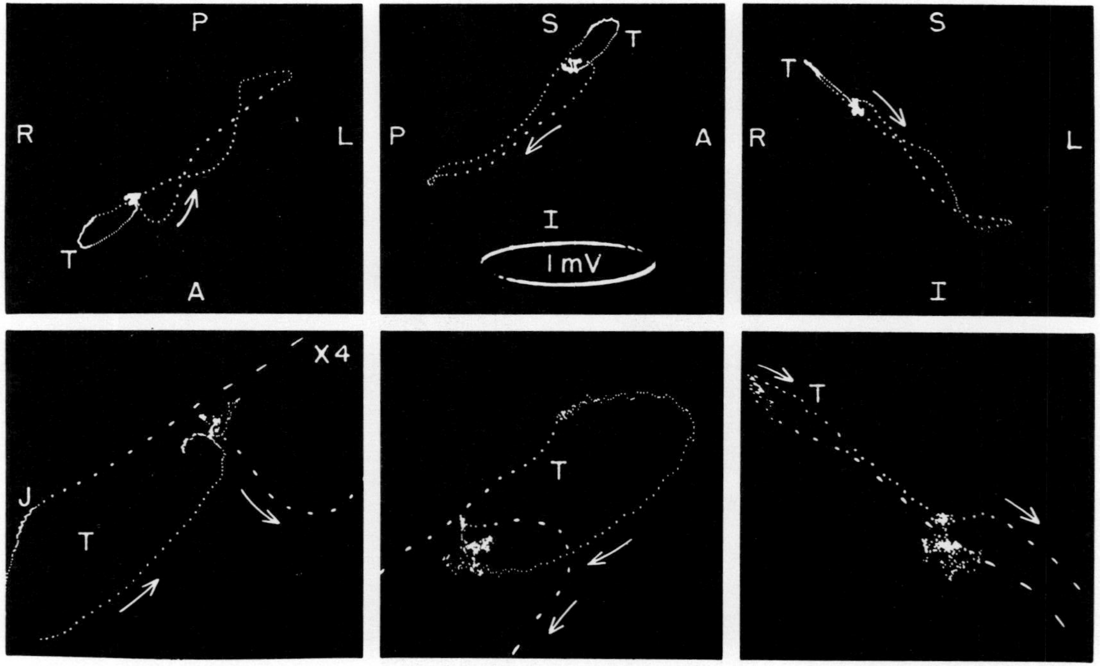

Frontal

Rt. Sagittal

Transverse

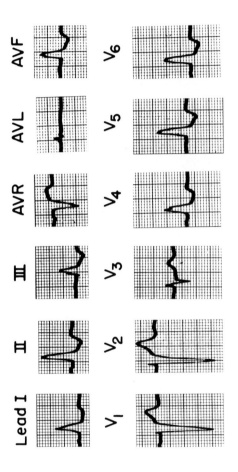

Fig. 8.4. Left bundle branch block. The vectorcardiogram and electrocardiogram were recorded from a 72-year-old woman with diabetes and arteriosclerotic heart disease. In the vectorcardiogram most of the characteristic findings of left bundle branch block as demonstrated in the previous illustrations are present. However, in this patient the QRS loop in the transverse and frontal planes presents a double figure-of-eight pattern.

C. H.   **dash interval 2 msec**

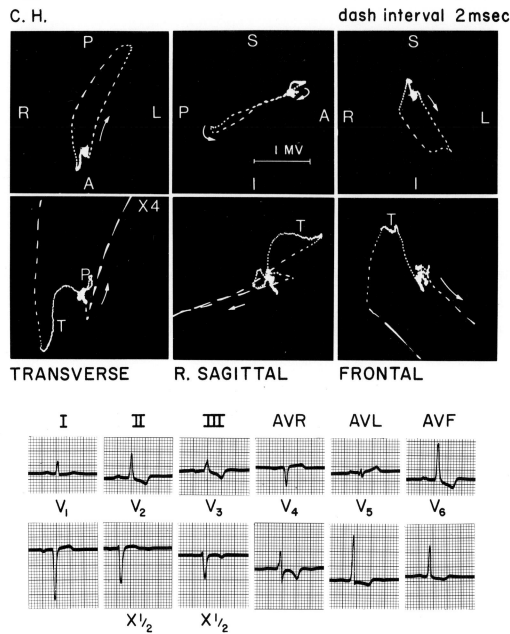

Fig. 8.5. (A) Intermittent left bundle branch block. See legend for Figure 8.5B.

posterior orientation of the initial forces is uncommon in patients with left bundle
branch block without myocardial infarction. However, the magnitude of the early
left anterior forces is often very small and this portion of the loop may not be
identified unless it is examined under magnification. From the initial deflection the
loop turns abruptly to a posterior direction to become the efferent limb of the body.
The afferent limb is usually located to the left of the efferent limb, and it proceeds
toward the J point without further distinctive change in its course. The duration of

C. H.

dash interval 2 msec

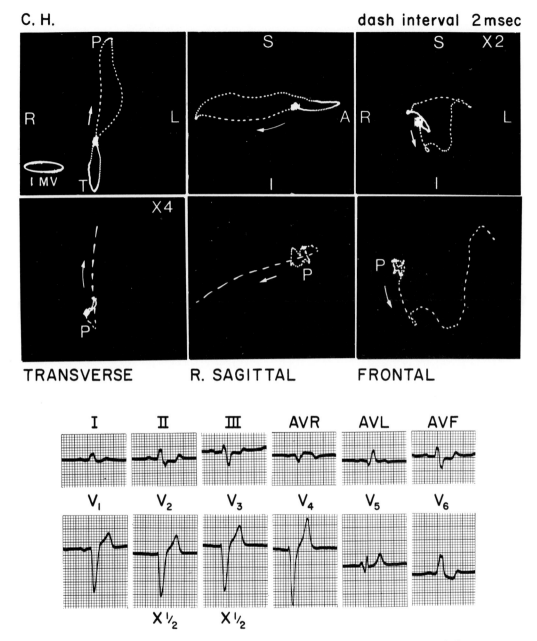

Fig. 8.5. (B) Intermittent left bundle branch block. The vectorcardiogram and electrocardiogram in Figure 8.5A and B were recorded from a 60-year-old man with primary myocardial disease. The two sets of tracings were obtained sequentially and the left bundle branch block pattern was observed when the heart rate increased. During normal intraventricular conduction the findings are consistent with left ventricular hypertrophy (Fig. 8.5A). With the development of complete left bundle branch block the QRS duration increases from 0.08 to 0.14 sec. The initial QRS forces are displaced slightly further to the left. The QRS loop in the transverse plane is now inscribed essentially clockwise instead of counterclockwise. In the frontal plane there is a superior displacement of the QRS loop which is inscribed counterclockwise instead of clockwise. The mid and late portions of the QRS loop are slowly inscribed and are best demonstrated in the transverse and sagittal projections.

123

the QRS loop is 0.12 sec or more. The evidence of a conduction delay, as indicated by the slowing of the speed of inscription, usually begins at about 0.04 sec after the onset of the QRS loop and involves the rest of the entire loop, but is most marked in its midportion.

The planar projection of the maximum spatial **QRS** vector is directed posteriorly and to the left. With few exceptions it is within the range of $-45°$ to $-80°$, thus being oriented more posteriorly than toward the left. Its magnitude often exceeds the normal upper limit (2 mV). In the typical case the time of occurrence of the maximum **QRS** vector is delayed (greater than 0.05 sec).

The leftward displacement of the initial deflection corresponds to the consistent absence of the Q wave in the left precordial leads (V_5 and V_6) of the scalar electrocardiogram. The reduced initial anterior forces are seen in lead V_1 as a small r wave. In cases in which the initial deflection is posterior to 25° and therefore projects on the negative side of the lead axis of V_1, the r wave will not be seen and a QS complex is recorded. Since the abnormally elongated body of the loop is oriented posteriorly and is more or less parallel to the negative side of the lead axis of V_1, the amplitude of the QS deflection in lead V_1 is usually increased. For the same reason the posterior displacement of the QRS loop also results in a relatively small or average-size R wave in lead V_6 since the loop subtends a rather large angle with its lead axis. The fact that the entire QRS loop is located on the left side, that is, on the positive side of the lead axis of V_6, explains the absence of an S wave in the left precordial leads in the uncomplicated case of left bundle branch block. The QRS complex in all the leads is abnormally wide because of the slow inscription of the QRS loop. The delay of the occurrence of the maximum **QRS** vector corresponds to the delay of the onset of the intrinsicoid deflection in the left precordial leads. The slurring and notching of the R wave in leads V_5 and V_6 and of the S wave in leads V_1 and V_2 have their counterparts in the vectorcardiogram as the marked reduction of the speed of inscription (especially in the mid portion) and the twisting of the distal portion of the QRS loop.

Sagittal plane QRS loop.   In the right sagittal projection the QRS loop is also elongated. Except for a small initial portion, the loop is oriented posteriorly with part of it located inferiorly and part superiorly. The loop is inscribed clockwise. In some instances there is a figure-of-eight pattern with the majority of the loop inscribed clockwise. The small initial deflection is directed anteriorly and usually inferiorly. The efferent limb proceeds posteriorly and inferiorly. The afferent limb is superior to the efferent limb. The increased duration of the QRS loop and the presence of a conduction delay in the mid and late portions are as have been described in the transverse plane projection. The projection of the maximum spatial **QRS** vector is often abnormally large in amplitude and is directed posteriorly, mostly inferiorly but occasionally superiorly, with a usual range of 155° to 190°.

Frontal plane QRS loop.   In the frontal plane projection the QRS loop appears small and slightly irregular in contour. This is related to the spatial loop being more or less directed posteriorly and perpendicular to the frontal plane. Any change in the course of the inscription will appear more abrupt and may result in a slight irregularity of the contour. Practically all of the QRS loop is located on the left side.

INCOMPLETE LEFT BUNDLE BRANCH BLOCK

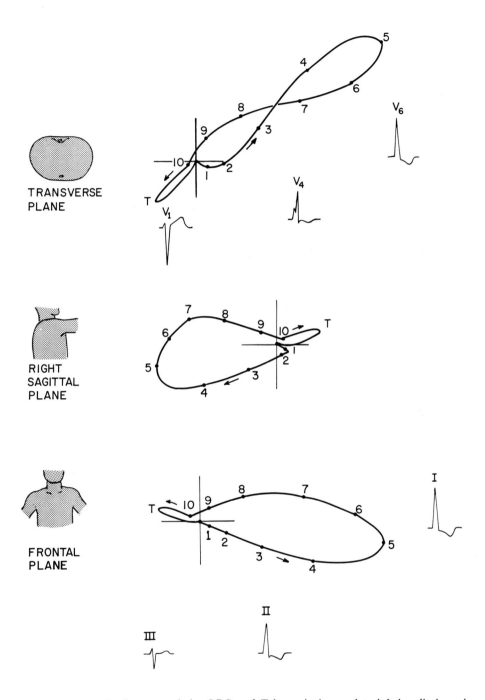

Fig. 8.6. Schematic diagrams of the QRS and T loops in incomplete left bundle branch block. The numerals indicate time in hundredths of a second after the beginning of the QRS loop. Representative scalar leads are given.

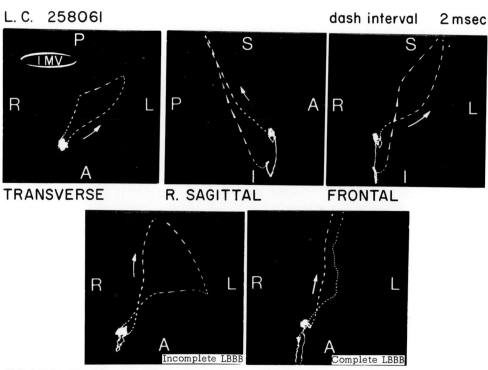

L.C. 258061   dash interval   2 msec

TRANSVERSE   R. SAGITTAL   FRONTAL

Incomplete LBBB   Complete LBBB

TRANSVERSE PLANE DURING CAROTID SINUS MASSAGE

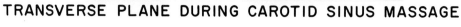

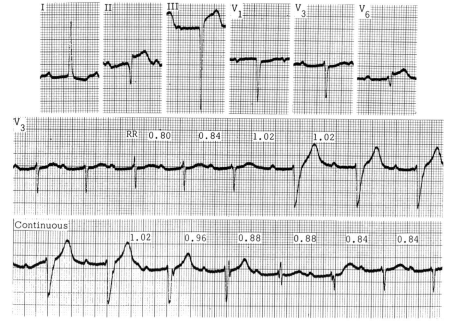

The initial deflection is directed leftward and inferiorly. The efferent limb continues the leftward and inferior direction and the loop is inscribed counterclockwise with the afferent limb more superior than the efferent limb. The beginning of the terminal deflection is usually not distinguishable. The projection of the maximum spatial **QRS** vector is directed to the left and has a usual range of $-20°$ to $55°$. Its magnitude may be normal or reduced.

The consistent leftward displacement of the initial deflection correlates with the absence of the Q wave in lead I of the scalar electrocardiogram (one of the diagnostic findings). Its inferior orientation is seen as an R wave in the inferior leads (II, III, and aVF). Occasionally, in a patient in whom the initial deflection is leftward and superior, a QS rather than an R wave will be seen in these leads. Since the entire loop is located on the left side, lead I records a monophasic R wave. As the portion of the loop located superiorly is variable, the depth of the negative deflection (S wave) in leads II, III, and aVF also varies. Slurring or notching of the R or S wave is seen in the limb leads for the same reason given previously when the transverse plane QRS loop was correlated with the precordial leads.

ST Vector and TsÊ Loop

The altered sequence of ventricular activation results in a secondary change of the recovery process. Before the abnormally prolonged depolarization process is completed, repolarization probably has already begun in the right ventricle and follows a similar pathway, that is, from right to left. The polarity of the resultant potential or vectors (**T** vectors) is therefore the reverse of the **QRS** vectors. The early initiation of the repolarization also displaces the terminal portion of the QRS loop and the J point in the same direction. In fact, the spatial **ST** vector and TsÊ loop in left bundle branch block are practically always $180°$ discordant to the spatial QRS loop.

Fig. 8.7.   Bradycardia-induced left bundle branch block. The vectorcardiogram and electrocardiogram were recorded from a 60-year-old man with hypertensive cardiovascular disease and acute myocardial infarction. The top panel of the vectorcardiogram and the 12-lead electrocardiogram (only 6 leads are shown) are suggestive of left ventricular hypertrophy, left anterior hemiblock, anterior myocardial infarction, and acute inferior myocardial infarction. These diagnoses are based on: (1) the abnormally large maximum **QRS** vector directed leftward and posteriorly (left ventricular hypertrophy); (2) superior displacement of the QRS loop with essentially counterclockwise inscription of the loop in the frontal plane (left anterior hemiblock); (3) the complete loss of the initial anterior QRS forces (anterior myocardial infarction); and (4) the superior displacement of the initial **QRS** vectors with initial clockwise inscription of the frontal plane QRS loop and abnormally large **ST** vector which is directed inferiorly (acute inferior myocardial infarction). In the lower panel of the vectorcardiogram the development of incomplete and complete left bundle branch block during carotid sinus massage and slowing of the heart rate is demonstrated. Note the increase of the QRS duration to 0.105 sec. and the appearance of the figure-of-eight loop in the transverse plane during incomplete left bundle branch block. There is further prolongation of the QRS duration to 0.15 sec with marked slowing of inscription of the late portion of the loop during complete left bundle branch block. The irregularity of the afferent limb is probably caused by myocardial infarction. The long strip of lead V_3 illustrates the relationship between the heart rate and the various degrees of left bundle branch block.

In the transverse plane the **ST** vector is directed to the right and anteriorly. Its magnitude is abnormally increased. The T loop points to the same direction as the **ST** vector. It is usually quite narrow and long. The initial portion is slowly inscribed as in the normal T loop. The direction of the inscription is counterclockwise. In our experience the occasional clockwise inscription of the T loop is mostly seen in patients with clinical evidence of myocardial infarction. In the right sagittal projection both the **ST** vector and the T loop are directed anteriorly and either superiorly or inferiorly. Their magnitudes are abnormally increased. The T loop is inscribed in a clockwise direction. In the frontal plane the **ST** vector and the T loop may be oriented either superiorly or inferiorly, but always to the right. Their magnitude may or may not appear to be abnormally large. With few exceptions the T loop is inscribed counterclockwise.

Since the spatial **QRS** and **ST-T** vectors are approximately 180° discordant to each other, it may be expected that ST segment depression and T wave inversion will be seen in the conventional leads with an R wave (as in leads I, V_5, and V_6) and elevation of the ST segment and an upright T wave in leads with predominantly negative QRS deflection (V_1, V_2). If the positive and negative deflections of the QRS complex are of equal amplitude, an isoelectric ST segment and a flat T wave will be recorded, as both the mean **QRS** and **ST-T** vectors are now perpendicular to the lead axis in question.

INCOMPLETE LEFT BUNDLE BRANCH BLOCK

In incomplete left bundle branch block the impulse conduction through the left bundle branch is not completely interrupted but occurs at a slower rate (Sodi-Pallares). Consequently, the area supplied by the right bundle branch system is activated first. The activation process spreads transseptally from right to left and activates the left septal mass to a varying extent, depending on the degree of the conduction delay in the left bundle branch system. After the impulse transmitted through the left bundle branch finally arrives, the rest of the left septal mass and the left ventricular free wall will be depolarized in the normal fashion. Therefore, during the initial phase, the sequence of ventricular activation in incomplete left bundle branch block is quite similar to that of the complete variety, but conduction during the later period is little affected.

In the vectorcardiogram (Figs. 8.6 and 8.7) the QRSsÊ loop is usually elongated and oriented posteriorly, to the left, and either slightly inferiorly or superiorly. The duration of the QRS loop is prolonged but does not exceed 0.11 sec. There is no evidence of a marked conduction delay in any particular portion of the loop. The maximum spatial **QRS** vector is increased in magnitude. Its time of occurrence may be slightly delayed. In the transverse plane the QRS loop is oriented to the left and posteriorly. The initial deflection is displaced to the left and anteriorly. The loop inscribes a figure-of-eight pattern with the proximal portion counterclockwise and the distal portion clockwise. In the right sagittal plane the initial deflection is directed anteriorly and inferiorly. The loop is inscribed clockwise. The later portion of the loop is usually superiorly located. In the frontal plane the loop is oriented to the left and either slightly inferiorly or superiorly. The initial deflection is directed to the left and inferiorly, and the loop is inscribed counterclockwise.

Both the **ST** vector and the T loop may be abnormally large in magnitude. Their directions are usually opposite to that of the QRS loop. Therefore, in the transverse plane both the **ST** vector and the T loop are oriented to the right and anteriorly. In the right sagittal plane they are directed anteriorly, either superiorly or slightly inferiorly, and in the frontal plane, to the right, either slightly superiorly or inferiorly.

In the scalar electrocardiogram the absence of a Q wave in leads I, V_5, and V_6 is related to the leftward displacement of the initial deflection. The increase of the magnitude of the maximum **QRS** vector with its leftward and posterior orientation is reflected in a tall R wave in the left precordial leads and limb lead I, and a deep S wave in the right precordial leads. The inferior leads (leads II, III, and aVF) show an R, RS, or rS complex depending on the degree of the superior displacement of the QRS loop as seen in the frontal plane. The QRS complex is slightly widened but the duration is less than 0.12 sec. A notching can often be seen in one or more of the precordial leads (especially the mid precordial leads) and is related to the figure-of-eight pattern of the QRS loop as viewed in the transverse plane projection. The ST segment deviation and the polarity of the T wave are opposite to the predominant direction of the QRS complex due to the discordancy of the QRSsÊ loop with the spatial **ST** vector and TsÊ loop.

Figure 8.7 is an example of bradycardia-dependent left bundle branch block in a patient with acute myocardial infarction. The development of incomplete and then complete left bundle branch block is demonstrated in the transverse plane vectorcardiogram.

Since most patients displaying the pattern of incomplete left bundle branch block also have evidence of anatomical left ventricular hypertrophy, increased left ventricular mass often contributes to the findings. In fact, when marked anatomical left ventricular hypertrophy is present, the pattern of incomplete left bundle branch block is encountered very frequently. Some examples were given in the chapter on left ventricular hypertrophy.

REFERENCES

1. Anselmi A, Montes O, Alvarez M: Participation of the free ventricular walls in the mechanism of production of bundle branch block. Their influence on the morphology of unipolar epicardial tracings. Am Heart J 61:387, 1961
2. Becker RA, Scher AM, Erickson RV: Ventricular excitation in experimental left bundle branch block. Am Heart J 55:547, 1958
3. Cabrera E, Garcia-Font R, Gaxiola A, Pileggi F: The vectorcardiogram of ventricular activation in chronic coronary heart disease. Am Heart J 55:557, 1958
4. Frimpter GW, Scherr L, Ogden D: The spatial vectorcardiogram in complete left bundle branch block with special reference to the initial component. Am Heart J 55:220, 1958
5. Gardberg M, Rosen IL: The electrocardiogram and vectorcardiogram in various degrees of left bundle branch block. Am J Cardiol 1:592, 1958
6. Kennamer R, Prinzmetal M: Depolarization of the ventricle with bundle branch block. Studies on the mechanism of ventricular activity. X. Am Heart J 47:769, 1954
7. Luna R, Jackson A: The vectorcardiogram in left bundle branch block. Am J Cardiol 7:638, 1961

8.   Rodriguez MI, Sodi-Pallares D: The mechanism of complete and incomplete bundle branch block. Am Heart J 44:715, 1952
9.   Sanchez C, Walsh TJ, Massie E: The vectorcardiogram in incomplete left bundle branch block. Am J Cardiol 7:629, 1961
10. Wallace AG, Estes EH, McCall BW: The vectorcardiographic findings in left bundle branch block. A study using the Frank lead system. Am Heart J 63:508, 1962

9

Right Bundle Branch Block

SEQUENCE OF VENTRICULAR ACTIVATION IN
RIGHT BUNDLE BRANCH BLOCK

In right bundle branch block the interruption of impulse conduction through the right bundle branch delays the activation of the right ventricle. The left ventricle is depolarized in the normal fashion by way of the intact left bundle branch. The activation begins at the septal surface and the impulse spreads in a rightward direction. While increasing portions of the left septum are being depolarized, the impulse is also propagated through the Purkinje network and activates the free wall of the left ventricle in an endocardium-to-epicardium direction. In contrast to the normal activation process, the septal depolarization in right bundle branch block depends entirely on the impulse coming from the left side instead of from both sides. Rodriguez and Sodi-Pallares maintain that there is a considerable delay of the conduction at the junction of the left and right septal mass, which is responsible for most of the prolongation of the QRS duration. However, Erickson and associates failed to demonstrate the presence of such a "barrier," and their experiments demonstrated a uniform, uninterrupted progression of the wave of depolarization across the septum. They believe that a significant factor in the prolongation of the QRS duration is the increase in the time required for septal activation by a single, rather than a double, enveloping wave front.

The earliest activity in the free wall of the right ventricle in right bundle branch block is at the junction of the free wall and the septum. The activating wave advances steadily through the rest of the free wall of the right ventricle. The last area to be depolarized is the pulmonary conus.

If the ventricular depolarization process in right bundle branch block is simplified, it may be divided into three phases and represented by three vectors (Fig. 9.1). During the initial phase part of the left septum is activated. The direction of spread is from left to right. As the position of the septum is such that its right surface is facing rightward, anteriorly and superiorly, the direction of the vector representing the initial phase (vector 1) is thus oriented in this same direction.

SEQUENCE OF VENTRICULAR ACTIVATION IN RBBB AND REPRESENTATIVE VECTORS

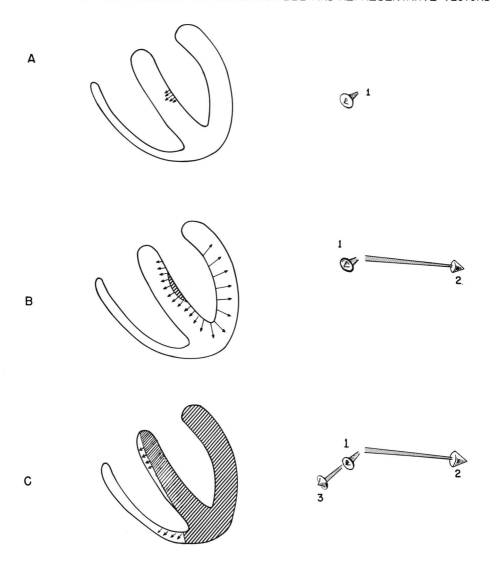

Fig. 9.1.   See text. The vectors are viewed in their transverse plane presentation.

During the second phase the activation involves the rest of the left septum and the free wall of the left ventricle. The resultant force is oriented in favor of the dominant force from the free wall of the left ventricle, and the vector (vector 2) is directed leftward, inferiorly, and either slightly anteriorly or posteriorly. It is apparent that the resultant vectors (vectors 1 and 2) thus far differ very little from those representing the normal process. When the activation of the free wall of the left ventricle is almost completed and the abnormal left-to-right activation of the right septum becomes the dominant event, the resultant force will be shifted again toward the right. Subsequently the free wall of the right ventricle is depolarized in a similar fashion. Thus the delayed and abnormal activation of the right septal mass and the free wall of the right ventricle can be expressed by a third vector representing the final phase. The vector (vector 3) is directed to the right, anteriorly, and either superiorly or inferiorly.

VECTORCARDIOGRAPHIC FINDINGS IN RIGHT BUNDLE BRANCH BLOCK

QRSsÊ Loop

The spatial QRS loop in right bundle branch block is usually normal in its overall magnitude. However, its configuration is typically deformed. The loop usually presents itself in two rather distinct portions. The major portion consists of the initial deflection, efferent and afferent limbs, and the smaller portion is represented by a finger-like terminal appendage. The course of the initial deflection and the efferent limb of the body do not differ significantly from that of the normal QRSsÊ loop. The afferent limb is, however, displaced anteriorly. The finger-like terminal appendage is the product of the delayed and abnormal depolarization of the right septal mass and the free wall of the right ventricle. It is directed to the right, anteriorly, and may be either slightly superior or slightly inferior in location. Most of the terminal appendage is slowly inscribed and the duration of the slowing is usually 0.03 sec or more. Indeed, the anteriorly, rightward oriented and slowly inscribed terminal appendage represents the most characteristic feature of right bundle branch block. The QRSsÊ loop ends either at, or slightly posterior and to the left of, the isoelectric point. The duration of the QRSsÊ loop is prolonged to 0.12 sec or more.

Planar Projections of the QRSsÊ Loop and Correlation with the Conventional Electrocardiogram (Figs. 9.2–9.5)

Transverse plane QRS loop. In the transverse plane projection the presentation of the QRS loop as two distinct portions is well demonstrated. The major portion of the loop is inscribed counterclockwise, although exceptions do occur and a figure-of-eight or clockwise rotation may be seen occasionally. The initial deflection is directed anteriorly and usually to the right. The efferent limb is inscribed to the left and anteriorly until the maximum leftward **QRS** vector is reached. Thus, the course of the initial deflection and the efferent limb closely resembles that of the normal person. In fact, when right bundle branch block is produced in a normal person during right heart catheterization, very little change can be detected in these segments. However, more obvious alterations can be seen in the afferent limb. This portion of the loop is usually inscribed abruptly toward the right and is displaced anteriorly. When the displacement is marked, it may cross the efferent limb, resulting in a figure-of-eight pattern, or even become entirely anterior to the efferent limb so that the main portion of the QRS loop is inscribed clockwise.

The terminal appendage is inscribed first to the right and anteriorly and then returns toward the origin of the loop. Most of the appendage is slowly inscribed as

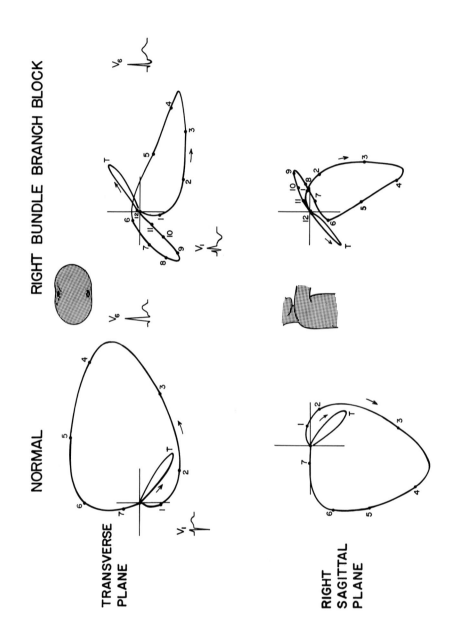

RIGHT BUNDLE BRANCH BLOCK

NORMAL

TRANSVERSE
PLANE

RIGHT
SAGITTAL
PLANE

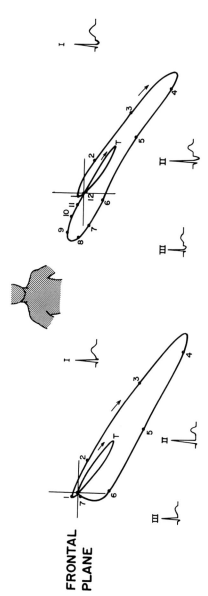

Fig. 9.2. Schematic diagrams of the QRS and T loops in right bundle branch block as compared with those of a normal person. The numerals indicate in hundredths of a second the time intervals after the beginning of the QRS loop. The representative leads of the conventional electrocardiogram are also outlined.

135

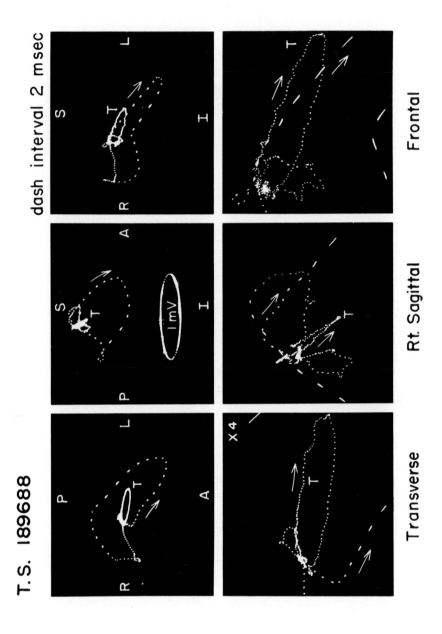

dash interval 2 msec

T.S. 189688

Frontal

Rt. Sagittal

Transverse

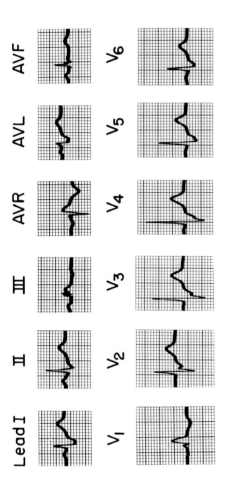

Fig. 9.3. Right bundle branch block. The vectorcardiogram and electrocardiogram were recorded from an 83-year-old man with arteriosclerotic heart disease. In the transverse plane there is a counterclockwise inscription of the QRS loop. The terminal appendage is directed to the right and anteriorly and is slowly inscribed. The T loop is oriented to the left and slightly anteriorly and is discordant to the terminal deflection of the QRS loop. It is inscribed clockwise. In the right sagittal plane the main portion of the QRS loop is displaced somewhat anteriorly as in the transverse plane. The terminal appendage, which is better seen in the magnified recording, is directed anteriorly and slightly superiorly. The T loop is inscribed counterclockwise but is rather narrow. In the frontal plane the QRS loop is located inferiorly and is inscribed clockwise. The terminal appendage is directed to the right and is slowly inscribed. The T loop is inscribed clockwise.

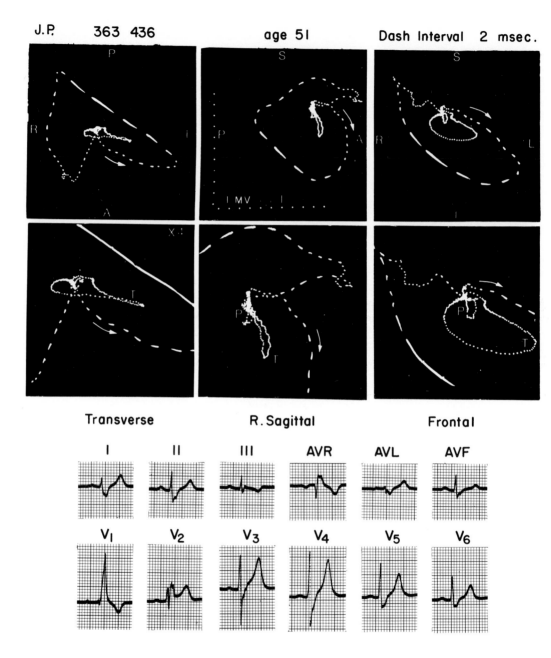

Fig. 9.4. Complete right bundle branch block. The vectorcardiogram and electrocardiogram were recorded from a 51-year-old man with coronary artery disease. In the vectorcardiogram the main portion of the QRS loop is inscribed counterclockwise in the transverse plane and clockwise in the sagittal and frontal projections. The terminal appendage is directed anteriorly, rightward, and superiorly. Its mid and late portions are slowly inscribed. The T loop is directed leftward, anteriorly, and inferiorly. As the T loop is not discordant to the terminal appendage additional primary T loop abnormalities may be present.

indicated by the close spacing of the dashes. The duration of this characteristic conduction delay ranges from 0.03 to 0.085 sec with an average value of 0.06 sec. The direction of inscription may be either clockwise or counterclockwise. The loop usually ends very close to the isoelectric point but may be slightly posterior and to the left of it. The duration of the entire QRS loop is prolonged to 0.12 sec or more.

The planar projection of the maximal spatial **QRS** vector is directed to the left, and usually anteriorly but occasionally posteriorly. Our data indicate that the average magnitude of the maximum **QRS** vector is smaller (1 mV versus 1.3 mV) and the average direction more anterior (20° versus −20°) than those of the normal individual. The time of its occurrence, however, is not significantly modified. The maximum vector of the terminal appendage is directed anteriorly and to the right with an average direction of 140°. The magnitude of the vector varies, and occasionally may approach that of the maximum **QRS** vector.

In the conventional electrocardiogram, the component deflections of the typical RSR′ complex in lead V_1 can readily be correlated with the initial deflection, body (efferent and afferent limbs), and terminal appendage of the transverse plane QRS loop, respectively. The anterior and rightward initial deflection is recorded as the initial small R wave and corresponds to the projection of the vector 1 described in the early part of this chapter. The depth of the S wave is variable and depends on the relative direction of the body of the loop, or vector 2, with respect to the lead axis of V_1. When the efferent and afferent limbs are posteriorly oriented, its projection on the negative side of the lead axis of V_1 results in a relatively deep S wave. However, if they are anteriorly located, the S wave may be small or even absent. The R′ wave corresponds to the anteriorly and rightward directed terminal appendage, or vector 3. The magnitude of the R′ is related to the amplitude of the maximum vector of the terminal appendage and the angle it subtends with the lead axis of V_1. Because of the slow inscription of the terminal appendage, the R′ is wide and slurred.

In the left precordial leads (V_5 and V_6) a small normal Q wave is usually seen because of the rightward direction of the initial deflection. Occasionally, in cases in which the initial orientation is anterior but leftward, the Q wave would be absent, and the initial deflection is seen as the beginning of an R wave. The upstroke and downstroke of the R wave have their counterparts in the efferent and afferent limbs of the QRS loop. The height of the R wave is related to the magnitude of the maximum **QRS** vector, and the angle it subtends with the lead axes. As the average magnitude of the maximum **QRS** vector in right bundle branch block is smaller than normal, the amplitude of the R wave in leads V_5 and V_6 is also reduced. (This observation may explain the difficulty in diagnosing left ventricular hypertrophy in the presence of right bundle branch block when the usual voltage criteria are applied.) As the terminal appendage is oriented to the right and toward the negative side of the lead axes of V_5 and V_6, an S wave is recorded in these leads. The slow inscription of this part of the QRS loop explains the increase in the width of the S wave.

The duration of the QRS complex in all leads is increased because of the slow inscription of the terminal appendage of the loop. The onset of the intrinsicoid deflection is delayed in the right precordial leads because of the secondary wide R′. It is normal in the left precordial leads as the time of occurrence of the maximum leftward **QRS** vector remains essentially normal.

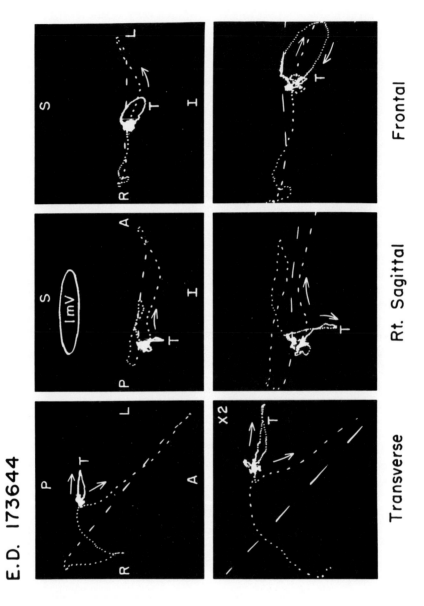

E.D. 173644

Frontal   Rt. Sagittal   Transverse

140

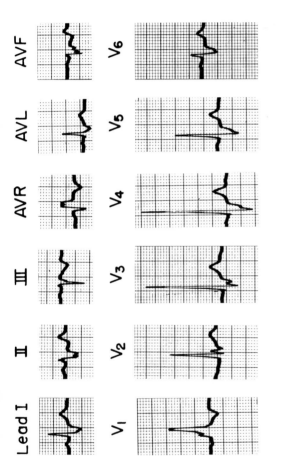

Fig. 9.5. Right bundle branch block. The patient is a 63-year-old man with mild hypertension and diabetes. In the transverse plane the main portion of the QRS loop presents a figure-of-eight pattern because of the rather marked anterior displacement of the afferent limb. The terminal appendage is directed anteriorly and to the right and is characteristically slowly inscribed. The T loop is directed to the left and is inscribed clockwise. In the right sagittal plane the QRS loop is displaced anteriorly and is inscribed counterclockwise except for a small distal portion. The terminal appendage is oriented anteriorly and is slowly inscribed. In the frontal plane the main portion of the QRS loop also presents a figure-of-eight pattern and is displaced slightly upward. The terminal appendage is directed to the right.

Sagittal plane QRS loop.   In the right sagittal projection the main portion of the QRS loop and the maximum **QRS** vector are directed inferiorly, and usually anteriorly. The direction of inscription of the loop is variable. The magnitude of the maximum **QRS** vector also varies a great deal, but the average value is smaller than that of the normal (0.8 mV versus 1.0 mV). The slowly inscribed terminal appendage is oriented anteriorly, and either slightly superiorly or inferiorly, the former being more frequently observed. The direction of inscription of this portion may be either clockwise or counterclockwise. The maximum vector of the terminal appendage has an average direction of $-25°$. The range of its magnitude is rather wide.

Frontal plane QRS loop.   In the frontal plane projection the main portion of the QRS loop (initial deflection, efferent and afferent limbs) is oriented to the left and inferiorly. It is usually relatively narrow and may be inscribed either clockwise or counterclockwise, the former being more common. The direction of the initial deflection varies a great deal as in normal subjects. It may be either superior or inferior, left or right. The efferent limb is inscribed to the left and inferiorly. The afferent limb then returns toward the right, either inferior or superior to the efferent limb. The maximum **QRS** vector is directed to the left with an average value of $25°$. The average magnitude is significantly smaller than that of the normal (1 mV versus 1.5 mV).

The presence of a terminal appendage is not as easily appreciated in this plane as in the other two projections. Its beginning may or may not be signaled by an abrupt change in the course of inscription. It is slowly inscribed and is always oriented to the right, but may be directed superiorly, inferiorly or horizontally. Its direction of inscription may be either clockwise or counterclockwise. The maximum vector of the terminal appendage has an average direction of $195°$ (or $-165°$). Its magnitude varies rather markedly as in the other projections.

The leftward orientation of the main portion of the QRS loop is represented in the conventional electrocardiogram as an R wave in lead I. In most instances a small Q wave is present because of the initial vectors which are directed to the right. Since the slowly inscribed terminal appendage is always directed to the right, a wide and slurred S wave is thus typically recorded in this lead. As the major portion of the loop is located inferiorly, a dominant R wave is seen in the inferior leads. Since the direction of the terminal appendage could be superior, horizontal, or inferior, the slurred terminal portion of the QRS complex in the inferior leads may thus be downward, isoelectric or upward. The reduction in the average magnitude of the maximum **QRS** vector has its counterpart in the lower amplitude of the R wave in lead I.

In right bundle branch block the apparent normality of the initial deflection and most of the efferent limb, which usually includes the initial 0.03 to 0.04 sec **QRS** vectors, is of both theoretical and clinical significance. It suggests that the contribution of the right ventricle to the resultant electrical potential during normal ventricular depolarization is indeed very small. It is only when the right ventricular activation is delayed and proceeds in an abnormal pathway that its potential manifests itself and modifies the later portion of the QRS loop. This fact also explains why abnormalities involving the early portion of the loop, as in most of the cases of myocardial infarction, will not be masked by the presence of right bundle branch block.

ST Vector and the TsÊ Loop

The alteration of the sequence of ventricular activation in right bundle branch block results also in secondary changes in the process of repolarization. Because of the delay of the right ventricular activation, recovery process probably has already begun in the left ventricle before right ventricular depolarization has completed. This may result in a displacement of the terminal **QRS** vectors and the appearance of an **ST** vector, which, however, is usually small. The repolarization of the right ventricle probably also follows an abnormal pathway similar to that of the wave of excitation. Since the polarity of the repolarization potential is opposite to that of the depolarization if the direction of the spread is the same, the abnormal repolarization of the right ventricle will rotate the **T** vectors away from the direction of the late **QRS** vectors which represent the delayed and abnormal depolarization of the right ventricle.

In the vectorcardiogram the spatial **ST** vector, if present, is usually small and directed to the left, either superiorly or inferiorly, anteriorly or posteriorly. The spatial T loop is oriented to the left, inferiorly, mostly posteriorly but occasionally anteriorly. Its direction is practically always opposite to that of the terminal **QRS** vectors. In the transverse plane projection the T loop is directed to the left and mostly posteriorly. It is usually oval in shape and retains the normal initial slowing of inscription. In most instances the direction of inscription is clockwise, which is abnormal. In the right sagittal projection the T loop is oriented inferiorly and mostly posteriorly. The direction of inscription is counterclockwise. In the frontal plane the loop is directed to the left and inferiorly, and the direction of incription may be either clockwise or counterclockwise.

As the **ST** vector is usually small, little ST segment displacement is seen in the conventional electrocardiogram. Occasionally, slight ST segment depression is seen in the right precordial leads because of the leftward direction of the **ST** vector. Since the T loop is discordant to the terminal slowly inscribed **QRS** vectors, an upright T wave is thus expected in the leads which display a wide S wave, and a negative T wave will be recorded in those leads which have a broad terminal upright deflection. Therefore, the T wave is inverted in the right precordial leads where a broad R' is present and is upright in the left precordial leads where a wide S wave is recorded. Similarly, the T wave in lead I is upright, and it may be upright or inverted in the inferior leads depending on the direction of the terminal **QRS** vectors.

INCOMPLETE RIGHT BUNDLE BRANCH BLOCK

In incomplete right bundle branch block the impulse transmission through the right bundle branch system is delayed but not totally interrupted. As a result the right septal mass and right ventricular free wall will be depolarized through impulses from both the right and the left bundle branches. The extent of the abnormal activation from the left depends upon the degree of conduction delay in the right bundle branch. As in the complete variety the alteration is manifested chiefly during the later period of the ventricular activation. During that period the wave of excitation spreads toward the right, anteriorly, and superiorly or inferiorly with the

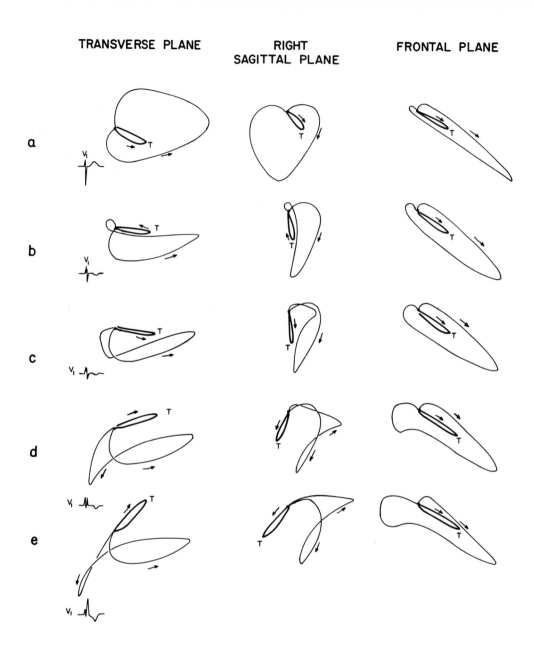

TRANSVERSE PLANE · RIGHT SAGITTAL PLANE · FRONTAL PLANE

Fig. 9.6. Schematic diagrams illustrating the changes of the QRS and T loops associated with increasing degree of right bundle branch block. (a) Normal QRS and T loops; (b,c, and d) increasing degree of incomplete bundle branch block; (e) complete right bundle branch block. The corresponding QRS-T complexes in the scalar lead V_1 are also presented (adapted from Penaloza et al). It should be mentioned here that in many cases of incomplete and complete right bundle branch block, the anterior displacement of the afferent limb of the QRS loop does not reach the degree illustrated in the diagrams.

144

resultant **QRS** vectors directed similarly. When the degree of right bundle branch block increases, these abnormal forces become more prominent.

In the vectorcardiogram the afferent limb and the terminal deflection of the QRSsÊ loop are displaced in the anterior and rightward direction. The extent of the displacement and the duration of the terminal conduction delay gradually increase in proportion to the degree of right bundle branch block. The total duration of the QRS loop is also prolonged, but, by definition, is less than 0.12 sec. However, it is obvious that this arbitrary value cannot always be expected to give an accurate separation of the complete and incomplete varieties on a physiologic basis.

Figure 9.6 illustrates the vectorcardiographic changes in various degrees of right bundle branch block as they are induced in a normal individual. In the transverse plane projection the gradual anterior and rightward displacement of the afferent limb and the terminal deflection can clearly be appreciated with finally the formation of a distinct, abnormal terminal appendage, which is slowly inscribed (the speed of inscription is not shown in the diagrams). The T loop is directed to the left and posteriorly and is inscribed clockwise in most cases when the block is severe. In the right sagittal plane projection the anteriorly directed terminal appendage increases progressively in its magnitude and may be slightly superiorly or inferiorly oriented. The T loop becomes more posterior and eventually is inscribed counterclockwise instead of clockwise. In the frontal plane projection the changes of the late **QRS** vectors are least apparent, and practically no changes in the T loop can be detected.

In the conventional electrocardiogram the typical findings of a wide S wave in lead I and V_6 and an R′ in lead V_1 correspond to the abnormal anteriorly and rightward directed terminal appendage, as has been similarly described in the complete variety. Both the amplitude and the width of the R′ in V_1 and the S wave in leads I and V_6 increase when the degree of conduction disturbance becomes more marked. The duration of the QRS complex does not exceed 0.11 sec. The changes in the T wave are related to the degree of the posterior displacement of the T loop, and it becomes isoelectric and eventually inverted in the right precordial leads. The T wave in the left precordial leads remains upright. No appreciable alteration of the T wave is seen in the limb leads, as the T loop in the frontal plane retains its normal orientation.

REFERENCES

1. Baydar ID, Walsh TJ, Massie E: A vectorcardiographic study of right bundle branch block with the Frank lead system. Clinical correlation in ventricular hypertrophy and chronic pulmonary disease. Am J Cardiol 15:185, 1965
2. Dodge HT, Grant RP: Mechanisms of QRS complex prolongation in man. Am J Med 21:534, 1956
3. Erickson RV, Scher AM, Becker RA: Ventricular excitation in experimental bundle-branch block. Circulation Res 5:5, 1957
4. Penaloza D, Gamboa R, Sime F: Experimental right bundle branch block in the normal human heart. Electrocardiographic, vectorcardiographic and hemodynamic observation. Am J Cardiol 8:767, 1961

5. Rodriguez MI, Sodi-Pallares D: The mechanism of complete and incomplete bundle branch block. Am Heart J 44:715, 1952

6. Scherlis L, Lee Y-C: Right bundle branch block following open heart surgery. Electrocardiographic and vectorcardiographic study. Am J Cardiol 8:780, 1961

7. Scherlis L, Lee Y-C: Transient right bundle branch block. An electrocardiograpaic and vectorcardiographic study. Am J Cardiol 11:173, 1963

10

The Hemiblocks, Bifascicular Block

THE HEMIBLOCKS

Normally, the left ventricle is activated by impulse conducted simultaneously through the two divisions of the left bundle branch system. The anterior (or superior) division sweeps anteriorly and superiorly across the outflow tract of the left ventricle toward the base of the anterior papillary muscle. Its fibers are continuous with the subendocardial Purkinje network which supplies the myocardium of the anterior and lateral wall of the left ventricle. The posterior (or inferior) division, which is anatomically thicker but shorter than the anterior division, proceeds inferiorly and posteriorly toward the base of the posterior papillary muscle. Its fibers are connected with the Purkinje network supplying the inferior and posterior wall of the left ventricle. The two divisions anastomose with each other at the periphery through the Purkinje system.

A failure or delay of impulse conduction through one of the divisions will result in asynchronous activation of the left ventricle. The associated electro and vectorcardiographic changes are quite distinctive. These conduction abnormalities are most commonly called the *left anterior* and *left posterior hemiblock*. Others prefer the terms *left anterior* and *left posterior fascicular block*. In either case, it is now generally agreed the intraventricular conduction network may be considered as a trifascicular system which includes the left anterior and posterior fascicles of the left bundle branch and the right bundle branch.

As mentioned previously in Chapter 8, simultaneous interruption of impulse conduction through both divisions have the same effect as interruption at the main left bundle branch level and the vectorcardiographic changes are identical.

LEFT ANTERIOR HEMIBLOCK (Figs, 10.1-10.6)

When the conduction through the left anterior division is interrupted activation impulse from the main stem of the left bundle branch travels distally through the posterior division (Fig. 10.1). The earliest left ventricular excitation occurs at the

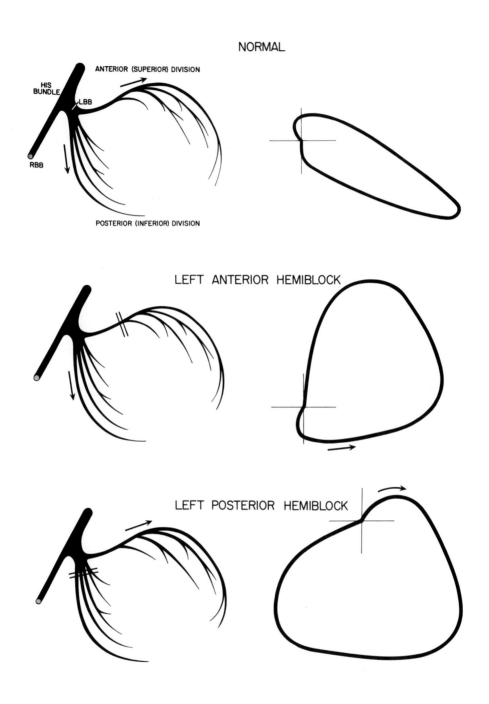

Fig. 10.1. Diagramatic representation of the trifascicular ventricular conduction system. The sequence of left ventricular activation and the frontal plane QRS loop in left anterior and left posterior hemiblock are compared with those of normal conduction.

subendocardial layer of the posterior paraseptal region. It is uncertain whether the initial left septal activation is now dependent entirely on the posterior division or is accomplished partly by fibers coming directly from the main stem left bundle branch.* The inferior and posterior portions of the left ventricular free wall are depolarized at the expected time. However, the activation of the anterolateral wall is delayed because of the failure of conduction through the anterior division. The impulse now has to arrive at this region in a retrograde manner through the network of anastomosis with the Purkinje fibers of the posterior division.

The ventricular activation process in left anterior hemiblock may be divided into three phases (Fig. 10.2). During the initial period of septal and paraseptal activation the normal component from the anterior paraseptal area is absent. Since the forces representing the endocardium-to-epicardium depolarization of this area are directed anteriorly, leftward, and superiorly, its absence allows the resultant vector to be displaced in the opposite direction. Although theoretically the initial QRS forces may be directed inferiorly, rightward, and posteriorly, these vectors are rarely oriented posteriorly as they are opposed by forces from the left midseptum and the right ventricle which are directed anteriorly. The early right ventricular forces may also be responsible for the occasional leftward orientation of the initial vectors.

LEFT ANTERIOR HEMIBLOCK

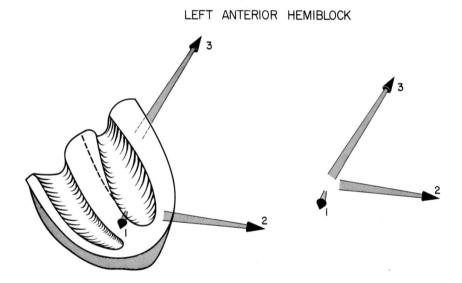

Fig. 10.2. Sequence of left ventricular activation and three representative spatial **QRS** vectors in left anterior hemiblock. See text.

* The excellent study by Durer et al on isolated human hearts has demonstrated three endocardial areas that are simultaneously activated in the initial phase of left ventricular excitation: an anterior, a posterior paraseptal area, and the midseptum. These authors believe the branches of the anterior division are responsible for the activation of the anterior paraseptal region and the midseptum. Rosenbaum and associates have presented evidence to suggest that the septum depends more on the posterior than the anterior division. A smaller central fascicle coming directly from the left bundle branch has also been described (Uhley). The recent finding of multiple simultaneous areas of initial left ventricular activation represents a significant and important departure from the traditional concept of a single site of early excitation at the midseptum.

During the next phase, the excitation involves the inferior wall and the apex of the left ventricle. The vectors are therefore directed inferiorly, leftward, and anteriorly. During the last period, the normal late activation of the posterobasal portion of the left ventricle and the delayed excitation of the anterolateral wall occur. The representative vectors are therefore directed posteriorly, leftward, and superiorly.

Vectorcardiographic Findings in Left Anterior Hemiblock

QRSsÊ loop.   In the absence of other associated abnormalities, the magnitude of the spatial QRS loop in left anterior hemiblock is within the normal range. One of the characteristic findings is its superior displacement and the majority of the spatial loop is located in the left superior-posterior octant. The initial deflection is inscribed inferiorly, usually to the right, and anteriorly. The efferent limb of the body of the loop proceeds leftward. The afferent limb is always superior to the efferent limb with most of its component being superior, leftward, and posterior. The terminal deflection is superior and posterior but may be either leftward or rightward. The end-point (J point) of the loop is usually anterior, inferior, and to the left of the origin of the loop. The duration of the QRS loop is usually slightly prolonged but does not exceed 0.10 sec, or 0.02 sec more than its duration during normal conduction. A slowing of the speed of inscription in the late portion of the loop suggesting conduction delay may be observed in a small percentage of cases. The maximum spatial **QRS** vector is invariably directed to the left and is usually posterior. It may be oriented either superiorly or inferiorly but is more superior than the maximum vector in the normal subjects. The time of its occurrence is not significantly changed.

Planar Projections of the QRSsÊ Loop and Correlation with the Conventional Electrocardiogram (Figs. 10.3–10.6)

Transverse plane QRS loop.   In the transverse plane projection the QRS loop does not present any characteristic finding. It is inscribed counterclockwise and its maximum vector is usually directed posteriorly and leftward. However, certain changes are often observed in the precordial leads of the conventional electrocardiogram. The transitional zone may be displaced to the left with a decrease of the amplitude of the R wave and an increase of the S wave in the left precordial leads (V_5 and V_6). This is related to the superior displacement of the QRS loop. The lead axes of leads V_5 and V_6 are not only directed leftward but also slightly downward. A superior displacement of the vector will result in a smaller projection on the lead axes. As the late **QRS** vectors are markedly superiorly oriented and sometimes slightly rightward they may therefore project on the negative side of the lead axes and a rather deep S wave is recorded in the left precordial leads. A less common but clinically important finding in anterior left hemiblock is the appearance of a small Q wave in the right or midprecordial leads to mimic anterior myocardial infarction. This is related to the changes in the orientation of the initial **QRS** vectors. They are now directed inferiorly and may project on the negative side of the lead axes of these leads. This explanation is supported by the fact that the Q wave is no longer present when these precordial leads are recorded one interspace below their routine locations.

LEFT ANTERIOR HEMIBLOCK

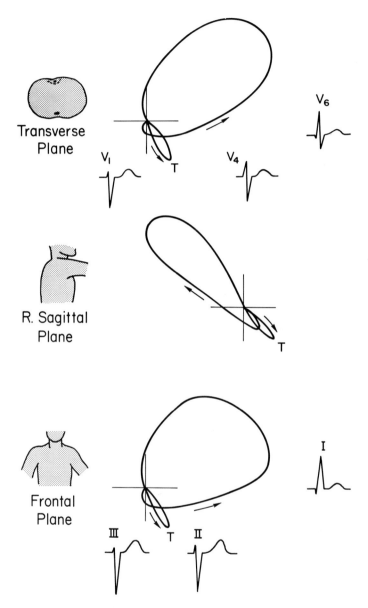

Fig. 10.3. Schematic diagram of the QRS and T loops in left anterior hemiblock. The representative conventional leads are given.

151

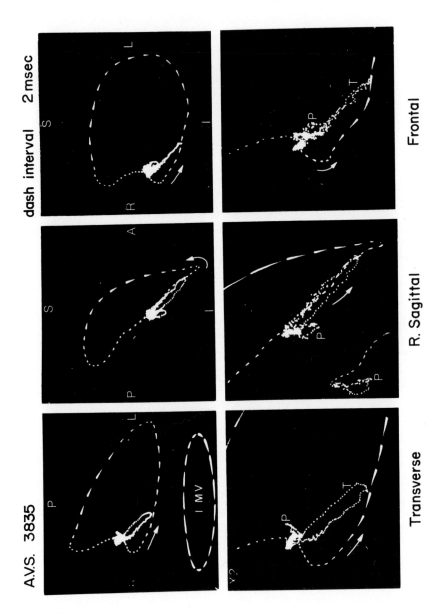

dash interval 2 msec

A.V.S. 3835

Frontal

R. Sagittal

Transverse

152

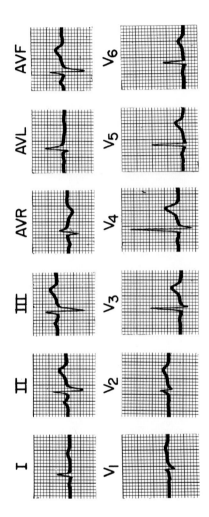

Fig. 10.4. Left anterior hemiblock. The tracings were recorded from a 72-year-old man with no other clinical evidence of heart disease. There is a superior displacement of the QRS loop. In the frontal plane the initial deflection is directed inferiorly and rightward. The loop is inscribed counterclockwise. The majority of the loop area is in the left upper quadrant. Note the counterclockwise inscription of the sagittal QRS loop. There is also a slight anterior displacement of the loop as indicated in the transverse and sagittal planes. The cause of this is unclear.

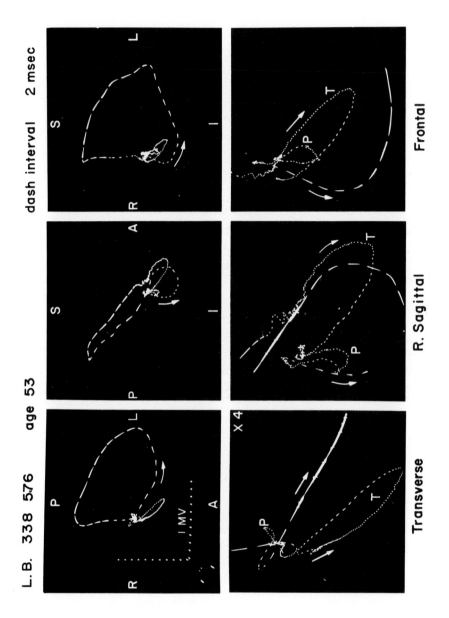

L.B. 338 576 age 53

dash interval 2 msec

Frontal

R. Sagittal

Transverse

154

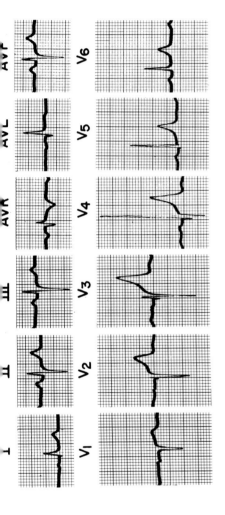

Fig. 10.5. Left anterior hemiblock and anterior myocardial infarction. The vectorcardiogram and electrocardiogram were recorded from a 53-year-old man with a documented previous anterior myocardial infarction. There is a superior displacement of the QRS loop. In the frontal plane the majority of the loop area is located in the left upper quadrant. The initial deflection is directed inferiorly and rightward and the loop is inscribed counterclockwise. In the sagittal projection the QRS loop is inscribed at first counterclockwise and then clockwise with most of the loop in the posterior-superior quadrant. The evidence of old anterior myocardial infarction is suggested by the posterior orientation of the initial forces as seen in the transverse and sagittal planes. The T loop is directed anteriorly, leftward, and inferiorly. In the electrocardiogram an abnormal Q wave is present in leads V_2 and V_3. In this patient it is most likely related to the previous myocardial infarction. However, a narrow Q wave may also be seen in these leads in the absence of myocardial infarction because of the altered initial vectors in left anterior hemiblock.

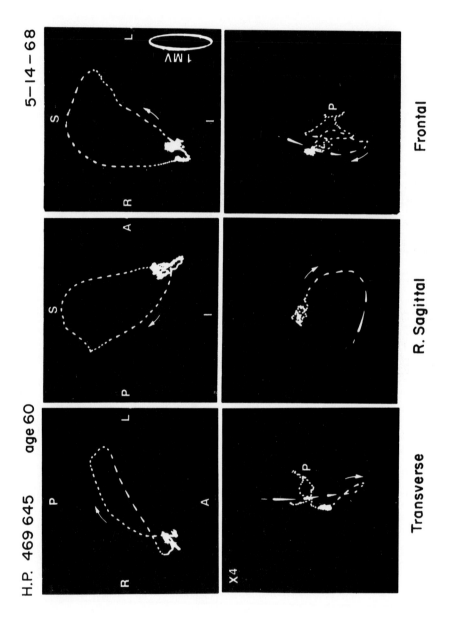

H.P. 469 645   age 60   5-14-68

Frontal   R. Sagittal   Transverse

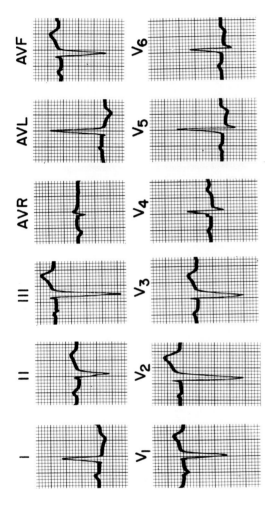

Fig. 10.6. (A) Intermittent left anterior hemiblock. See also Figure 10.6B. The tracings were recorded from a 60-year-old man with coronary artery disease. In the transverse plane there is a posterior displacement of the efferent limb of the QRS loop. Most of the loop is inscribed clockwise. The 0.02-sec vector is directed posteriorly. These findings suggest anterior wall myocardial infarction. The frontal and sagittal projections reveal the superior displacement of the QRS loop. In the frontal plane the initial deflection is directed inferiorly and leftward. A small initial part of the QRS loop is inscribed clockwise which is atypical for uncomplicated left anterior hemiblock. The rest of the loop is inscribed counterclockwise. The maximum **QRS** vector and the majority of the loop are located in the left superior quadrant. The T loop is directed rightward, anteriorly, and inferiorly. The rightward orientation of the T loop is probably due to lateral wall myocardial ischemia.

157

H.P.   469 645

7-12-68

Lead II

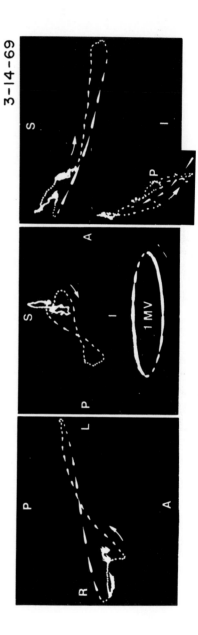

3-14-69

158

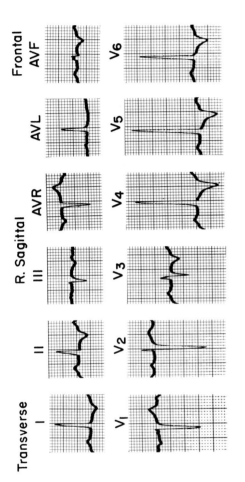

Fig. 10.6. (B) Intermittent left anterior hemiblock. The tracings were recorded from the same patient as those in Figure 10.6A. The lead II electrocardiogram recorded on 7/12/68 demonstrates the intermittent nature of the left anterior hemiblock shown in Figure 10.6A. In the vectorcardiogram and electrocardiogram recorded on 3/14/69 the left anterior hemiblock is no longer present. The QRS loop is consistent with anterior myocardial infarction. It is inscribed in a figure-of-eight pattern in the transverse and sagittal planes. Note that the maximum **QRS** vector is now directed inferiorly. The QRS loop in the frontal plane is inscribed narrowly clockwise. The T loop is directed to the right and superiorly. It is inscribed clockwise in the transverse plane, counterclockwise in the sagittal plane. The changes are consistent with anterolateral and inferior myocardial ischemia.

159

Sagittal plane QRS loop. In the right sagittal projection most of the QRS loop is located in the posterior-superior quadrant. In the majority of instances the loop is inscribed clockwise. However, a figure-of-eight or counterclockwise inscription is also seen in the absence of other associated abnormalities such as inferior myocardial infarction. The initial deflection is directed anteriorly and inferiorly. The early course of the efferent limb is variable but is most often in the posterior-inferior quadrant. The rest of the body and the terminal deflection are in the posterior-superior quadrant.

Frontal plane QRS loop. In the frontal plane projection the changes are most characteristic. The loop is wide and most of the loop area is located in the left superior quadrant. One of the diagnostic findings is the counterclockwise inscription of the loop. The initial deflection is always directed inferiorly, most often to the right, but may be leftward. The efferent limb proceeds more or less horizontally to the left and then rather rapidly in the superior direction to become the afferent limb of the loop. The terminal deflection is superior and either slightly leftward or slightly rightward. The planar projection of the maximum **QRS** vector is directed leftward, either superiorly or slightly inferiorly. In the latter case the direction is usually superior to 10°. The magnitude of the maximum **QRS** vector is not increased in the absence of left ventricular hypertrophy. As the major part of the loop area is in the left upper quadrant the half-area or mean **QRS** vector is invariably directed leftward and superiorly. As mentioned previously, the total duration of the QRS loop may be increased but seldom exceeds 0.10 sec in the absence of additional ventricular conduction defect. Slow inscription of the terminal part of the QRS loop may be seen in cases with longer duration.

Since the majority of the QRS loop is located in the left upper quadrant and projects on the positive side of the lead axis of lead I and the negative side of the lead axes of the inferior leads, a predominant R wave will therefore be recorded in lead I and a deep S wave in leads II, III, and aVF. When the initial deflection is directed inferiorly and rightward, a small Q wave will be recorded in lead I resulting in a qR complex in this lead. A monophasic R wave may be seen if the initial deflection is leftward. Since the initial deflection is invariably directed inferiorly, a small R wave (therefore an rS complex) is always present in leads II, III, and aVF. The consistent superior displacement of the QRS loop has its counterpart in the abnormal left axis deviation of between −30° to −90°.*

ST vector and TsÊ loop. The orientation of the spatial **ST** vector and T loop and its maximum vector in left anterior hemiblock is often within normal limits. However, there is a tendency for the T loop to be displaced anteriorly and inferiorly. In the transverse plane the T loop is directed anteriorly and leftward. The loop is inscribed counterclockwise. In the right sagittal plane it is directed anteriorly and inferiorly and is inscribed clockwise. In the frontal plane the loop is directed leftward

* Because of the lack of adequate electrocardiographic and anatomic correlation the quantitative criteria for the diagnosis of left anterior hemiblock has not been definitely established. It is generally agreed that an axis deviation beyond −45° is strongly indicative of left anterior hemiblock. Some investigators consider a QRS axis of −30° to −45° to represent only a partial block. In this text the description is based on the findings of 100 cases with a mean QRS axis of −30° to −90° as determined from the conventional electrocardiogram.

and inferiorly. The direction of the maximum **T** vector is often more inferior than the normal limit of 55°. The direction of inscription of the T loop is variable but mostly counterclockwise.

In the conventional electrocardiogram, the T wave is upright in all leads except lead aVR and sometimes leads aVL and V_1. Because of the inferior displacement of the T loop the T wave in the inferior leads is usually taller than that in leads I and aVL.

LEFT POSTERIOR HEMIBLOCK (Figs. 10.1, 10.7-10)

Left posterior hemiblock is less common than left anterior hemiblock. Rosenbaum attributes the lower incidence to the following characteristics of the posterior division of the left bundle branch:

1. It is short and thick.
2. It has a dual blood supply from the anterior and posterior descending arteries.
3. It belongs to the less turbulent left ventricular inflow tract.
4. It is the first group of fibers to leave the bundle of His.

When there is an interruption or delay of impulse conduction through the posterior division of the left bundle branch left ventricular excitation begins in the area normally supplied by the anterior division, that is, the subendocardium of the anterior paraseptal region and perhaps the mid septum. From there the impulse

LEFT POSTERIOR HEMIBLOCK

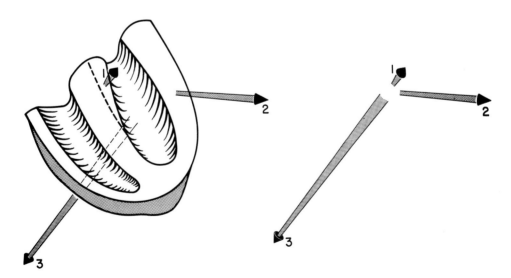

Fig. 10.7. The sequence of left ventricular activation and three representative spatial **QRS** vectors in left posterior hemiblock. See text.

spreads to the anterior and anterolateral wall of the left ventricle. The excitation of the inferior and posterior wall is delayed because of the failure of impulse conduction through the posterior division. The activation of this area now depends on the retrograde conduction of impulse from the anterior division (Fig. 10.1).

As previously mentioned, the endocardium-to-epicardium activation of the anterior paraseptal region of the left ventricle generates forces directed anteriorly, leftward, and superiorly. In the presence of left posterior hemiblock the opposing forces from the simultaneous activation of the posterior paraseptal region is no longer present. Therefore, the initial phase of the left ventricular activation will be dominated by the potential from the anterior paraseptal region (Fig. 10.7). During the next phase the activation of the anterior and anterolateral wall of the left ventricle occurs at the expected time. The representative vectors are directed leftward and anteriorly but become gradually more inferior and posterior as excitation is proceeding in that direction. The last area to be depolarized is the inferior and posterior wall of the left ventricle. The rightward spread of the impulse from the anterolateral wall toward this area results in late vectors which are oriented inferiorly, rightward, and posteriorly.

Vectorcardiographic Findings in Left Posterior Hemiblock

QRSsÊ loop. The characteristic changes of the spatial QRS loop in left posterior hemiblock is its inferior and rightward displacement. An abnormally large percentage of the loop is located in the right, inferior, posterior octant. The extent of the rightward displacement may depend on the degree of the block. The loop has a smooth contour and is rather wide. Its overall magnitude is usually within the normal range. The duration of the QRS loop may be slightly prolonged up to 0.10 sec, or 0.02 sec longer than the duration before the block in the absence of other conduction defect. In some cases there is a slowing of the speed of inscription in the late portion of the loop. The maximum spatial **QRS** vector is directed posteriorly and inferiorly, either leftward or rightward. Frequently two "maximum" vectors are present, one directed to the left, and the other to the right. In either event the presence of prominent rightward, inferior, and posterior vectors is always observed.

Planar Projections of the QRSsÊ Loop and Correlation with the Conventional Electrocardiogram (Figs. 10.8–10.10)

Transverse plane QRS loop. In this projection the QRS loop may appear wide or narrow. The majority of the loop area is located posteriorly. The loop is displaced rightward, the degree of which varies. The loop area in the right posterior quadrant is always greater than 20 percent of the total. The loop is inscribed counterclockwise.

The initial deflection is inscribed anteriorly and leftward. The efferent limb of the body of the loop continues leftward but turns posteriorly. The afferent limb proceeds rightward and posteriorly, and may form a rather acute angle with the terminal deflection before the latter returns toward the E point. The maximum QRS vector is directed posteriorly, either to the left or to the right.

The QRS complex in the right precordial leads of the conventional electrocardiogram may be normal as the initial vectors are directed anteriorly and the late forces

LEFT POSTERIOR HEMIBLOCK

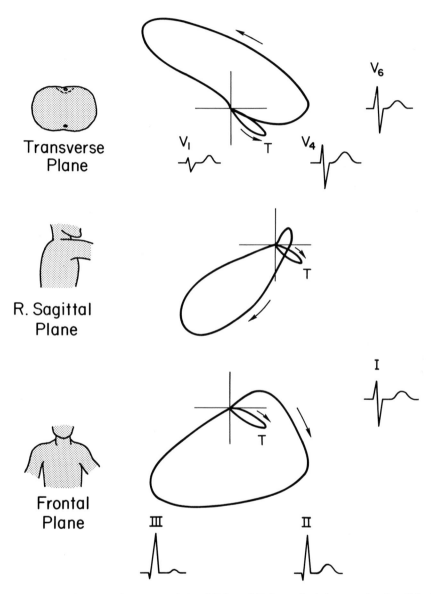

Fig. 10.8. Schematic diagrams of the QRS and T loops in left posterior hemiblock. The representative conventional leads are also illustrated.

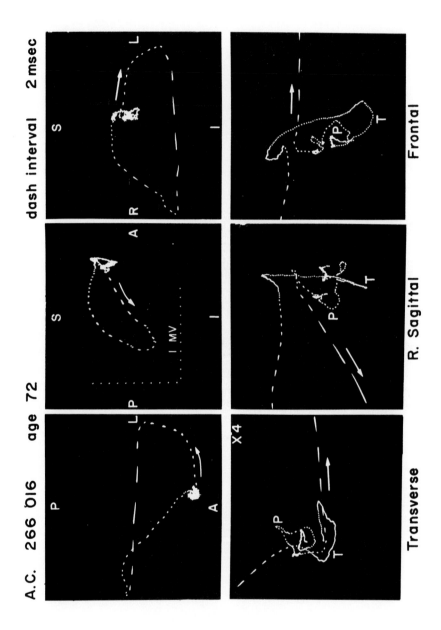

A.C. 266 016 age 72 dash interval 2 msec

Frontal R. Sagittal Transverse

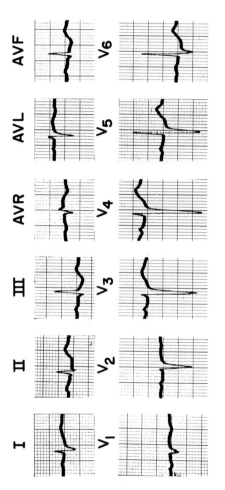

Fig. 10.9. Left posterior hemiblock. The vectorcardiogram and electrocardiogram were recorded from a 72-year-old man with diabetes mellitus and angina pectoris. There was clinical and radiological evidence of left ventricular hypertrophy but no right ventricular hypertrophy or pulmonary emphysema. In the vectorcardiogram there is a rightward and inferior displacement of the QRS loop. In the transverse plane the QRS loop is inscribed mostly counterclockwise. In the right sagittal plane it is at first counterclockwise and then clockwise. In the frontal plane the initial forces are directed superiorly and the loop is inscribed clockwise. The loop is wide with more than 50 percent of the loop area located in the right inferior quadrant. The duration of the QRS loop is 0.09 sec. The T loop is abnormally small and irregular in configuration. Additional primary T loop abnormalities are probably present. Part of the changes may be attributed to digitalis which the patient was receiving.

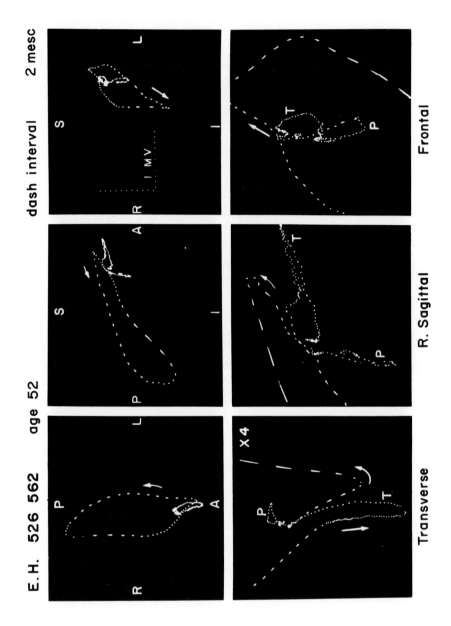

dash interval   2 mesc

E.H. 526 562   age 52

Frontal

R. Sagittal

Transverse

166

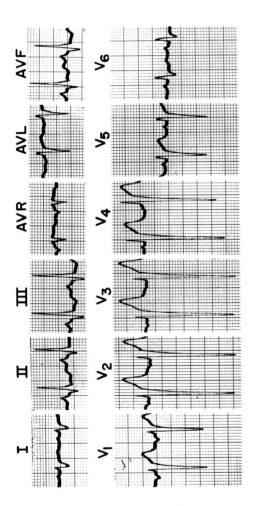

Fig. 10.10. Left posterior hemiblock and inferior myocardial infarction. The vectorcardiogram and electrocardiogram were recorded from a 52-year-old man with a history of previous myocardial infarction. Coronary arteriogram revealed a total occlusion of the proximal right coronary artery and 70 percent narrowing of the anterior descending branch of the left coronary artery. The ventriculogram showed akinesis of the inferior wall and the apex. In the vectorcardiogram the QRSsÉ loop is displaced posteriorly, rightward, and inferiorly. The QRS loop is inscribed counterclockwise in the transverse and right sagittal planes and clockwise in the frontal plane. In the frontal plane the direction of the maximum **QRS** vector is 110°. The major portion of the QRS loop area is in the right inferior quadrant. There is also an increase in the duration of the initial superior QRS forces to exceed 0.03 sec to suggest inferior myocardial infarction. The counterclockwise inscription of the early part of the QRS loop in the sagittal plane is probably also related to the inferior myocardial infarction. The T loop is directed anteriorly, slightly leftward, and superiorly. The superior orientation is probably related to the inferior myocardial infarction. The P loop is consistent with left atrial enlargement.

167

posteriorly. However the S wave in lead V_1 is often small because of the reduction of the left posterior forces. For the same reason the amplitude of the R wave in leads V_5 and V_6 may be reduced. The leftward orientation of the initial deflection accounts for the absence of a Q wave in the left precordial leads. The prominent late rightward forces have their counterpart in the rather deep S wave in leads V_5 and V_6.

Sagittal plane QRS loop. In the right sagittal projection the QRS loop is located mostly in the inferoposterior quadrant. The exceptions are the initial deflection which is directed anteriorly and superiorly, and the early part of the efferent limb which is inscribed in the anterior quadrants. The direction of inscription of the loop is clockwise.

Frontal plane QRS loop. In this projection the findings are most characteristic. The loop is smoothly inscribed. Its configuration may be wide or narrow. The major part of the QRS loop is inferior with an abnormally large portion of the loop area (over 20 percent) located in the right inferior quadrant. The extent of the rightward displacement varies and may be related to the degree of block. The projection of the maximum spatial **QRS** vector is always directed inferiorly and often rightward.

The initial deflection is directed superiorly and leftward. The efferent limb proceeds inferiorly and leftward and the amplitude of the leftward forces is often reduced. The afferent limb is inscribed toward the right. The terminal deflection is directed inferiorly and rightward. The direction of inscription of the loop is practically always clockwise which is one of the important diagnostic findings in left posterior hemiblock. As mentioned previously, the duration of the QRS loop may be prolonged up to 0.10 sec. Slowing of inscription may be observed in some cases in the late portion of the loop.

Because of the leftward orientation of the initial deflection, an initial R wave is recorded in lead I of the conventional electrocardiogram. As the amplitude of the leftward forces is reduced, the R wave in this lead is usually small. The abnormal rightward displacement of the late **QRS** vectors accounts for the deep S wave in this lead. A qR pattern is consistently observed in the inferior leads II, III, and aVF because the initial forces are always directed superiorly and the main body of the loop is always inferior. The rightward displacement of the QRS loop has its counterpart in the right axis deviation. Although in the conventional electrocardiogram the mean QRS axis in left posterior hemiblock is usually between 90° and 130°, in the vectorcardiogram the area of the QRS loop in the right lower quadrant is often less than 50 percent of the total. This is explainable in that the true electrical axis of lead I is not horizontal but is directed toward the left shoulder. A vector recorded with the corrected orthogonal lead system with a direction of less than 90° may project on the negative side of the lead I axis and display a negative deflection in this lead.

TsÊ loop. The spatial T loop in left posterior hemiblock is directed anteriorly, leftward, and inferiorly. It is inscribed counterclockwise in the transverse plane and clockwise in the right sagittal and frontal projections.

Differential diagnosis of left posterior hemiblock and type C right ventricular hypertrophy. It is apparent from the above description that the vectorcardiographic findings in left posterior hemiblock simulate closely those of type C right ventricular hypertrophy. Indeed, electrocardiographic and vectorcardiographic differentiation of these two entities are often impossible. It must be emphasized that the diagnosis of left posterior hemiblock can only be made after right ventricular hypertrophy, pulmonary emphysema, a vertical heart, and extensive lateral wall myocardial infarction are excluded on clinical grounds.

BIFASCICULAR BLOCK

The intraventricular conduction system may be considered as a trifascicular system consisting of the anterior and posterior divisions of the left bundle branch and the right bundle branch. Conduction abnormalities involving two of the three fascicles may present themselves as right bundle branch block with left anterior hemiblock, right bundle branch block with left posterior hemiblock, or combined left anterior and left posterior hemiblocks. As previously stated, the combined effect of complete left anterior and posterior hemiblocks cannot be distinguished from complete main-stem left bundle branch block. In clinical practice, the term *bifascicular block* is generally used to indicate the failure of conduction in one of the divisions of the left bundle branch in addition to right bundle branch block. The interruption of impulse conduction in both divisions or the main stem of the left bundle branch and the right bundle branch will result in complete AV block. The combination of partial block in one or two fascicles and complete block in the rest of the trifascicular system causes many varieties of AV and intraventricular conduction abnormalities which are beyond the scope of the present discussion.

RIGHT BUNDLE BRANCH BLOCK WITH LEFT ANTERIOR HEMIBLOCK

This is the more common type of bifascicular block. It has been also called the "variant," "classic," or "uncommon" type of right bundle branch block in the past. The sequence of ventricular activation and the vectorcardiographic and electrocardiographic changes reflect the combined effect of the failure of conduction in the two component fascicles. As both the right bundle branch block and the hemiblocks have already been discussed, the following description will be relatively brief.

In the presence of right bundle branch block and left anterior hemiblock the excitation impulse is conducted through the third fascicle—the posterior division of the left bundle branch. The earliest ventricular depolarization occurs at the posterior paraseptal region of the left ventricle and perhaps also the midleft septum. The initial QRS forces are directed inferiorly, anteriorly, and rightward. As the impulse spreads through the inferior wall and the apex of the left ventricle the QRS forces are directed inferiorly, leftward, and anteriorly. This is followed by the normal late activation of the posterobasal region and the abnormal delayed excitation of the anterolateral wall. The representative vectors are oriented posteriorly, leftward, and superiorly. However, at this time the abnormal left-to-right activation of the right septum has begun and generates forces in the anterior and rightward direction. As the left ventricular excitation is being completed and the delayed activation of the right septum and the free wall of the right ventricle becomes the dominant event the resultant vectors are oriented rightward, anteriorly, and either superiorly or inferiorly.

Vectorcardiographic Findings in Right Bundle Branch Block with Left Anterior Hemiblock (Figs. 10.11-10.14)

QRSsÊ loop. The spatial QRS loop in this bifascicular block may be divided into two parts, the main portion of the loop and the finger-like terminal appendage. The main portion of the loop is located mostly to the left, superior, and usually anterior to the E point. Its initial deflection and the efferent limb reveal changes essentially identical to those of left anterior hemiblock alone. The afferent limb is modified by the combined effect of the bifascicular involvement. The characteristics of the slowly inscribed terminal appendage are similar to those of the uncomplicated right bundle branch block. The maximum spatial **QRS** vector is directed leftward, superiorly, and usually anteriorly. The magnitude of this vector is usually reduced in the absence of left ventricular hypertrophy. The total duration of the QRS loop is 0.12 sec or longer.

Transverse plane. In the transverse plane projection the findings are essentially the same as those of the uncomplicated right bundle branch block. A counterclockwise, clockwise, as well as a figure-of-eight, inscription of the main portion of the QRS loop may be seen. The clockwise inscription is frequently observed in the absence of coexisting right ventricular hypertrophy or true posterior myocardial infarction. The conventional electrocardiogram records an RSR' pattern in lead V_1. The S wave is often small or absent because of marked anterior displacement of the afferent limb of the QRS loop. The left precordial leads record a relatively small R wave with a broad, slowly inscribed S wave.

Sagittal plane. The right sagittal plane projection reveals the superior displacement of the main body of the QRS loop. The initial deflection is inscribed anteriorly and downward. Most of the efferent and afferent limbs are located in the anterior-superior quadrant. Counterclockwise, clockwise, or a figure-of-eight inscription of the loop may be seen; the former is the most common finding. It is in this projection the loop often presents a rather confusing picture because of its irregular course.

Frontal plane. In the frontal plane projection the changes of the main portion of the QRS loop resemble closely those seen in the isolated left anterior hemiblock. The loop appears wide and is displaced superiorly with the majority of the loop area located in the left upper quadrant. The initial deflection is inscribed inferiorly, either rightward or leftward. The direction of inscription of the loop is counterclockwise. The projection of the maximum spatial **QRS** vector is leftward and superior but occasionally leftward and slightly inferior. Its magnitude is often reduced. The slowly inscribed terminal appendage is directed rightward and is most often located in the right upper quadrant. In the conventional electrocardiogram lead I records a

Right Bundle Branch Block
With Left Anterior Hemiblock

A

B

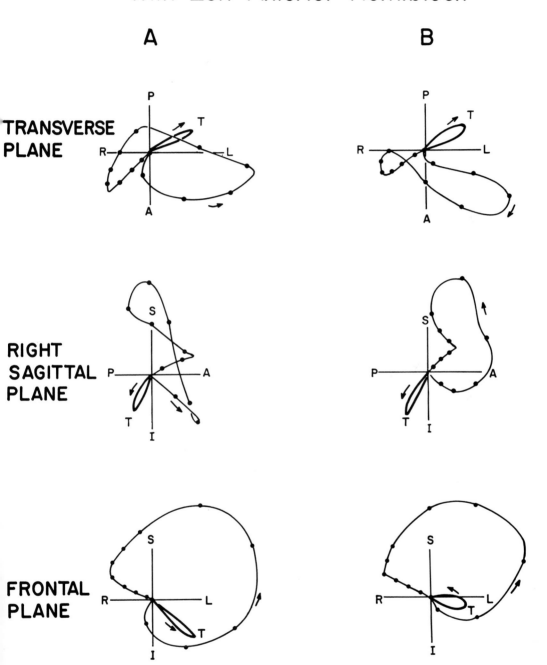

TRANSVERSE PLANE

RIGHT SAGITTAL PLANE

FRONTAL PLANE

Fig. 10.11. Schematic diagram of the QRS and T loops in right bundle branch block with left anterior hemiblock. Note in A the transverse plane QRS loop is inscribed counterclockwise. In B its main body is inscribed clockwise.

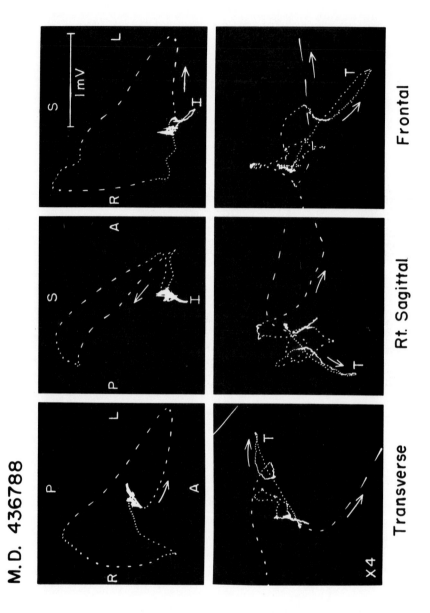

M.D. 436788

Frontal

Rt. Sagittal

Transverse

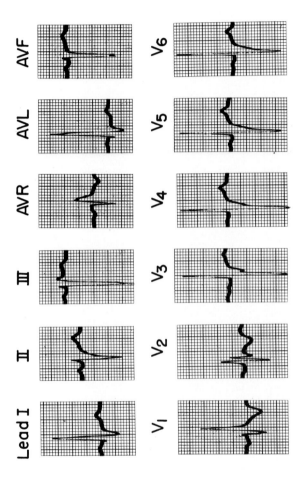

Fig. 10.12. Right bundle branch block with left anterior hemiblock. The vectorcardiogram and electrocardiogram were recorded from a 68-year-old woman with hypertension. The transverse plane QRS loop is typical for right bundle branch block. The sagittal and frontal planes reveal the superior displacement of the QRS loop. In the frontal plane the initial deflection is directed inferiorly and rightward and the QRS loop is inscribed counterclockwise. These findings are consistent with left anterior hemiblock. A large portion of the QRS loop in the frontal projection is in the right superior quadrant. The rightward displacement is caused by right bundle branch block.

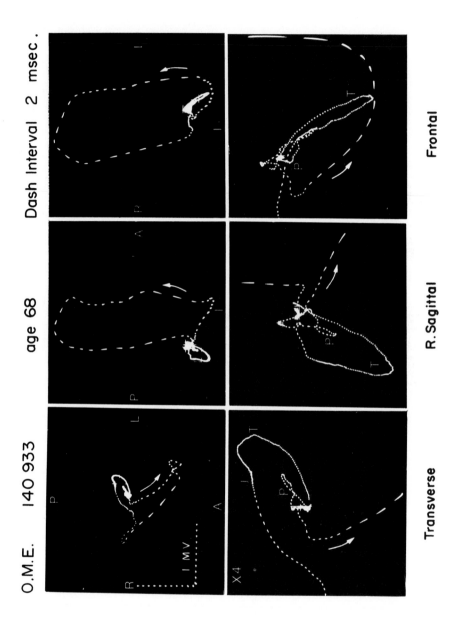

O.M.E.   140 933   age 68   Dash Interval 2 msec.

Transverse   R.Sagittal   Frontal

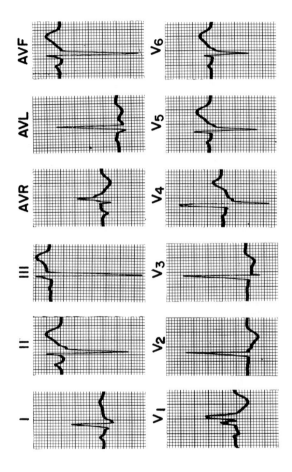

Fig. 10.13. Right bundle branch block with left anterior hemiblock. The tracings were recorded from a 68-year-old woman with hypertensive cardiovascular disease. Cardiac fluoroscopy revealed left ventricular hypertrophy. In the vectorcardiogram the QRS loop is abnormally large and is displaced anteriorly and markedly superiorly. The main portion of the QRS loop is inscribed clockwise in the transverse plane and counterclockwise in the sagittal and frontal planes. The slowly inscribed terminal appendage is best seen in the transverse plane. In the frontal plane the initial deflection is directed inferiorly and rightward. As in Figure 10.12 a large portion of the QRS loop is in the right superior quadrant.

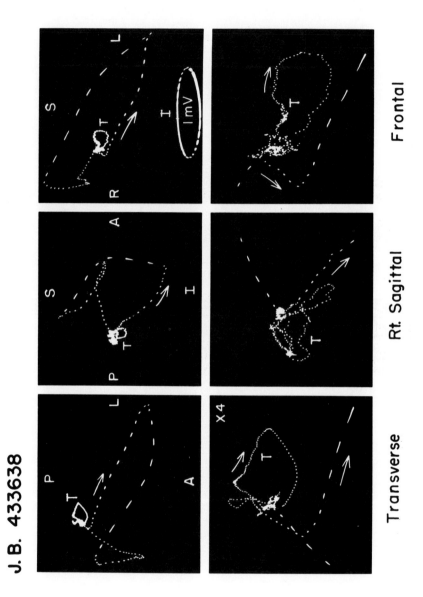

J.B. 433638

Frontal

Rt. Sagittal

Transverse

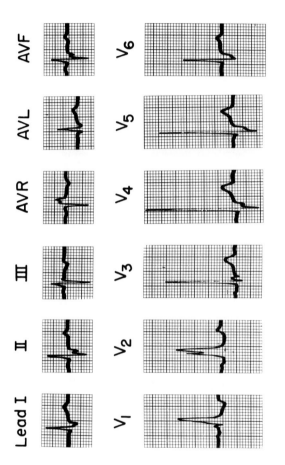

Fig. 10.14. Right bundle branch block with possible left anterior hemiblock. The patient is a 65-year-old man with borderline cardiomegaly on x-ray examination but no other evidence of heart disease. The vectorcardiogram shows right bundle branch block with clockwise inscription of the main portion of the QRS loop in the transverse plane. In the frontal plane there is a counterclockwise inscription with some superior displacement of the QRS loop. However, the majority of the loop area is still in the left inferior quadrant. The conventional electrocardiogram reveals a QRS axis of $-30°$ based on the first 0.06-sec portion of the QRS complex.

qRS or an RS complex. The small Q wave is the result of the projection of the inferiorly and usually rightward directed initial deflection on the negative side of lead I axis. The R wave in lead I is taller than normal because of the superior displacement of the efferent and afferent limbs of the loop. The corresponding vectors are now more parallel to the true electrical axis of lead I (which points more or less toward the left shoulder). For the same reason a taller R wave is also recorded in lead aVL. The broad and slurred S wave is the equivalent of the rightward oriented terminal appendage as in the case of uncomplicated right bundle branch block. An rS complex is recorded in the inferior leads II, III, and aVF because of the left anterior hemiblock. The late portion of the S wave is slurred and slowly inscribed because of the usually superiorly oriented terminal appendage. If the mean QRS axis is determined by using the first part of the QRS complex which is rapidly inscribed, there is an abnormal left axis deviation of $-30°$ to $-90°$.

The ST vector and TsÊ loop. The spatial **ST** vector and T loop in right bundle branch block with left anterior hemiblock are similar to those of uncomplicated right bundle branch block. Their directions are practically always opposite to the terminal appendage. They are therefore oriented to the left, posteriorly, and usually inferiorly. The **ST** vector is usually small. The T loop is inscribed clockwise in the transverse plane, counterclockwise in the right sagittal and frontal projections in the majority of cases. Their counterparts in the conventional electrocardiogram are also similar to those of the uncomplicated right bundle branch block.

RIGHT BUNDLE BRANCH BLOCK WITH LEFT POSTERIOR HEMIBLOCK

This type of bifascicular block is uncommon. The initial ventricular activation begins at the region supplied by the anterior division of the left bundle branch. The activation of the anterior paraseptal area is accompanied by initial forces which are directed anteriorly, superiorly, and leftward. This is followed by activation of the anterior and anterolateral wall of the left ventricle which results in forces that are oriented anteriorly, leftward, and superiorly. As the impulse spreads in a retrograde fashion to the areas normally supplied by the posterior division, the inferior and posterobasal part of the left ventricle are depolarized and the generated forces are directed accordingly. However, at this time the abnormal left-to-right excitation of the right septal mass and the free wall of the right ventricle also has begun. The associated forces are oriented anteriorly and rightward. Consequently, the resultant vectors are directed inferiorly and turning rightward, and may be either anterior or slightly posterior. As the left ventricular activation is being completed the delayed activation of the right ventricle becomes the dominant event and the late QRS forces are directed anteriorly and rightward.

Vectorcardiographic Findings in Right Bundle Branch Block with Left Posterior Hemiblock (Figs. 10.15-10.16)

QRSsÊ loop. As in right bundle branch block with left anterior hemiblock the spatial QRS loop in the right bundle branch block with left posterior hemiblock may likewise be divided into the main portion of the loop and the terminal appendage.

The main body of the loop is displaced inferiorly and rightward, and anteriorly. Its initial deflection and efferent limb resemble those of isolated left posterior hemiblock. The afferent limb is altered by the combined effect of the bifascicular involvement. The terminal appendage is similar to that seen in uncomplicated right bundle branch block. The maximum spatial **QRS** vector is always directed inferiorly but may be either leftward or rightward, anterior or posterior. The total duration of the QRS loop is 0.12 sec or longer.

Transverse plane.   In the transverse plane projection the QRS loop is similar to that of uncomplicated right bundle branch block in its general configuration. The main portion of the loop is inscribed either clockwise or counterclockwise, or in a figure-of-eight pattern. The initial deflection is directed anteriorly and usually to the left. The maximum leftward **QRS** vector is oriented anteriorly and its magnitude,

RIGHT BUNDLE BRANCH BLOCK WITH
LEFT POSTERIOR HEMIBLOCK

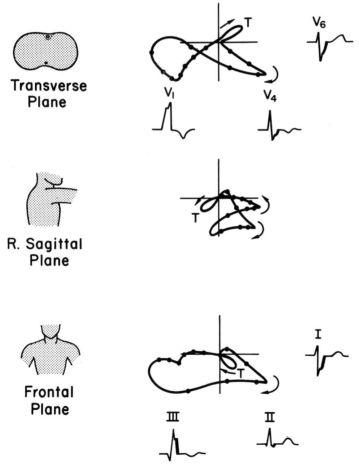

Fig. 10.15.   Schematic diagrams of the QRS and T loops in right bundle branch block with left posterior hemiblock. Representative scalar complexes are also shown.

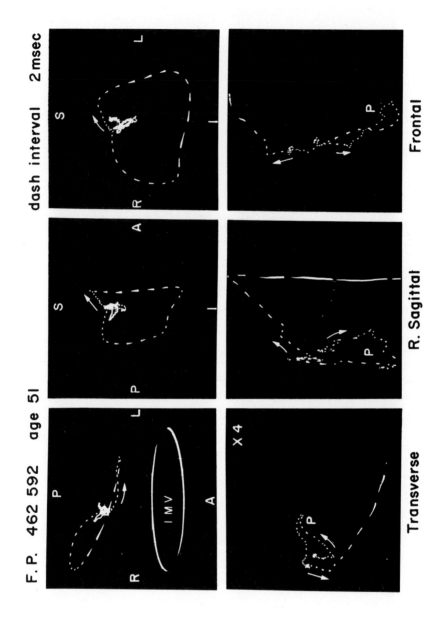

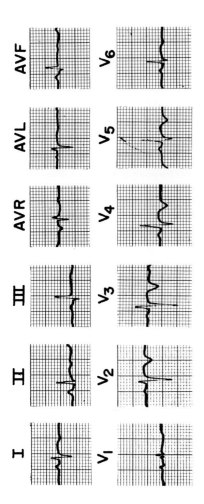

Fig. 10.16. (A) True posterior myocardial infarction with left posterior hemiblock. The tracings were obtained from a 51-year-old woman with severe coronary artery disease. Coronary arteriogram demonstrated 90 percent obstruction of the right coronary artery near its origin, 50 percent of the anterior descending artery and the left circumflex artery distal to a large marginal branch. A Vineburg procedure was performed 2 weeks prior to the recording of these tracings. The QRS complex is similar to that before surgery. In the vectorcardiogram the QRSsÊ loop is displaced anteriorly, rightward, and inferiorly. In the transverse plane there is a loss of the left posterior QRS forces consistent with true posterior myocardial infarction. The frontal plane QRS loop is inscribed clockwise. The loop is wide and an abnormally large portion of the loop area is located in the right inferior quadrant. These changes are consistent with left posterior hemiblock, especially since there is no clinical evidence to suggest right ventricular hypertrophy or chronic lung disease. The TsÊ loop is directed posteriorly, rightward, and superiorly. This is probably due to postoperative pericarditis. See Figure 10.16B for the development of right bundle branch block in this patient.

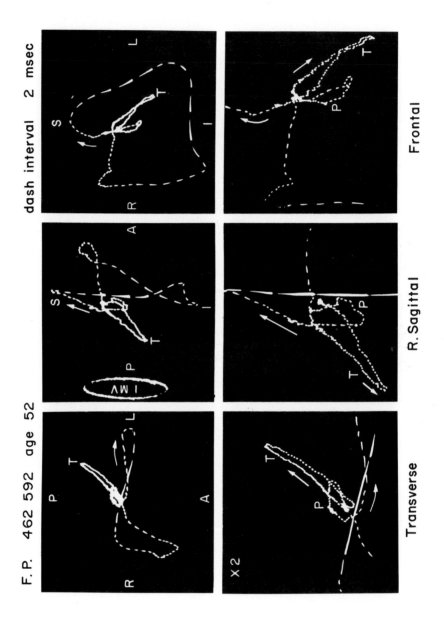

dash interval 2 msec

F.P. 462 592 age 52

Frontal

R.Sagittal

Transverse

182

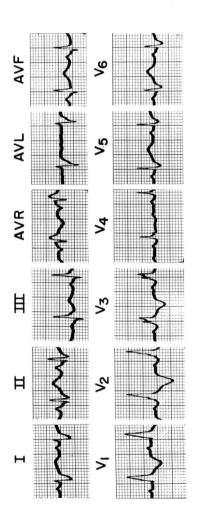

Fig. 10.16. (B) Posteroinferior myocardial infarction with right bundle branch block and left posterior hemiblock. The vectorcardiogram and electrocardiogram were recorded from the same patient 10 months after Figure 10.16A was obtained. Right bundle branch block has developed in addition to the left posterior hemiblock. A slowly inscribed terminal appendage has appeared and is directed anteriorly, rightward, and superiorly. There is also a slight increase in the duration of the initial superior forces as seen in the sagittal and frontal projections. Inferior wall myocardial infarction is suspected. The diagnosis of posterior myocardial infarction is based on the previous tracing because the anterior displacement of the QRS loop in the present trace may be the result of the conduction abnormalities alone. Note the spatial T loop is now directed leftward, posteriorly, and inferiorly, and is opposite to the terminal appendage of the QRS loop.

however, is further reduced when compared with that of the uncomplicated right bundle branch block. The afferent limb proceeds further to the right before it continues with the terminal appendage. Similarly, in the conventional electrocardiogram an RSR′ pattern is recorded in the right precordial leads with the S wave being usually small and often absent. In the left precordial leads (V_5 and V_6) the amplitude of the R wave is much reduced and the S wave is prominent with its late part being slurred and slowly inscribed.

Sagittal plane.   In the right sagittal plane projection the majority of the loop is located inferiorly. The direction of inscription of the main portion of the loop is variable. The slowly inscribed terminal appendage is similar to that of the uncomplicated right bundle branch block.

Frontal plane.   In the frontal plane projection the effect of the left posterior hemiblock is best displayed. The main part of the QRS loop is located in the inferior quadrants. There is also an abnormal rightward displacement of the loop so that frequently more than half of the loop area is in the right inferior quadrant. The loop is often wide. The direction of inscription of this portion is practically always clockwise even though a figure-of-eight pattern may be seen. The initial deflection is directed superiorly and usually leftward but may be to the right. The efferent limb proceeds leftward and inferiorly. The afferent limb continues rightward to be connected with the terminal appendage. The characteristics of the slowly inscribed terminal appendage are similar to those of uncomplicated right bundle branch block. The projection of the maximum **QRS** vector is always directed inferiorly, either to the left or to the right. The magnitude of the leftward forces is reduced. In the conventional electrocardiogram lead I records a small R wave followed by a deep S wave which is abnormally broad. The first part of the S wave is written rapidly and is related to the abnormal rightward displacement of the afferent limb of the QRS loop. The late part of the S wave is slurred and slowly inscribed and is the counterpart of the terminal appendage in the vectorcardiogram. In the inferior leads a qR or qRS pattern is present. The equivalent of the terminal appendage may present itself as a slurring of the end of the R wave or as a wide S wave depending on the orientation of the terminal appendage. If the mean QRS axis is determined from the first part of the QRS complex before the slurring there is an abnormal right axis deviation of 90° to 130°.

ST vector and TsÊ loop.   The spatial **ST** vector in right bundle branch block with left posterior hemiblock is usually quite small. The spatial T loop is directed leftward, posteriorly, and inferiorly. In the transverse plane it is inscribed clockwise; in the right sagittal plane, counterclockwise; and in the frontal plane, usually clockwise.

REFERENCES

1.   Benchimol A, Barreto EC, Pedraza A: The Frank vectorcardiogram in left anterior hemiblock. J Electrocardiol 4:116, 1971
2.   Benchimol A, Desser KB: The Frank vectorcardiogram in left posterior hemiblock. J Electrocardiol 4:129, 1971

3. Castellanos A Jr, Chapunoff E, Lemberg L, Portillo B: The vectorcardiogram in left posterior hemiblock. Proc XIth Int Vectorcardiography Symp. Amsterdam and London, North-Holland, 1971, p 264

4. Cohen SI, Lau SH, Stein E, Young MW, Damato AN: Variations of aberrant ventricular conduction in man: Evidence of isolated and combined block within the specialized conduction system. An electrocardiographic and vectorcardiographic study. Circulation 38:899, 1968

5. Durrer D, van Dam RT, Freud GE, Janse MJ, Meijler FL, Arzbaecher RC: Total excitation of the isolated human heart. Circulation 41:895, 1970

6. Fernandez F, Scebat L, Lenegre J: Electrocardiographic study of left intraventricular hemiblock in man during selective coronary arteriography. Am J Cardiol 26:1, 1970

7. Hecht HH, Kossmann CE, Childers RW, Langendorf R, Lev M, Rosen KM, Pruitt RD, Truex RC, Uhley HN, Watt TB Jr: Atrioventricular and intraventricular conduction. Revised nomenclature and concepts. Am J Cardiol 31:232, 1973

8. Kulbertus H, Collignon P, Humblet L: Vectorcardiographic study of the QRS loop in patients with left anterior focal block. Am Heart J 79:293, 1970

9. Kulbertus H, Collignon P, Humblet L: Vectorcardiographic study of QRS loop in patients with left superior axis deviation and right bundle-branch block. Br Heart J 32:386, 1970

10. McHenry PL, Phillips JF, Fisch C, Corya BR: Right precordial qrS pattern due to left anterior hemiblock. Am Heart J 81:498, 1971

11. Medrano GA, Brenes C, DeMicheli A, Sodi-Pallares D: Clinical electrocardiographic and vectorcardiographic diagnosis of the left anterior subdivision block isolated or associated with RBBB. Am Heart J 83:447, 1972

12. Pryor R, Blount SG Jr: The clinical significance of true left axis deviation. Left intraventricular blocks. Am Heart J 72:391, 1966

13. Pryor R: Fascicular blocks and the bilateral bundle branch block syndrome. Editorial. Am Heart J 83:441, 1972

14. Rosenbaum MB, Elizari MV, Levi RJ, Nau GJ, Pisani N, Lazzari JO, Halpern MS: Five cases of intermittent left anterior hemiblock. Am J Cardiol 24:1, 1969

15. Rosenbaum MB, Elizari MV, Lazzari JO, Nau GJ, Levi RJ, Halpern MS: Intraventricular trifascicular blocks. Review of the literature and classification. Am Heart J 78:450, 1969

16. Rosenbaum MB, Elizari MV, Lazzari JO: The Hemiblocks. Oldsmar, Fla., Tampa Tracings, 1970

17. Rosenbaum MB: The hemiblocks: Diagnostic criteria and clinical significance. Modern Concepts Cardiovas Dis 39:141, 1970

18. Saltzman P, Linn H, Pick A: Right bundle-branch block with left axis deviation. Br Heart J 28:703, 1966

19. Uhley HN: Some controversy regarding the peripheral distribution of the conduction system. Editorial. Am J Cardiol 30:919, 1972

20. Varriale P, Kennedy RJ: Right bundle branch block and left posterior fascicular block. Vectorcardiographic and clinical features. Am J Cardiol 29:459, 1972

21. Watt TB, Murao S, Pruitt RD: Left axis deviation induced experimentally in a primate heart. Am Heart J 70:381, 1965

22. Watt TB Jr, Freud GE, Durrer D, Pruitt RD: Left anterior arborization block combined with right bundle branch block in canine and primate hearts. An electrocardiographic study. Circulation Res 22:57, 1968

11

Myocardial Infarction, Injury and Ischemia

The instantaneous vector of ventricular depolarization represents the sum and balance of the numerous forces generated from the various areas of the myocardium at a given moment. The reduction or loss of a portion of the component forces will, therefore, modify the characteristics of the resultant vector. In myocardial infarction the involved area becomes electrically inert and allows the opposing forces to become more prominent. Consequently, the postinfarction resultant vector tends to point away from the direction of the infarcted area. The extent of the alteration of the resultant vector depends on the size and relative importance of the infarcted area before the infarction. To illustrate, in Figure 11.1A the forces generated by the anterior wall of the myocardium during a certain period are represented by vector **I**, the remaining leftward forces are represented by vector **L**, and the rightward forces, vector **R**. The summation of all the forces gives a resultant vector which is directed to the left and anteriorly. After infarction of the anterior myocardium with the loss of potential represented by vector **I**, the balance of the remaining forces (vectors **L** and **R**) will now be directed to the left and posteriorly (Fig. 11.1B). Therefore, the net result of the anterior myocardial infarction is the posterior displacement of the resultant vector. Similarly, in the presence of an inferior wall myocardial infarction the mean instantaneous vector will be displaced in the superior direction.

As the various portions of the myocardium assume different degrees of importance during the various phases of the ventricular activation process, the location of the infarction also determines the time of appearance of the abnormal **QRS** vectors. For instance, the potential of the septal activation normally manifests itself in the initial phase of the ventricular depolarization; therefore, a septal infarction will alter the initial vectors. The posterobasal portion of the left ventricle is activated in the later phase of the ventricular depolarization, during which its potential becomes the dominant force. Infarction of this area will thus modify chiefly the late **QRS** vectors. By the same token, as the inner one-third to two-thirds of the free wall of the left ventricle probably contribute very little to the resultant vector, subendocardial infarction of this region may not result in any changes of the **QRS** vectors.

A. BEFORE INFARCTION

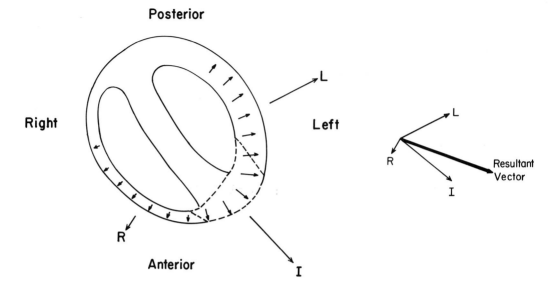

B. AFTER INFARCTION

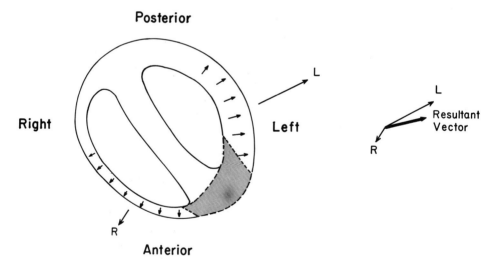

Fig. 11.1. Schematic diagrams illustrating the effect of an anterior myocardial infarction on the resultant **QRS** vector. (See text.)

The term *infarction vector* has been used to represent the force that is equal in magnitude but opposite in direction to that normally generated by the infarcted myocardium before the infarction occurs (Fig. 11.2). It is the hypothetical force which is responsible for the alteration of the normal resultant vector. By simple vectoral addition, the direction and magnitude of the postinfarction vector may be estimated when the preinfarction vector and the "infarction vector" are known. Similarly, the infarction vector may be derived by subtracting the preinfarction vector from the postinfarction vector.

In the following sections the characteristic findings of the QRSsÊ loop in the various types of myocardial infarction will be described. The changes in the **ST** vector and TsÊ loop during the acute, subacute and old phases of the infarction will be discussed in association with myocardial injury and ischemia. It should be emphasized that the classification of the site of infarction is rather arbitrary and is based on manifested electrical changes. The location of the infarct may not

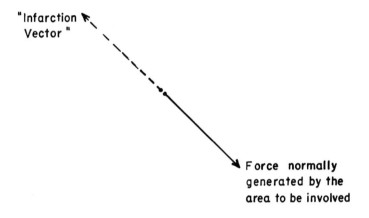

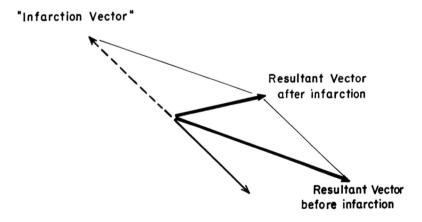

Fig. 11.2. "Infarction vector" and derivation of the postinfarction vector from the preinfarction and infarction vectors.

necessarily correlate closely with the anatomical finding. The alteration of the vectorcardiogram may be insufficient to indicate the presence of myocardial damage, especially when previous records are not available for comparison. Furthermore, the diagnostic accuracy of infarction may be impaired by the presence of complicating factors such as ventricular hypertrophy and conduction disturbances.

CLASSIFICATION OF MYOCARDIAL INFARCTION

Anteroseptal Myocardial Infarction (Figs. 11.3–11.5)

In anteroseptal myocardial infarction the area of involvement includes the anterior portion of the interventricular septum and the adjacent anterior wall of the left ventricle. As the ventricular activation begins at the interventricular septum and spreads to the adjacent anterior wall of the left ventricle shortly afterward, infarction of the anteroseptal region would therefore affect the initial **QRS** vectors. The normal septal forces are directed anteriorly, rightward and usually superiorly. Septal infarction results in either reduction or absence of these initial vectors. The loss of potential from the adjacent anterior wall of the left ventricle tends to reduce or abolish the succeeding normal anterior forces. Thus the total effect of anteroseptal infarction is to displace the early **QRS** vectors posteriorly and to the left. Since the changes are mostly in the anteroposterior and left-to-right directions, they can be seen best in the transverse plane, and to a lesser extent, in the other two projections.

Transverse plane QRS loop.   In the transverse plane there is an absence of the normal anterior and rightward initial deflection. The QRS loop begins its course in the left posterior direction. In certain instances, when the septal forces are reduced but not abolished, there is a small initial deflection inscribed to the right but posteriorly. In either event the early anterior convexity of the normal efferent limb is replaced by an anterior concavity with often clockwise inscription of this segment of the QRS loop. The afferent limb and the terminal deflection are usually not affected significantly. They are inscribed in the normal counterclockwise direction. The speed of inscription and the duration of the loop are normal unless the infarction is complicated by a conduction defect.

The orientation of the 0.02-sec instantaneous vector is consistently abnormal. In the normal person this vector may be directed either to the left or right but is always anterior. In the presence of anteroseptal myocardial infarction it is displaced posteriorly and to the left in the direction of a 0 to $-60°$ range. The magnitude of the vector may or may not be reduced. There is also a tendency for the 0.04-sec and maximum **QRS** vector to be displaced posteriorly. However, in most instances they are still within the normal range. There is no significant change of the 0.06-sec instantaneous vector.

The absence of the normal initial deflection to the right and anteriorly explains the loss of the R wave over the right precordial leads (V_1 and V_2) of the conventional electrocardiogram, and a QS complex instead is recorded. For the same reason the normal "septal" Q wave is no longer seen in the left precordial leads (V_5 and V_6).

A QS or QR pattern may be recorded in leads V_3 and V_4, depending on the degree of the posterior displacement of the efferent limb.

Right sagittal plane QRS loop. In the right sagittal plane there is a similar loss of the normal early convexity of the loop. The QRS loop begins its course in the inferior and posterior direction and most of the efferent limb is often inscribed counterclockwise. The remaining part of the loop is not significantly altered and is inscribed in the normal clockwise direction.

The 0.02-sec instantaneous **QRS** vector is consistently displaced posteriorly. Although the directions of the 0.04-sec and maximum **QRS** vectors tend to be more

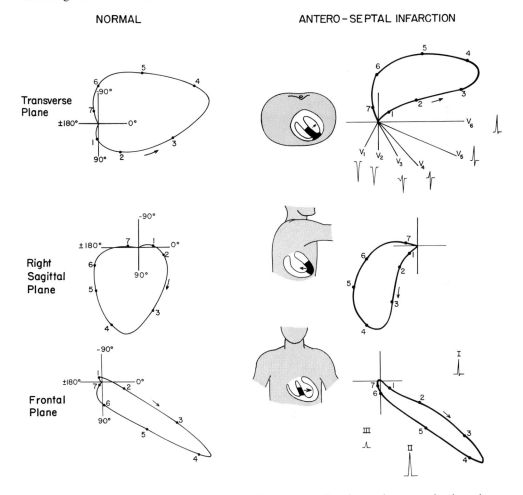

Fig. 11.3. Schematic diagrams of the QRS loop in the three planar projections in anteroseptal myocardial infarction as compared with those of the normal. In this and other similar diagrams in this chapter the time intervals of the QRS loop are indicated by the numerals which represent the time in hundredths of a second after the beginning of the QRS loop. The representative scalar lead QRS complexes are given. In the diagrams depicting the anatomical location of the infarction in the three planar views the arrow indicates the direction of the "infarction vector."

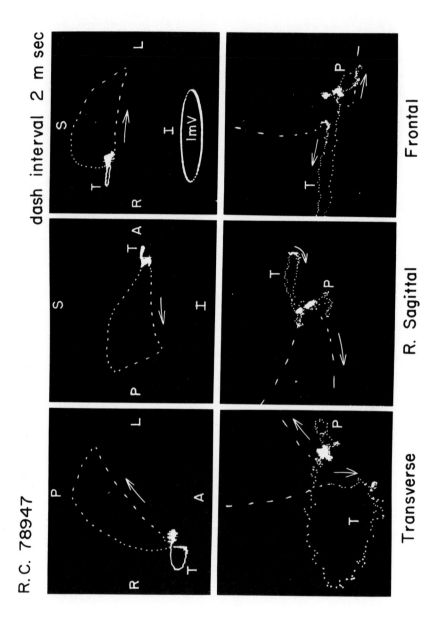

dash interval 2 m sec

R.C. 78947

Frontal

R. Sagittal

Transverse

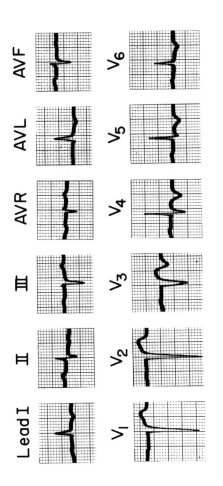

Fig. 11.4. Anteroseptal myocardial infarction. In the transverse plane there is a loss of the initial anterior QRS forces and the QRS loop begins its inscription in the left posterior direction. The loss of forces can also be seen in the right sagittal plane. The QRS loop is also displaced superiorly and is inscribed counterclockwise in the frontal plane to suggest left anterior hemiblock. The TsÉ loop is displaced to the right and slightly superiorly, suggesting myocardial ischemia. In the electrocardiogram a QS deflection is recorded in leads V_1, V_2, and V_3 with symmetrical T-wave inversion in the mid and left precordial leads as well as leads I and aVL.

R.F. 199301

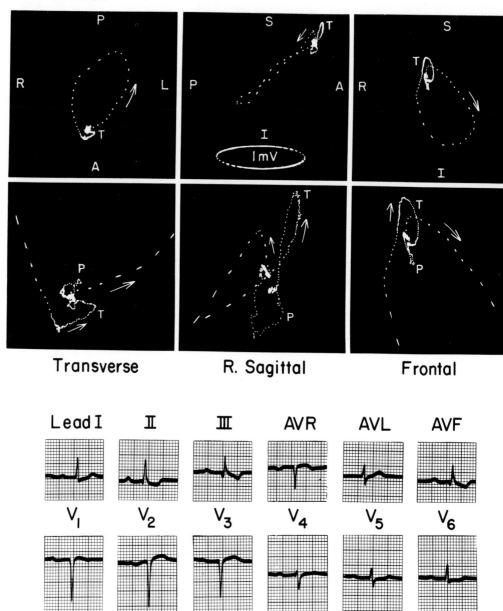

Fig. 11.5. Anteroseptal myocardial infarction. In the vectorcardiogram the loss of the initial anterior QRS forces is seen in the transverse and sagittal planes. In the right sagittal plane the early part of the QRS loop is superior and is inscribed counterclockwise, which may represent some coexisting involvement of the inferior wall. This is further supported by the superior displacement of the T loop which is evident in the sagittal and frontal planes. In the electrocardiogram a QS deflection is present in leads V_1 through V_3. A Q wave is recorded in the inferior leads but is neither abnormally wide nor deep. The T-wave inversion in these leads correlates with the superior displacement of the T loop in the vectorcardiogram.

posterior than those of the normal persons, they usually remain within the normal range. The 0.06-sec vector is unchanged.

Frontal plane QRS loop.   In this projection the initial part of the QRS loop is written to the left, either inferiorly or superiorly. As a significant number of the normal individuals exhibit a similar finding, the absence of the initial rightward forces alone cannot be considered as a diagnostic sign. The more characteristic posterior displacement of the initial vectors in anteroseptal myocardial infarction is not apparent in the frontal plane projection, which does not include the anteroposterior lead. Consequently, the standard and unipolar limb leads of the conventional electrocardiogram also fail to display any diagnostic abnormalities.

Localized Anterior Myocardial Infarction (Figs. 11.6 and 11.7)

When the infarction is limited to the anterior aspect of the left ventricle, the normal initial right anterior septal forces are preserved. As the depolarization of the anterior wall of the left ventricle follows closely that of the interventricular septum, the effect of the infarction is seen mostly during the early part of the QRSsÊ loop. The loss of the normal anterior forces during that period allows the opposing forces to dominate and displace the vectors posteriorly. Since the changes occur in the anteroposterior direction, the abnormalities associated with a localized anterior myocardial infarction can only be detected in the transverse and right sagittal planes in which the anteroposterior component of the spatial vectors is displayed.

Transverse plane QRS loop.   In the transverse plane the initial deflection of the QRS loop remains essentially normal and is inscribed anteriorly and to the right. However, the efferent limb is displaced posteriorly. Depending on the size of the infarction and thus the degree of the displacement, the first portion of the efferent limb may be either anterior or posterior to the initial deflection as it proceeds posteriorly and leftward. In the latter instance a clockwise inscription of the early part of the QRS loop will be seen, which is distinctly abnormal. The afferent limb and terminal deflection usually do not show significant changes.

The 0.02-sec instantaneous **QRS** vector is oriented posteriorly and to the left and serves as a useful diagnostic sign.* The maximum and 0.04-sec vectors are often displaced more posteriorly, but usually still remain in the normal range. The 0.06-sec vector is essentially unchanged. The duration of the QRS loop and the speed of inscription of the QRS loop are normal in the absence of complicating conduction disturbance.

In the conventional electrocardiogram an abnormal Q wave is seen in one or more of the mid precordial leads (V_3 and V_4). This is related to the posterior displacement of the efferent limb so that the corresponding vectors are now directed toward the negative side of the lead axes of these leads. A normal r wave is recorded in leads V_1 and V_2 because the septal forces are preserved. For the same reason a small q wave is present in lead V_6.

---

* It should be mentioned that when left ventricular hypertrophy or pulmonary emphysema is present the 0.02-sec vector may occasionally be directed posteriorly in the absence of anterior myocardial infarction.

LOCALIZED ANTERIOR MYOCARDIAL INFARCTION

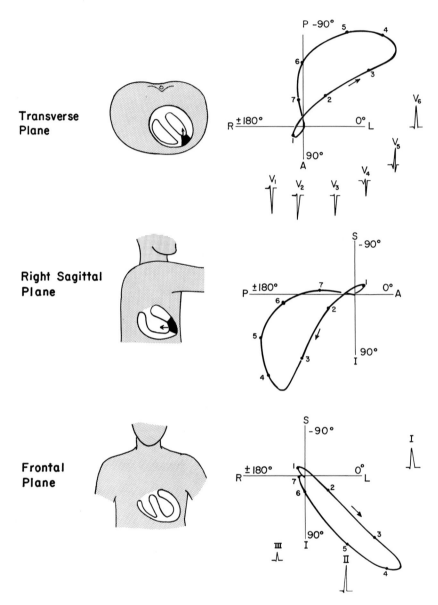

Fig. 11.6. Localized anterior myocardial infarction. The diagrams depict the anatomic location, the direction of the "infarction vector," and the QRS loop in the three planar views. Representative scalar leads are also shown. (See text.)

Right sagittal plane QRS loop.   In the right sagittal plane the initial deflection is directed anteriorly and superiorly, and is similar to that of the normal individual. However, the efferent limb is displaced posteriorly so that its normal anterior convexity is lost. If the posterior displacement is marked, the early part of the QRS loop may be inscribed counterclockwise.* The afferent limb may or may not be more

---

* According to some investigators, counterclockwise inscription of the right sagittal plane QRS loop in the presence of other signs of anterior infarction strongly suggests coexisting inferior wall infarction.

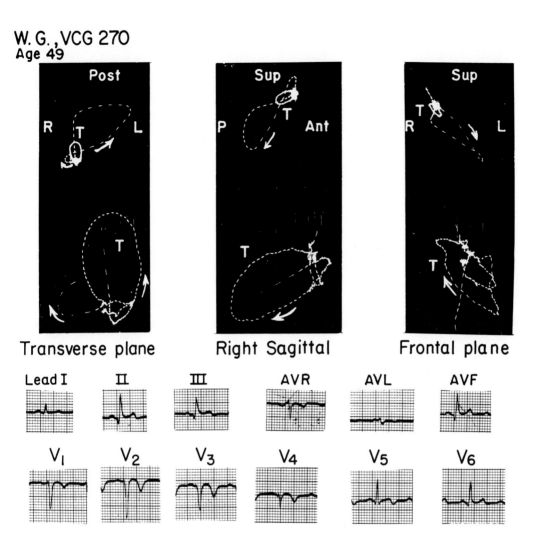

W. G., VCG 270
Age 49

Post — Transverse plane

Sup / P / Ant — Right Sagittal

Sup / R / L — Frontal plane

Lead I II III AVR AVL AVF

V_1 V_2 V_3 V_4 V_5 V_6

Fig. 11.7. Localized anterior myocardial infarction. In the vectorcardiogram the initial deflection of the QRS loop in the transverse plane is directed to the right and slightly anteriorly. The loop is at first inscribed briefly clockwise and then counterclockwise throughout the remaining portion. The posterior displacement of the efferent limb is indicative of an anterior wall myocardial infarction. The presence of the right anterior initial deflection suggests that the septal forces are preserved. In the right sagittal plane there is an initial counterclockwise inscription of the QRS loop which may indicate some involvment of the inferior wall. The TsÊ loop is displaced posteriorly as revealed in the transverse and right sagittal planes and is consistent with ischemia of the anterior wall. Note that the TsÊ loop is inscribed at a uniform speed and is abnormally wide. In the electrocardiogram a small R wave is present in leads V_1 and V_2. A QS deflection is recorded in leads V_3 and V_4. The T-wave inversion in most of the precordial leads correlates with the posterior orientation of the TsÊ loop. (From Chou TC, et al: The significance of a wide TsÊ loop, Circulation 30:400, 1964, with permission of the American Heart Association. In the vectorcardiogram the loops are interrupted every 2.5 instead of 2.0 msec as is usually the case.)

posteriorly located. The terminal deflection usually remains unchanged. The 0.02-sec instantaneous **QRS** vector is directed posteriorly and inferiorly. As in the transverse plane its posterior orientation represents one of the most useful signs for the diagnosis of anterior infarction.

Frontal plane QRS loop. Since anterior wall myocardial infarction only alters the spatial **QRS** vectors in the anteroposterior direction, no abnormality is demonstrated in the frontal plane projection. For the same reason the standard and unipolar limb leads remain normal.

Anterolateral Myocardial Infarction (Figs. 11.8-11.11)

The anterolateral portion of the free wall of the left ventricle begins to depolarize later than the interventricular septum. Infarction of this area does not alter the initial forces but affects the succeeding instantaneous vectors which inscribe the efferent limb and perhaps also part of the afferent limb of the QRSsÊ loop. Since the anterolateral wall normally generates forces that are directed anteriorly and to the left, an infarction of the area allows the opposing forces to dominate and displace the **QRS** vectors rightward and posteriorly. As the changes are in the anteroposterior and left-to-right directions, the abnormalities can therefore be best observed in the transverse plane projection even though some signs of the infarction can also be seen in the sagittal and frontal planes.

Transverse plane QRS loop. In the transverse plane the initial deflection of the QRS loop is inscribed normally, that is, anteriorly and to the right. The efferent limb is, however, displaced posteriorly and to the right. In the typical case the efferent limb becomes more posterior and rightward than the afferent limb so that the QRS loop is inscribed clockwise. In other instances when the displacement is less, the efferent limb may be inscribed clockwise but the rest of the QRS loop, counterclockwise, or the entire loop retains its counterclockwise rotation. The duration of the initial rightward forces is often abnormally prolonged and exceeds the normal upper limit of 0.022 sec. (The duration is measured from the beginning of the QRS loop to the point where the loop crosses the anteroposterior axis to the left side, see Fig. 11.9.) The changes in the afferent limb and terminal deflection are usually not diagnostically significant.

The 0.02-sec vector is directed to the right, either anteriorly or posteriorly. The maximum **QRS** vector tends to be more posteriorly oriented than that of the normal subject.

In the conventional electrocardiogram the right precordial leads (leads V_1 and V_2) record a normal rS complex because the initial right anterior septal forces are intact and the rest of the loop projects on the negative side of their lead axes. The rightward and posterior displacement of the efferent limb results in a deep and wide Q wave in the left precordial leads as both the initial deflection and part of the efferent limb are now on the negative side of the axes of derivation of leads V_5 and V_6. The R wave in these leads becomes smaller as the maximum **QRS** vector is now oriented more posteriorly and less leftward. For the same reason the displacement of the efferent limb may result in an rS, QS, or QR complex in leads V_3 and V_4, depending more or less on the size of the infarction and the extent of the

ANTERO-LATERAL MYOCARDIAL INFARCTION

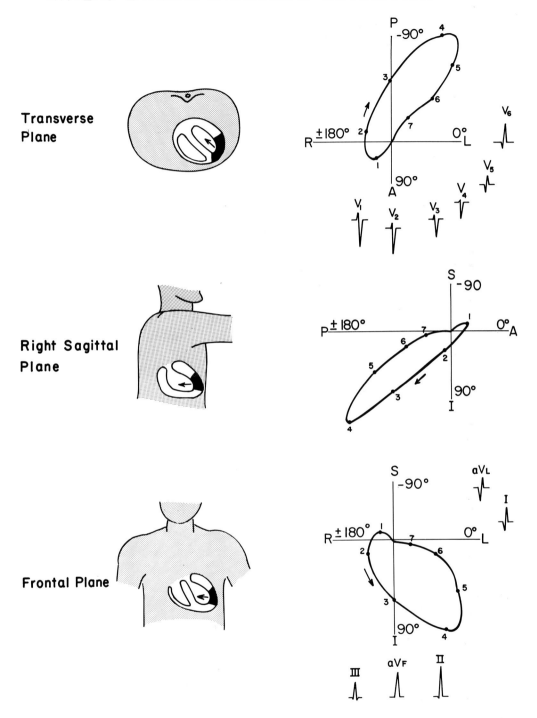

Fig. 11.8. Anterolateral myocardial infarction. The diagrams depict the anatomical location, the direction of the "infarction vector" and the QRS loop in the three planar views. Representative scalar leads are also shown. (See text.)

A. Initial rightward forces

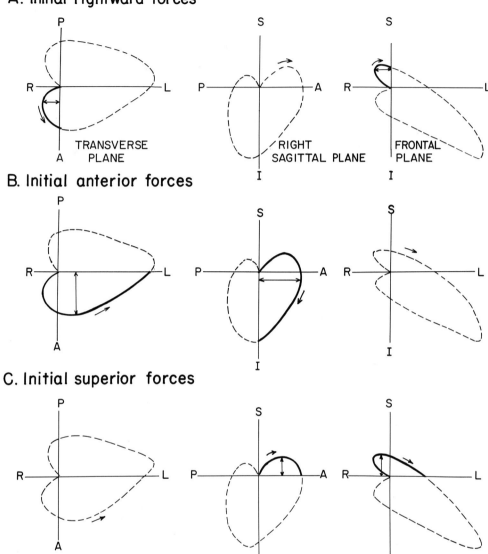

B. Initial anterior forces

C. Initial superior forces

Fig. 11.9. Some of the measurements of the QRS loop which are useful for the recognition of myocardial infarction. The solid line in the diagram represents the forces in question. The time interval from the beginning to the end of the solid line gives the duration of the forces. The distance between the most outward point of the segment and the coordinate axis it embraces represents the maximum magnitude of the forces.

displacement. Frequently, a rather typical vectorcardiographic pattern of anterolateral infarction is accompanied by a QS or QR complex in leads V_3 and V_4, but an abnormal Q wave is not observed in leads V_5 and V_6. A probable explanation is that the conventional unipolar leads V_5 and V_6 have lead axes which are directed somewhat inferiorly and therefore record some of the inferior components of the spatial **QRS** vectors, and the initial negative potential may not be realized.

Right sagittal plane QRS loop. In this projection only the anteroposterior component of the abnormalities is observed. The initial deflection is inscribed normally, that is, anteriorly and usually superiorly. The efferent limb is displaced posteriorly, and depending on the degree of displacement, it may be anterior or posterior to the afferent limb. The direction of inscription of the QRS loop may thus remain clockwise or become counterclockwise. A figure-of-eight pattern may also be seen. The 0.02-sec instantaneous vector is directed either anteriorly or posteriorly. The maximum **QRS** vector is often more posterior than the average normal direction, but the change is usually not diagnostically helpful.

Frontal plane QRS loop. In the frontal plane projection the left-to-right component of the changes is displayed. The inscription of the initial deflection is normal. The efferent limb is displaced rightward and the duration of the initial rightward forces often exceeds the normal limit of 0.022 sec. As the efferent limb is now to the right of the afferent limb, the loop is inscribed counterclockwise. The 0.02-sec instantaneous vector is directed to the right and inferiorly. The maximum **QRS** vector is oriented more inferiorly and less leftward. The counterclockwise inscription of a more or less vertical QRS loop represents a rather characteristic finding of infarction involving the lateral wall of the left ventricle. (As discussed in Chapter 5, in the normal person when the frontal plane maximum **QRS** vector is more vertical than 40°, the direction of inscription of the QRS loop is practically always clockwise.)

In the conventional electrocardiogram the rightward initial deflection and early part of the efferent limb have their counterpart in the abnormally wide and deep Q wave in leads I and aVL. These segments of the loop are now projecting on the negative side of the lead axes of these leads. The R wave in these same leads is often reduced in amplitude. This is related to the medial displacement of the maximum **QRS** vector toward the vertical axis, and consequently the magnitude of its projection on leads I and aVL will be smaller.

Extensive Anterior Myocardial Infarction (Fig. 11.12)

When the infarction is massive and involves the entire aspect of the anterior wall of the left ventricle including the anterior part of the interventricular septum, the vectorcardiographic changes resemble the sum of the effect of anteroseptal and anterolateral infarctions. There is a total loss of the anteriorly oriented forces. In the transverse plane projection the QRS loop begins its course in the posterior and rightward direction, and it is usually inscribed clockwise. In the right sagittal plane the entire QRS loop is also located posteriorly. It may be inscribed clockwise or counterclockwise. In the frontal plane there is usually a counterclockwise loop with an abnormally prolonged initial rightward portion.

Inferior Myocardial Infarction (Figs. 11.13–11.18)

In this text, as well as in most of the recent publications, inferior myocardial infarction means infarction of the diaphragmatic aspect of the left ventricle. The term *posterior infarction* is reserved for involvement of the posterobasal region. When the inferior wall of the left ventricle becomes electrically inert, its effect is

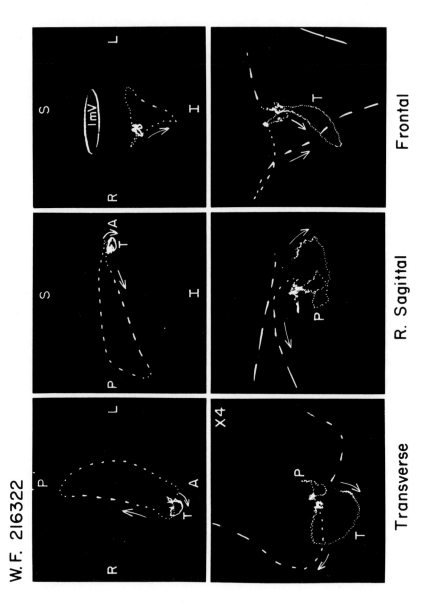

W.F. 2I6322

Frontal

R. Sagittal

Transverse

202

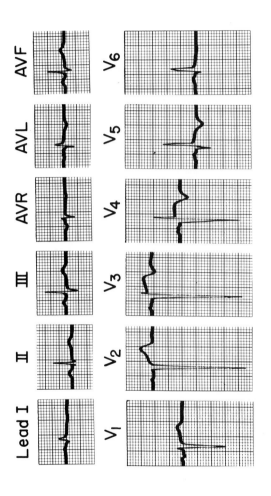

Fig. 11.10. Old anterolateral myocardial infarction. The record was obtained 10 months after the occurrence of the acute episode. Note the QRS loop is inscribed clockwise in the transverse plane and counterclockwise in the frontal plane. The frontal plane maximum **QRS** vector is directed at 80°. The TsÊ loop is displaced rightward and posteriorly with a rather uniform speed of inscription. The transverse plane T loop is inscribed clockwise.

203

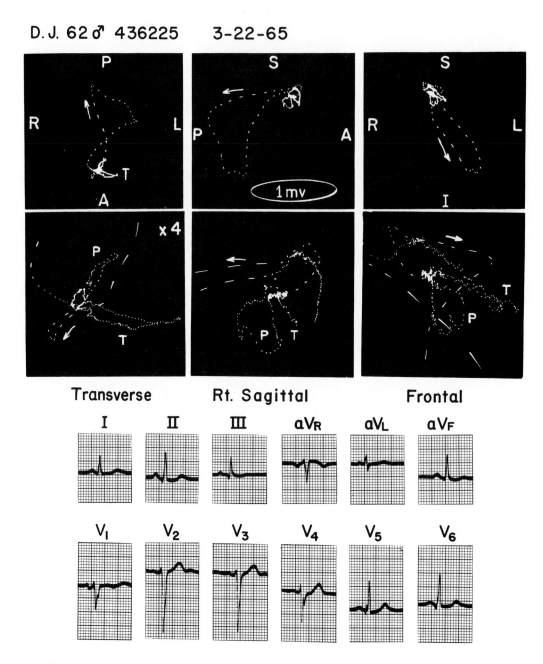

D.J. 62 ♂ 436225   3-22-65

Transverse   Rt. Sagittal   Frontal

I   II   III   aV$_R$ aV$_L$ aV$_F$

V$_1$ V$_2$ V$_3$ V$_4$ V$_5$ V$_6$

Fig. 11.11. Old anterolateral and inferior myocardial infarction. The patient is a 62-year-old man who had a well-documented acute anterior myocardial infarction 3 years prior to the recording of the vectorcardiogram and electrocardiogram illustrated above. In the vectorcardiogram the essential findings diagnostic of anterolateral myocardial infarction are the rightward displacement of the efferent limb of the QRS loop in the transverse and frontal planes. There is also an increase in the duration of the initial superior forces (0.034 sec) as indicated in the right sagittal and frontal planes to suggest an inferior infarction. The QRS loop presents a figure-of-eight pattern in the transverse and frontal planes and is inscribed counterclockwise in the sagittal plane. In the electrocardiogram the changes are minimal and rather nonspecific. The notching of the QRS complex in leads V$_1$, V$_4$, and V$_5$ may suggest some myocardial damage.

manifested mostly during the early part of the ventricular depolarization process. The initial septal forces, however, are usually not changed as most of the septum is spared, even though occasionally exceptions do occur. As the vectors representing the potential generated by the inferior wall are directed inferiorly, the loss of these forces allows the opposing forces to dominate and displace the resultant vector in the superior direction.

Since the alteration is in the superior-inferior direction, the vectorcardiographic abnormalities are demonstrated in the sagittal and frontal plane projections. No significant change can be seen in the transverse plane if the infarction is limited to the inferior wall.

Transverse plane QRS loop. The transverse plane QRS loop is normal when the infarction is restricted to the inferior wall. Similarly, the precordial lead electro-cardiogram also remains unchanged.

Right sagittal plane QRS loop. The characteristic feature of inferior myo-cardial infarction in the right sagittal plane is the superior displacement of the initial **QRS** vectors. In the typical case the duration of the initial superior forces exceeds 0.025 sec, that is, the 0.025-sec vector lies above the 0° to 180° axis. In contrast, such a finding occurs in less than 5 percent of the normal persons. The magnitude of the initial superior forces may also increase and exceed the normal limit of 0.2 mV. However, it is not unusual to find either the duration or the magnitude to be within normal range in a proved case of myocardial infarction.

The initial deflection is directed anteriorly and superiorly. The efferent limb may be inscribed clockwise so that the QRS loop in the sagittal plane retains its normal sense of rotation. However, frequently it is inscribed counterclockwise, and depending on the extent of its superior displacement in relation to the afferent limb, the entire QRS loop may be counterclockwise or present a figure-of-eight pattern. Hugenholz et al, maintain that a reversal of the direction of inscription of the QRS loop in the sagittal plane is practically always associated with an infarction of the adjacent anterior wall.

The projection of the maximum spatial **QRS** vector tends to be directed more posteriorly and less inferiorly. The duration and the speed of the inscription of the QRS loop remain normal in the absence of a conduction defect.

Frontal plane QRS loop. In the frontal plane projection the abnormal su-perior displacement of the early portion of the QRS loop is well displayed. The duration of the initial superiorly oriented forces is greater than 0.025 sec (Fig. 11.17A). The magnitude of the superior forces often exceeds that of the normal individuals (0.2 mV).

The initial deflection is directed superiorly, either to the left or right. Both the initial deflection and the efferent limb are characteristically inscribed in a clockwise direction. In fact, if the maximum **QRS** vector in the frontal plane lies above 10°, the clockwise inscription of these portions of the QRS loop in this plane is highly sug-gestive of inferior myocardial infarction even in the absence of abnormal duration and magnitude of the initial superior forces (Fig. 11.17B).

The afferent limb and terminal deflection of the QRS loop are usually inferior to the efferent limb. The direction of the maximum **QRS** vector tends to be less inferior than that of the average normal subject.

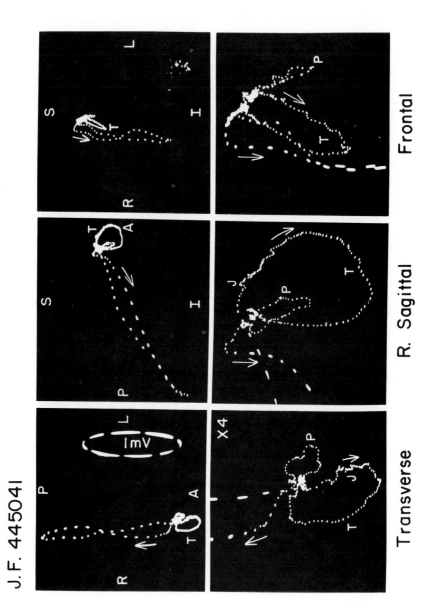

J.F. 445041

Frontal

R. Sagittal

Transverse

206

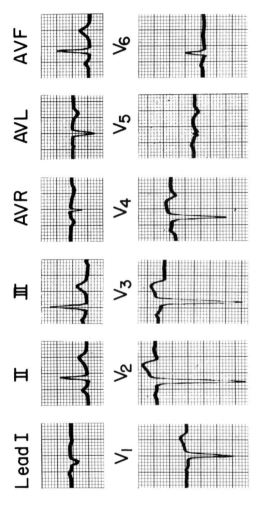

Fig. 11.12. Extensive anterior myocardial infarction. The vectorcardiogram and electrocardiogram were recorded from a 40-year-old man 10 days after the onset of an acute myocardial infarction. The loss of the anterior, leftward, as well as the initial septal forces are well displayed in the transverse plane. The entire QRS loop is displaced posteriorly and slightly to the right. The loss of the anterior forces can also be seen in the sagittal plane and the rightward displacement of the loop in the frontal plane. There is a small **ST** vector directed anteriorly and slightly to the left. The TsE loop is displaced toward the right and is inscribed clockwise in the transverse plane. There is some loss of the normal initial slow inscription of the TsE loop and the spatial loop is abnormally wide. The electrocardiogram reveals QS deflection in leads I, aVL, and V_1 through V_5. The T wave is inverted in leads I, V_4 and V_5.

207

INFERIOR MYOCARDIAL INFARCTION

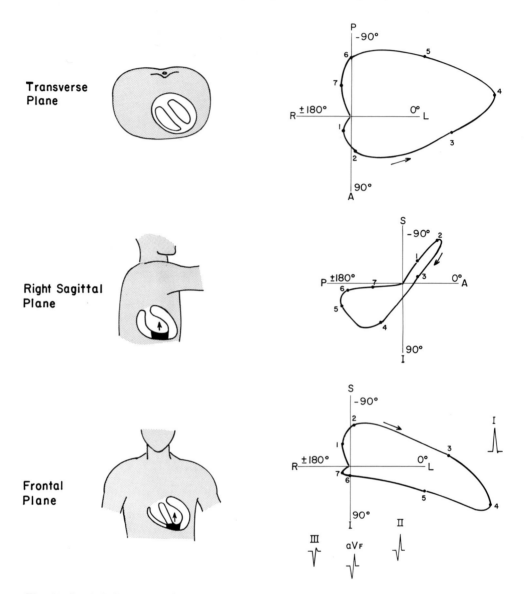

Fig. 11.13. Inferior myocardial infarction. The diagrams depict the anatomic location, the direction of the "infarction vector," and the QRS loop in the three planar projections. The representative scalar leads are also illustrated.

Young and Williams have described other less typical changes. They have suggested the following additional criteria for the diagnosis of inferior myocardial infarction (Fig. 11.17):
1. The duration of the initial superior forces is 0.025 sec or longer, but this portion of the loop is not completely clockwise (Fig. 11.17C).
2. The duration of the initial superior forces is 0.02 sec or longer and is accom-

panied by an increase of the maximum left superior force to more than 0.25 mV. This portion of the loop is inscribed completely clockwise (Fig. 11.17D).

3. The initial QRS forces are directed inferiorly, but the subsequent efferent limb of the loop is located superiorly and is inscribed clockwise. The duration of these early superior forces is 0.025 sec or longer with the magnitude of the maximum left superior force greater than 0.25 mV (Figs. 11.17E and 11.17F).

4. The initial forces are directed inferiorly but the subsequent efferent limb is inscribed clockwise and the maximum **QRS** vector lies above 10° (Figs. 11.17G and 11.17H).

Young and associates also call attention to the mid-to-late QRS abnormalities seen in the frontal plane of patients with inferior myocardial infarction. These include a localized sharp reversal of the direction of inscription of the afferent limb of the QRS loop (the equivalent of a "bite") (Fig. 11.17I). Three other deformities are described but their definitions are rather complicated. In the author's experience they are relatively uncommon. Young and associates give a detailed description in their original article.

In the conventional electrocardiogram the superior displacement of the initial forces results in an abnormal Q wave in the inferior leads (leads II, III, and aVF). The prolongation of the duration of the superior forces corresponds to the increase of the width, and the larger magnitude to the depth, of the abnormal Q wave in these leads. The scalar equivalents of the less typical vectorcardiographic changes are often difficult to detect. Figure 11.18 gives an example of proved inferior myocardial infarction. Although the vectorcardiogram is suggestive of the infarct, the electrocardiogram is unrevealing.

Inferolateral Myocardial Infarction (Figs. 11.19-11.21)

When the myocardial damage includes not only the inferior but also the adjacent lateral wall of the left ventricle, there is a loss of both the inferior and leftward forces. Consequently the QRSsÊ loop, particularly its early segments, will be displaced toward the opposite direction, that is, superiorly and rightward. Although changes may be seen in all the planar projections, the frontal plane reveals the abnormalities most clearly as it contains both the superior-inferior and right-left components.

Transverse plane QRS loop. There is an increase of the loop area to the right, and a decrease to the left of the −90° to 90° axis. The duration of the initial rightward forces is often prolonged (normal upper limit—0.022 sec). The magnitude of the maximum initial rightward force becomes greater (normal upper limit—0.16 mV).

The direction of inscription of the QRS loop remains counterclockwise. The initial deflection is written to the right and anteriorly. Although its direction is normal, its magnitude is increased. The efferent limb proceeds leftward but to a lesser degree than the normal. The afferent limb and terminal deflection are the least affected or may not be affected at all.

Examination of the instantaneous **QRS** vectors reveals that the 0.02-sec vector is usually directed anteriorly and to the right. The leftward component of the 0.04-sec and maximum vectors is reduced in amplitude. The 0.06-sec vector is essentially unchanged.

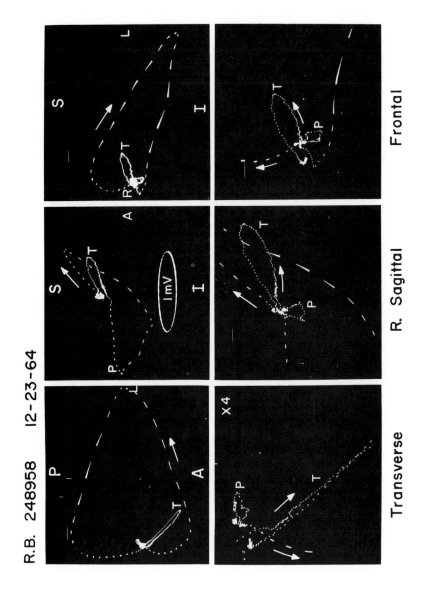

R.B. 248958 12-23-64

S L

T

R

A

S A

T

P I

ImV

P L

T

A

T

Frontal

T

P I

T

P I

X4

P

T

R. Sagittal

Transverse

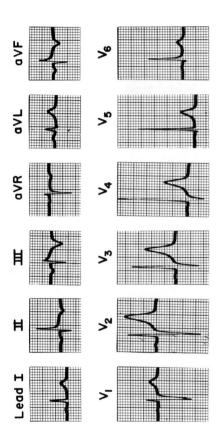

Fig. 11.14. Recent inferior myocardial infarction. The vectorcardiogram and electrocardiogram were recorded from a 54-year-old male hospital attendant. The transverse plane vectorcardiogram is normal. Both the right sagittal and frontal planes show the abnormal increase in the duration of the initial superior forces (0.03 sec). The magnitude of the maximum superior force measures 0.5 mV. The T loop is displaced superiorly and is inscribed counterclockwise in both the right sagittal and frontal projections. The electrocardiogram reveals abnormal Q wave with T-wave inversion in leads II, III, and aVF. The inverted P wave in these leads indicates an ectopic atrial pacemaker which was not present during the recording of the vectorcardiogram.

211

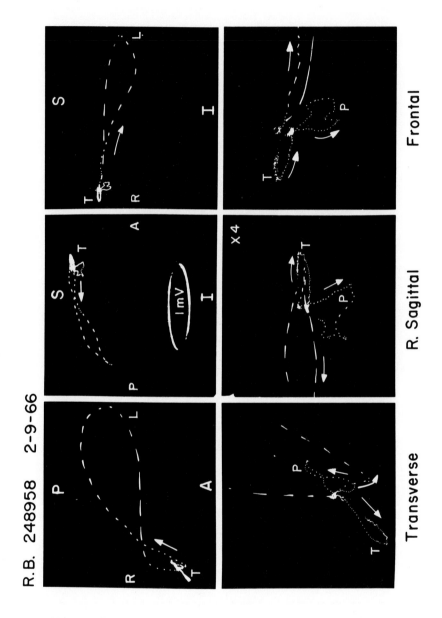

R.B. 248958 2-9-66

Frontal

R. Sagittal

Transverse

212

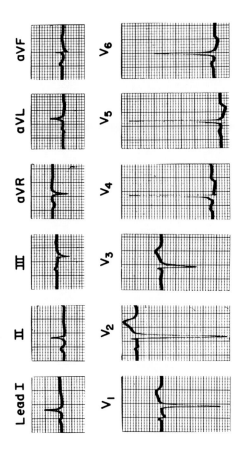

Fig. 11.15. Fourteen months later, the vectorcardiogram and electrocardiogram of the same patient as illustrated in Fig. 11.14. During the interval he developed cardiomegaly. Both the vectorcardiogram and electrocardiogram are now consistent with left ventricular hypertrophy and incomplete left bundle branch block. Note that the findings diagnostic of inferior myocardial infarction are no longer present.

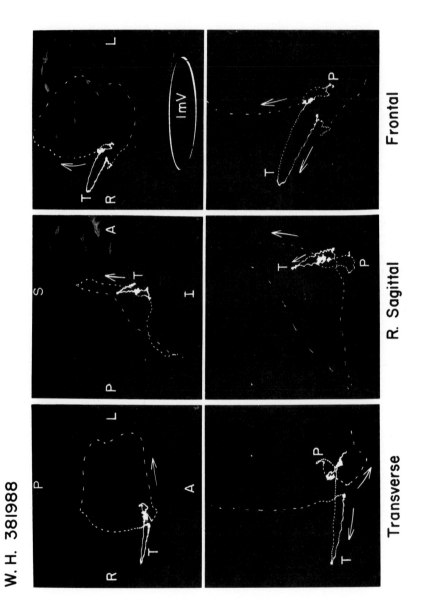

W. H. 381988

214

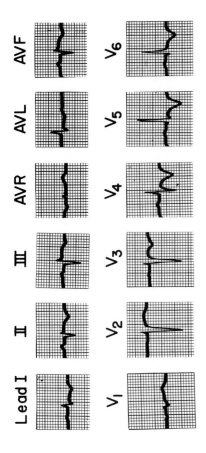

Fig. 11.16. Recent inferior wall myocardial infarction. In the vectorcardiogram there is a marked superior displacement of the efferent limb of the QRS loop as seen in the sagittal and frontal planes. The duration of the initial superior forces increases to 0.044 sec. The magnitude of the maximum superior force is increased to 0.6 mV. The efferent limb is inscribed counterclockwise in the sagittal plane and clockwise in the frontal plane. The TsÊ loop is displaced to the right and superiorly, suggesting that the ischemic process involves also the lateral wall of the left ventricle.

INFERIOR MYOCARDIAL INFARCTION

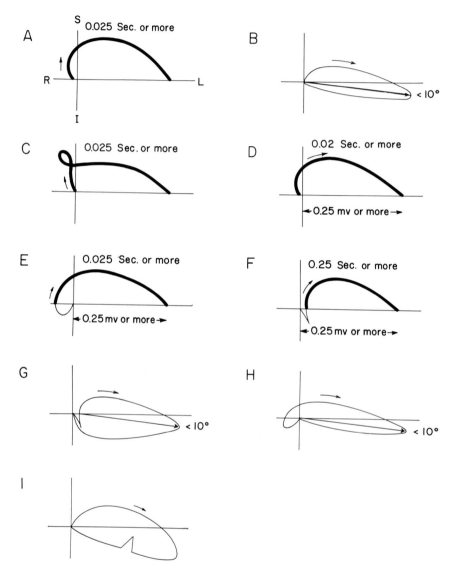

Fig. 11.17. Schematic diagrams of the frontal plane QRS loop in inferior myocardial infarction. In A, C, D, E, and F only the early part of the QRS loop is depicted. The portion of the QRS loop for which the duration is labeled is drawn in heavy line. See text.

In the conventional electrocardiogram the Q wave in leads V_5 and V_6 is abnormally wide and deep and is related to the increase in the duration and magnitude of the initial rightward forces which project on the negative side of the lead axes. The reduction of the amplitude of the R wave in these leads has its counterpart in the decrease of the leftward forces.

Right sagittal plane QRS loop. The alterations of the QRS loop in this projection are similar to those of inferior myocardial infarction described previously. There is an increase of the duration and amplitude of the initial superior forces. The loop may be inscribed clockwise, counterclockwise, or present a figure-of-eight pattern.

Frontal plane QRS loop. In the frontal plane projection both the superior and rightward displacement of the loop are displayed. The duration and magnitude of the initial rightward forces are increased; so are those of the initial superior forces.

The initial deflection is directed superiorly and rightward. The efferent limb proceeds leftward and the loop characteristically is inscribed clockwise.

The 0.02-sec **QRS** vector is directed superiorly and usually rightward. The 0.04-sec and maximum vectors are oriented leftward and reduced in magnitude. The late **QRS** vectors usually show very little change.

In the limb leads of the electrocardiogram a wide and deep Q wave is present in leads I, II, III, and aVF and is related to the abnormal initial superior and rightward vectors which are oriented toward the negative side of the lead axes of derivation. The same vectors project on the positive side of lead aVR and an initial R wave is recorded (i.e., lead aVR displays an RS instead of QS complex). The R wave in lead I is smaller and is caused by the reduction of the maximum leftward forces.

True Posterior Myocardial Infarction (Figs. 11.22-11.24)

By true posterior myocardial infarction we mean that the area of myocardium involved is the posterobasal or dorsal aspect of the left ventricle. It is called "true posterior" infarction to avoid confusion with "posterior" infarction which has often been used in the past to indicate the involvement of the diaphragmatic or inferior wall. The term *strictly posterior myocardial infarction* has also been used.

Normally the posterobasal region of the left ventricle is the last portion of the ventricle to be activated. When it becomes electrically inert, the effect manifests itself mostly in the alteration of the late **QRS** vectors. As the vectors representing the electrical potential generated from this area are normally directed posteriorly, the result of the infarction is to allow the opposing forces to become dominant and displace the vectors in the anterior direction. Consequently, the changes in the vectorcardiogram are best seen in the transverse and sagittal planes, in which the anterior and posterior components of the spatial vectors are displayed. Frequently, there is also involvement of the adjacent inferior or lateral wall of the left ventricle and additional abnormalities will be observed.

Transverse plane QRS loop. In the transverse plane projection there is anterior displacement of the QRS loop. The portion of the loop located anterior to the 0° to 180° axis may exceed 70 percent of the total loop area. Hoffman and associates found that in the great majority of true posterior infarction the half area **QRS** vector (i.e., the vector which divides the QRS loop into two equal areas) is anterior to 10°.

The initial deflection is inscribed normally to the right and anteriorly. The efferent limb proceeds leftward and usually remains anterior throughout its course. The anterior displacement of the afferent limb and the terminal deflection is, however, the most consistent finding. The extent of the displacement varies.

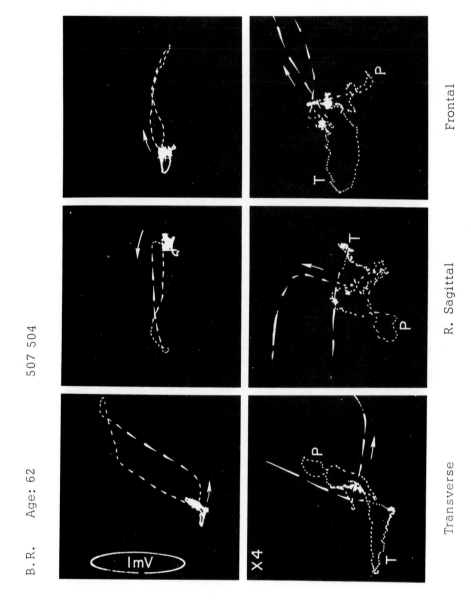

B.R.　　Age: 62

507 504

1mV

X4

Frontal

R. Sagittal

Transverse

218

B.R.   Age: 62   507 504

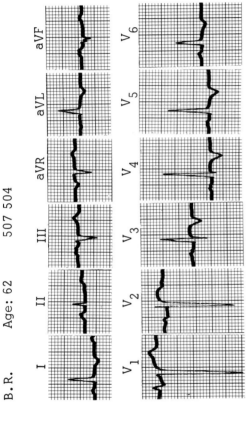

I   II   III   aVR   aVL   aVF

V₁   V₂   V₃   V₄   V₅   V₆

Fig. 11.18. Inferior wall myocardial infarction. The tracings were obtained from a 62-year-old man with autopsy-proved inferior myocardial infarction. Left ventricular hypertrophy was also demonstrated. In the vectorcardiogram the frontal plane maximum **QRS** vector is directed at 5°. The very early part of the QRS loop is directed inferiorly. But the efferent limb is mostly superior and is inscribed clockwise. In the right sagittal plane the efferent limb of the QRS loop is inscribed counterclockwise which also supports the diagnosis of inferior myocardial infarction. In the transverse plane the QRS loop is inscribed in a figure-of-eight pattern and is directed rather posteriorly. Although the configuration of the loop is abnormal, no specific diagnosis can be made. The voltage criteria for the diagnosis of left ventricular hypertrophy are not met. The T loop is displaced rightward and is inscribed clockwise in the transverse plane. This is probably caused by the combined effect of left ventricular hypertrophy and lateral wall myocardial ischemia. Note that in the electrocardiogram the diagnosis of inferior myocardial infarction cannot be made. However, the voltage criteria for left ventricular hypertrophy are present.

219

INFERO-LATERAL INFARCTION

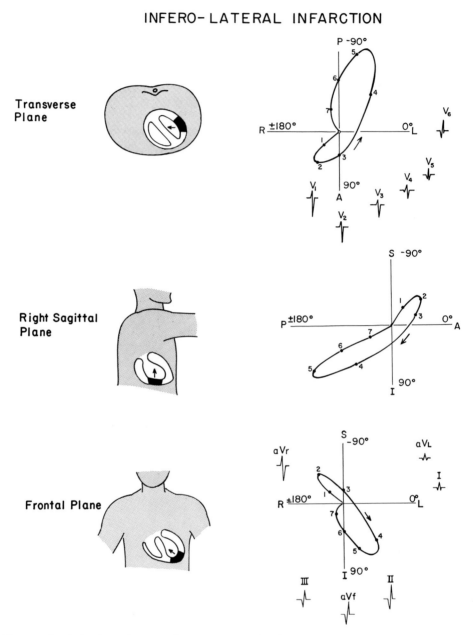

Fig. 11.19. Inferolateral myocardial infarction. The diagrams depict the anatomical location, the direction of the "infarction vector," and the QRS loop in the three planar projections. The representative scalar leads are also illustrated.

Depending on its relationship with the efferent limb, the QRS loop may be inscribed counterclockwise or clockwise or present a figure-of-eight pattern. The counterclockwise rotation is most commonly observed.

The magnitude and direction of the early **QRS** vectors (e.g., 0.02-sec vector) are little affected. The maximum and 0.04-sec vectors are oriented more anteriorly. The former may exceed the normal limit of 20°. The predominant changes occur in the late **QRS** vectors. The 0.06-sec vector may lie anterior to the 0° to 180° axis, a finding not observed in the normal persons.

The anterior displacement of the loop also results in an increase of the duration of the anterior forces which often exceeds the normal upper limits of 0.05 sec. The maximum anterior voltage, measuring from the 0° to 180° axis to the most anterior point of the QRS loop, increases and may be equal or greater than 0.6 mV. It is to be emphasized that in many of the proved cases of true posterior myocardial infarction, some or all of these measurements remain within the normal range. The use of less stringent criteria, however, would result in higher incidence of false-positive diagnoses.

In the conventional electrocardiogram the voltage of the R wave recorded in the right precordial leads (leads V_1 and V_2) increases and that of the S wave decreases as the QRS loop is displaced anteriorly. The R/S ratio in these leads often becomes greater than 1. The increase in the duration of the anterior forces has its counterpart in the increase of the width of the R wave. A notching or slurring of the R wave may be seen in lead V_1 when the normal relationship of the components of the QRS loop is disturbed, especially when there is a figure-of-eight pattern.

Right sagittal plane QRS loop. The anterior displacement of the QRS loop is also well seen in the right sagittal projection. The initial deflection usually remains normal. The efferent limb may or may not be significantly altered. The afferent limb is more consistently displaced in the anterior direction. In most of the instances the loop is inscribed in the normal clockwise direction. However, occasionally a counterclockwise loop is also observed.

Frontal plane QRS loop. Since the effect of a true posterior infarction is to modify the spatial **QRS** vectors in the anterior and posterior direction which is perpendicular to the frontal plane, no appreciable changes are detectable in this projection. However, frequently there is also involvement of the adjacent inferior or lateral aspect of the left ventricle. Accordingly, some abnormalities may be seen owing to the associated muscle damage.

In the conventional electrocardiogram the QRS complex in the limb leads is likewise normal unless there is coexisting infarction of the adjacent region.

HIGH LATERAL MYOCARDIAL INFARCTION (Fig. 11.25)

Myocardial infarction localized in the lateral wall of the left ventricle near the base is relatively uncommon. As the forces normally generated from this region are directed superiorly and slightly to the left, the resultant **QRS** vector after infarction would therefore be displaced in the opposite direction, that is, inferiorly and slightly to the right.

In the vectorcardiogram the changes are best seen in the frontal plane projection. The initial deflection and efferent limb are inscribed inferiorly and slightly to the right. Although the loop is usually oriented more or less vertically with the maximum **QRS** vector directed more inferior than 40°, the loop is inscribed counterclockwise.

In the conventional electrocardiogram an abnormal Q wave is seen in leads I and aVL because the initial vectors are now oriented toward the negative side of the lead axes of these leads.

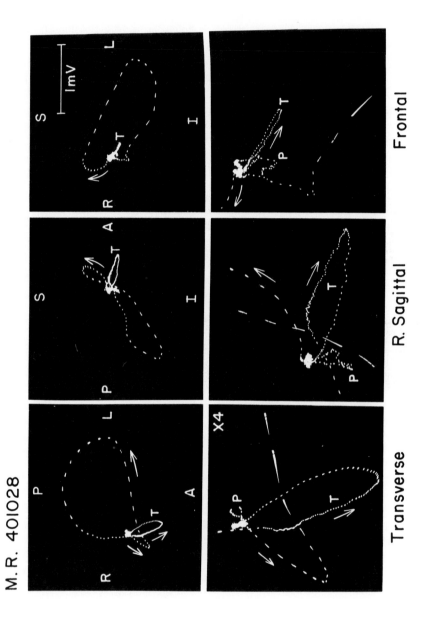

M.R. 40I028

Frontal

R. Sagittal

Transverse

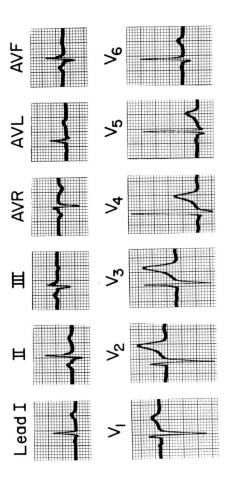

Fig. 11.20. Old inferolateral myocardial infarction. In the vectorcardiogram there is an increase of the initial rightward and superior QRS forces. The duration of the initial rightward forces, as seen in the transverse and frontal planes, measures 0.03 sec. The duration of the initial superior forces in the sagittal and frontal planes is 0.034 sec. The magnitude of the maximum superior forces is also increased. The T loop is normal. In the electrocardiogram a rather wide Q wave is seen in leads V_5 and V_6, and a wide and deep Q wave is seen in the inferior leads.

223

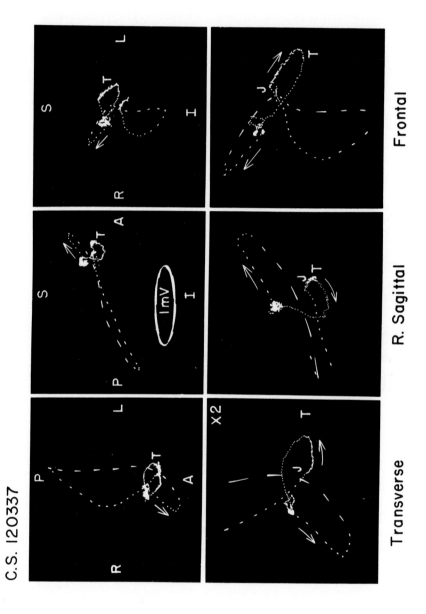

C.S. 120337

Frontal

R. Sagittal

Transverse

224

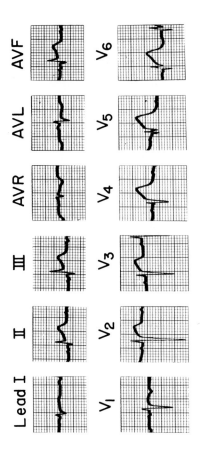

Fig. 11.21. Acute inferolateral myocardial infarction. In the vectorcardiogram the transverse plane projection shows the rightward displacement of the initial deflection and the efferent limb of the QRS loop. The duration of the initial rightward forces (0.022 sec) is at the upper limit of normal. The magnitude of the maximum initial rightward forces is increased. In the right sagittal plane both the duration and magnitude of the initial superior forces are at the upper limits of normal. The loop is inscribed in a figure-of-eight pattern. The rightward and superior displacement of the initial forces and the rightward displacement of the efferent limb are all demonstrated in the frontal plane. There is an abnormally large **ST** vector directed to the left, inferiorly and slightly anteriorly. The electrocardiogram shows abnormal Q waves and ST segment elevation in the inferior leads and the left precordial leads.

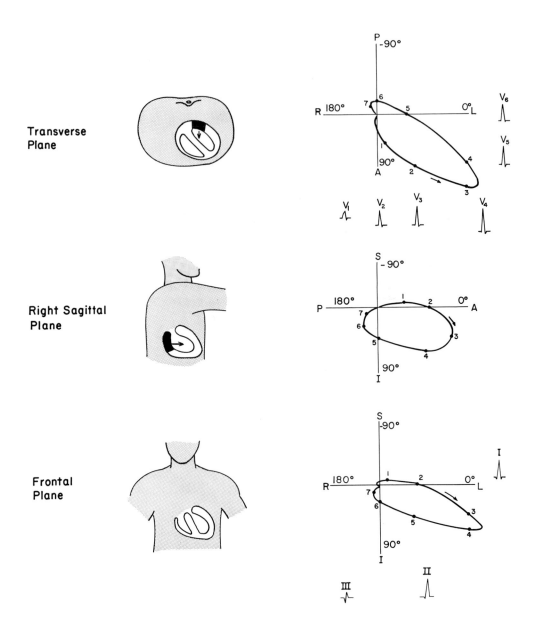

Fig. 11.22. True posterior myocardial infarction. The diagrams depict the anatomic location, the direction of the "infarction vector," and the QRS loop in the three planar projections. The representative scalar leads are also illustrated.

Subacute True Posterior Myocardial Infarction

M. B. 435080   10-15-64

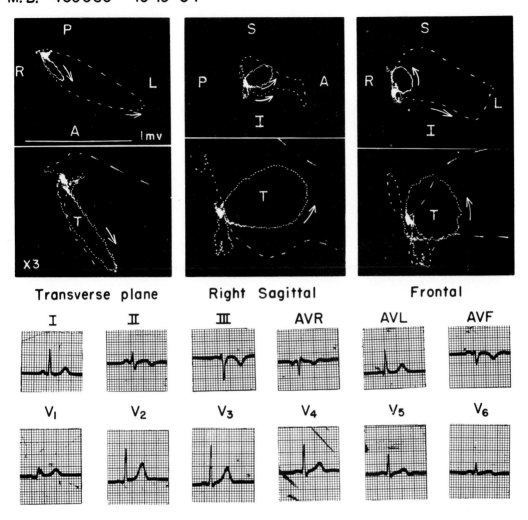

Transverse plane   **Right Sagittal**   **Frontal**

Fig. 11.23. True posterior myocardial infarction, subacute stage. The diagnostic features include the anterior displacement of the QRS loop as seen in the transverse and right sagittal planes. There is an increase of both the duration and magnitude of the anterior forces. The TsÊ loop is wide and inscribed at a relatively uniform speed. It is displaced superiorly. The T loop is inscribed clockwise in the transverse plane and counterclockwise in the sagittal and frontal planes. In the electrocardiogram there is a notched R wave in lead V_1 and monophasic tall R wave in lead V_2. The T wave is upright in both of these leads. The T wave is inverted in the inferior leads suggesting ischemia of the adjacent inferior wall, and correlates with the superior displacement of the TsÊ loop.

H.I. 41850

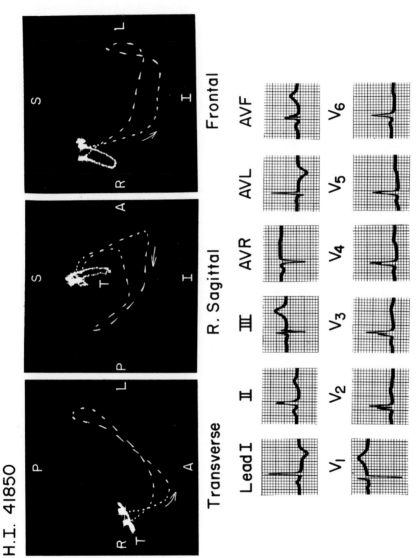

Transverse   R. Sagittal   Frontal

Fig. 11.24. True posterior myocardial infarction. In the vectorcardiogram the transverse and sagittal planes show marked anterior displacement of the afferent limb and terminal deflection of the QRS loop. The loop presents a figure-of-eight pattern in the transverse plane. The TsE loop is directed inferiorly, to the right and slightly anteriorly. The rightward displacement of the TsE loop suggests lateral wall myocardial ischemia. The electrocardiogram demonstrates a monophasic, tall, and notched R wave in leads V_2 and V_3 with an upright T wave in the right precordial leads and inverted T wave in leads I and aVL.

MULTIPLE INFARCTIONS (Fig. 11.26)

When myocardial infarction involves more than one area, its effect on the vectorcardiogram is the sum of that from the individual infarcts. The **QRS** vector will be displaced in a direction represented by an "infarction vector," which is the resultant force of the individual component "infarction vectors." Each area of myocardial damage can usually be recognized by the same criteria outlined previously.

SUMMARY OF VECTORCARDIOGRAPHIC CRITERIA FOR THE DIAGNOSIS OF MYOCARDIAL INFARCTION

Anteroseptal Myocardial Infarction (1 and 2)*

1.   Absent initial anterior QRS forces
2.   0.02-sec **QRS** vector directed posteriorly

Localized Anterior Myocardial Infarction (1, 2, and 3)

1.   Initial anterior septal forces present
2.   0.02-sec **QRS** vector directed posteriorly
3.   Absence of voltage criteria for left ventricular hypertrophy

Anterolateral Myocardial Infarction (1, 2, and 3)

1.   Normal initial anterior septal forces
2.   Initial rightward QRS forces > 0.022 sec
3.   Efferent limb of transverse plane QRS loop inscribed clockwise
4.   Initial rightward QRS forces > 0.16 mV
5.   Maximum frontal plane **QRS** vector $> 40°$, QRS loop inscribed counter-clockwise

Extensive Anterior Myocardial Infarction (1 and 2)

1.   Absent initial anterior QRS forces
2.   Transverse plane QRS loop inscribed clockwise

Inferior Myocardial Infarction (one or more)

1.   Initial superior QRS forces > 0.025 sec
2.   Initial superior QRS forces $\lessgtr 0.02$ sec, maximum left superior force $\lessgtr 0.25$ mV
3.   Maximum frontal plane **QRS** vector $< 10°$, efferent limb of frontal QRS loop inscribed clockwise
4.   Bites in afferent limb of frontal QRS loop

Inferolateral Myocardial Infarction (1 and 2)

1.   Initial rightward QRS forces > 0.022 sec
2.   Initial superior QRS forces > 0.025 sec

* The numbers in parenthesis after each infarction location indicate the minimum requirements for the diagnosis.

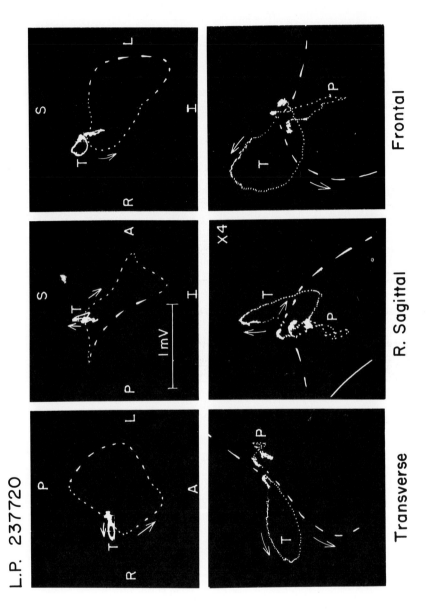

L.P. 237720

Frontal

R. Sagittal

Transverse

230

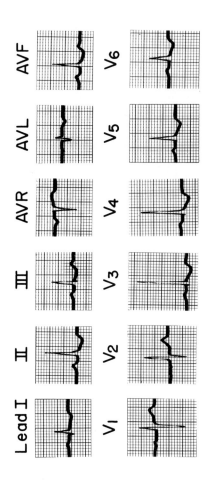

Fig. 11.25. Recent high lateral myocardial infarction. In the vectorcardiogram the frontal plane shows the displacement of the early part of the QRS loop inferiorly and to the right. The loop is inscribed counterclockwise even though the maximum **QRS** vector is directed at 50°. The electrocardiogram records a qR complex in leads I and aVL. The diagnosis of high lateral infarction is supported by serial electrocardiographic changes.

M.G. 439681

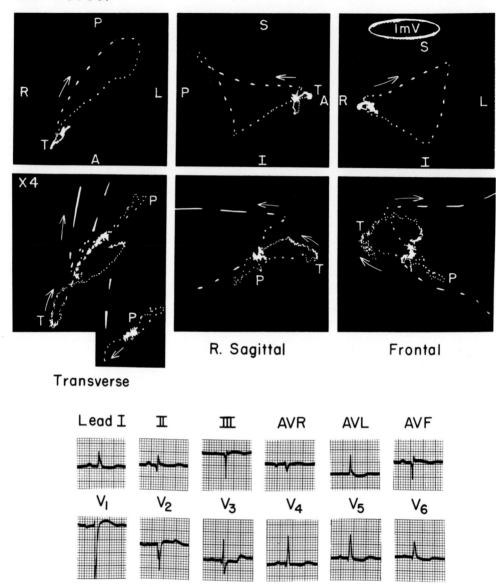

Transverse   R. Sagittal   Frontal

Fig. 11.26. Anterolateral and inferior myocardial infarction. In the vectorcardiogram the transverse plane QRS loop displays the posterior and rightward displacement of the efferent limb, and the loop is inscribed clockwise. These changes are indicative of anterolateral myocardial infarction. The evidence for inferior myocardial infarction includes the increase in the duration and magnitude of the superior forces as seen in the sagittal and frontal planes. The QRS loop is inscribed counterclockwise in the right sagittal plane and clockwise in the frontal plane. The electrocardiogram reveals definite signs of inferior infarction, but the extent of the anterior wall damage is not as extensive as is indicated in the vectorcardiogram.

3.   Efferent limb of frontal plane QRS loop inscribed clockwise
4.   Initial rightward QRS forces > 0.16 mV

True Posterior Myocardial Infarction (one or more)
  In the transverse plane

1.   Anterior loop area > 70 percent of total QRS area
2.   Maximum **QRS** vector anterior to 20°
3.   Duration of anterior QRS forces > 0.05 sec
4.   Half-area **QRS** vector anterior to 10°
5.   Maximum anterior QRS voltage $\lessgtr$ 0.6 mV

High Lateral Myocardial Infarction (1 and 2)

1.   Maximum frontal plane **QRS** vector > 40°, QRS loop inscribed counter-
     clockwise
2.   No specific changes in transverse plane QRS loop

The experience of many investigators including the author indicates that the vectorcardiogram is more sensitive than the conventional electrocardiogram in the recognition of
myocardial infarction. However, it is not more sepcific. A significant number of false-positive
diagnoses of myocardial infarction may be made when the previously described criteria are
used. This is especially true when ventricular hypertrophy or chronic obstructive lung disease
is present. Replacement of the myocardium by other electrically inert tissues may also result
in a pseudoinfarction pattern. As in electrocardiographic interpretation, the importance of
other clinical information and serial tracings cannot be overemphasized.

MYOCARDIAL INFARCTION AND CONDUCTION DISTURBANCES

Myocardial Infarction in the Presence of
Right Bundle Branch Block (Fig. 11.27)

In uncomplicated right bundle branch block, the alterations of the QRSsÊ loop
primarily involve the afferent limb and terminal deflection. The initial deflection and
efferent limb are essentially unchanged. Since most myocardial infarctions result in
abnormalities of the initial **QRS** vectors, the presence of right bundle branch block
does not interfere with the diagnosis of the infarction. The criteria described
previously for the recognition of the various types of infarction should apply equally
well under this circumstance. The only exception is in true posterior infarction in
which the major changes occur in the later portion of the QRSsÊ loop. Doucet and
associates, however, have indicated that true posterior myocardial infarction may be
recognized in the presence of right bundle branch block by the anterior displacement
of both the efferent and afferent limbs. Additional observation is required to
determine the reliability of this sign.

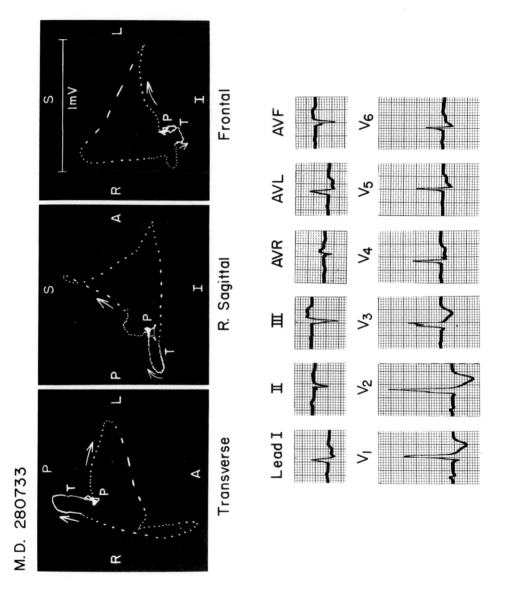

M.D. 2807633

Transverse   R. Sagittal   Frontal

Lead I   II   III   AVR   AVL   AVF

V1   V2   V3   V4   V5   V6

Fig. 11.27. Right bundle branch block with left anterior hemiblock and inferior and anteroseptal myocardial infarction. Note the slowly inscribed anterior and rightward terminal appendage which is diagnostic of right bundle branch block. The superior displacement and counterclockwise inscription of the afferent limb and terminal deflection of the frontal plane QRS loop are consistent with left anterior hemiblock. The superior and posterior displacement of the early part of the QRS loop is indicative of myocardial damage of the inferior and anteroseptal areas.

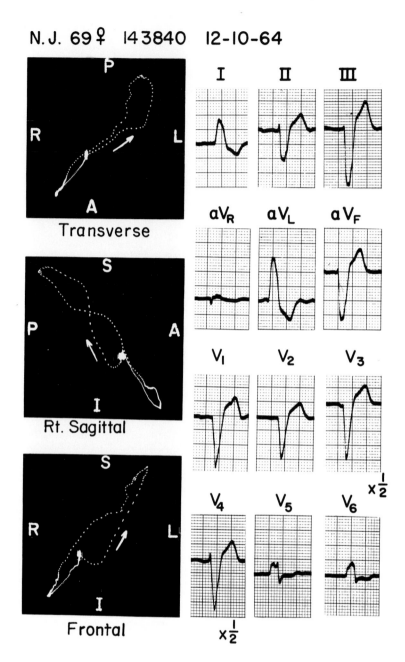

Fig. 11.28.   Left bundle branch block with myocardial infarction. The patient was a 69-year-old woman who had symptoms suggestive of myocardial infarction with serum enzyme elevation. The vectorcardiogram reveals that the QRSsÊ loop is oriented to the left, posteriorly, and superiorly. The loop is slowly inscribed, especially the returning portion. The TsÊ loop is discordant to the QRS. These findings are consistent with left bundle branch block. However, there is a total absence of the initial anterior QRS forces. The transverse plane QRS loop is inscribed counterclockwise. There are also gross irregularities of the afferent limb of the QRS loop as displayed in the transverse and frontal planes. Myocardial damage is therefore probably present. The electrocardiogram shows left bundle branch block. A QS complex is present in leads V_1 through V_3.

Myocardial Infarction in the Presence of
Left Bundle Branch Block (Figs. 11.28-11.30)

It is generally agreed that the diagnosis of myocardial infarction is difficult when left bundle branch block is present. In left bundle branch block the changes in the sequence of ventricular activation result in abnormalities of both the early and

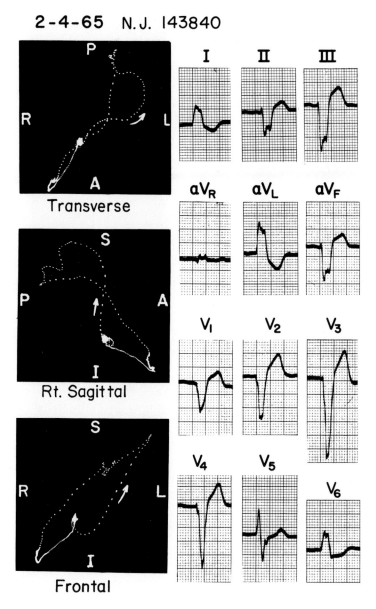

Fig. 11.29. Left bundle branch block with myocardial infarction. The record was taken from the same patient (Fig. 11.28) about 2 months later, after another episode of severe chest pain with serum enzyme elevation. The vectorcardiogram now shows further increase in the distortion of the QRS loop. There is also increased slurring and notching of the QRS complexes in some of the leads in the conventional electrocardiogram.

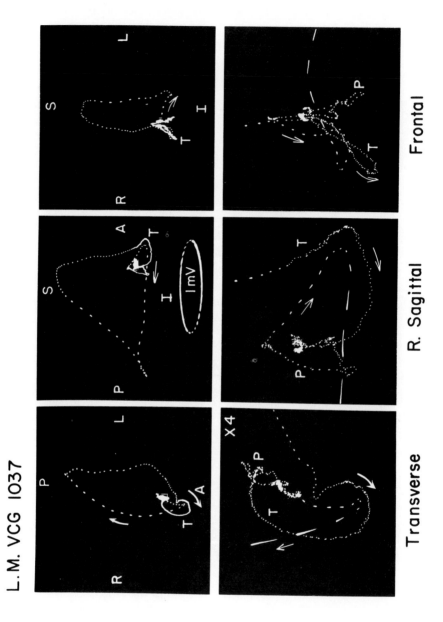

L.M. VCG 1037

Frontal

R. Sagittal

Transverse

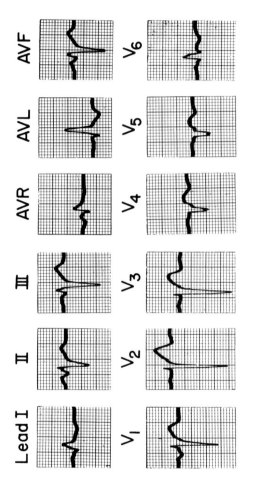

Fig. 11.30. Left bundle branch block with myocardial infarction. The patient is a 65-year-old man with typical clinical manifestations and serial electrocardiographic changes of acute myocardial infarction a few months before the recording of the above vectorcardiogram and electrocardiogram. The vectorcardiogram shows that the QRSsÊ loop is directed to the left, posteriorly and superiorly. It is inscribed clockwise in the transverse plane and counterclockwise in the frontal plane projection. The afferent limb is slowly inscribed. The TsÊ loop is essentially opposite to the QRS loop. These findings are quite consistent with the diagnosis of left bundle branch block. However, in the transverse plane the initial deflection of the QRS loop is directed anteriorly and to the right, which is atypical for left bundle branch block and strongly suggests septal infarction. The clockwise inscription of the T loop in the transverse plane is also atypical. The electrocardiogram reveals a Q wave in leads I, aVL, and V₆ and a QS deflection in leads V₄ and V₅. Otherwise the tracing is consistent with left bundle branch block.

late **QRS** vectors. The usual criteria for the diagnosis of infarction are no longer applicable. However, certain signs which are atypical for uncomplicated left bundle branch block suggest the probable existence of an infarction:

1. The complete absence of the initial anterior QRS forces.
2. The initial deflection of the QRS loop in the transverse plane is inscribed anteriorly and to the right instead of anteriorly and leftward.
3. Displacement of the afferent limb to the right so that the loop in the transverse plane is inscribed counterclockwise.
4. Marked distortion or irregularity of the contour of the QRSsÊ loop which is evident in all planar projections.

Signs 1 and 2 are suggestive of infarction of the interventricular septum and signs 3 and 4, the free wall of the left ventricle. In the author's experience sign 4 has been most useful.

Myocardial Infarction with Hemiblock, Bifascicular Block

Because of the anatomical location of the anterior division of the left bundle branch and the right bundle branch, anterior myocardial infarction, especially anteroseptal infarction, is often accompanied by left anterior hemiblock alone or left anterior hemiblock with right bundle branch block. The diagnosis of the myocardial infarction and the associated conduction abnormalities is usually not difficult. The usual criteria still apply (see Figs. 10.5 and 10.6A in Chapter 10; Figs. 11.4 and 11.27).

When inferior myocardial infarction and left anterior hemiblock coexist the significant vectorcardiographic changes are seen in the frontal and sagittal planes. The initial deflection and efferent limb of the QRS loop display the signs of inferior myocardial infarction, whereas the afferent limb and terminal deflection retain the characteristics of left anterior hemiblock (Fig. 11.31). There is a superior displacement of the initial QRS forces. The duration of the early superior forces is usually longer than 0.025 sec. Occasionally, the very early **QRS** vectors may be directed inferiorly, but the subsequent efferent limb is displaced upward. In the frontal projection the initial deflection and efferent limb are inscribed clockwise. The afferent limb and terminal deflection are more superiorly displaced and are inscribed counterclockwise. The great majority of the loop area is therefore in the left upper quadrant. In the right sagittal plane the superior orientation in the loop is also seen, but the direction of inscription is quite variable. In the electrocardiogram a QS complex with or without notching or a QrS complex is recorded in the inferior leads because of the superior orientation of the loop. The small r wave is occasionally seen in the midportion of the complex if a small midsegment of the loop is still in the left inferior quadrant. When leads II, III, and aVF reveal a QS complex, it is sometimes difficult to determine whether left anterior hemiblock coexists with the infarction. On the other hand, in some cases when the very early QRS vectors are directed inferiorly, an rS deflection is seen in the inferior leads. The recognition of the inferior infarction in addition to the more obvious left anterior hemiblock may also be difficult.

The association of myocardial infarction and left posterior hemiblock is less common. When present, the area of infarction is usually the inferior or posterior wall owing to the anatomic relationship of the posterior division of the left bundle branch and the region of involvement. In inferior myocardial infarction the frontal plane QRS loop reveals the most characteristic changes (see Fig. 10.10). The diagnosis of inferior infarction is based on the abnormalities of the initial deflection and efferent limb. The same criteria described earlier for the uncomplicated inferior myocardial infarction still apply. However, there is a marked rightward displacement of the afferent limb and terminal deflection of the QRS loop as seen in patients with isolated left posterior hemiblock (Fig. 11.32A). The changes in the transverse plane QRS loop resemble those of the left posterior hemiblock alone. In the electrocardiogram there is an abnormal right axis deviation, with an RS complex in lead I and a QR in the inferior leads. In contrast to uncomplicated left posterior hemiblock, the Q wave in leads II, III, and aVF is abnormally wide and deep.

If true posterior myocardial infarction is complicated by left posterior hemiblock, there will be a rightward and inferior displacement of the mid and late QRS forces (Fig. 10.16A). Therefore, in the transverse plane the afferent limb and terminal deflection are not only displaced anteriorly because of the infarction but also rightward because of left posterior hemiblock. The leftward forces are reduced. The rotation of the loop is variable. The changes are indistinguishable from those of right ventricular hypertrophy. In the frontal plane the QRS loop reveals the findings of left posterior hemiblock only. In the electrocardiogram an RsR' or RR' complex

Frontal Plane

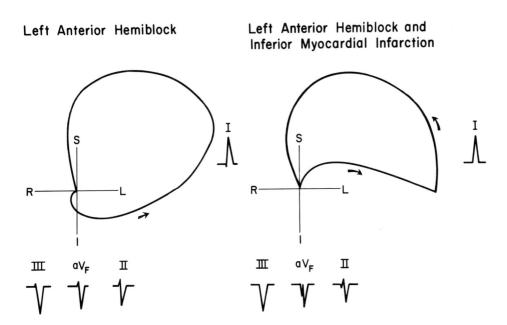

Fig. 11.31. Schematic diagrams of the frontal plane QRS loop in left anterior hemiblock with and without inferior myocardial infarction.

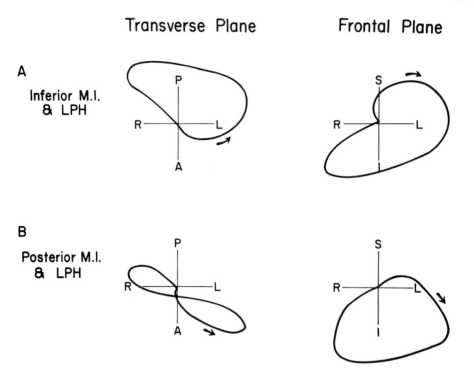

Fig. 11.32. Schematic diagrams of the transverse and frontal plane QRS loops. (A) Inferior myocardial infarction with left posterior hemiblock. (B) True posterior myocardial infarction with left posterior hemiblock.

is recorded in lead V_1. The S wave in leads V_5 and V_6 is abnormally deep. The limb leads are similar to those of the uncomplicated left posterior hemiblock.

When right bundle branch block is superimposed on left posterior hemiblock in the presence of inferior infarction, prolongation of the QRS duration and the development of a slowly inscribed terminal appendage is seen. The vectorcardiographic signs of inferior infarction are not affected. This is, however, not true in true posterior myocardial infarction. Marked anterior displacement of the afferent limb of the QRS loop may occur because of the conduction abnormalities without the presence of posterior myocardial damage. The usual diagnostic criteria for the latter can no longer apply and its recognition is unattainable from the single record alone.

Periinfarction Block (Fig. 11.33)

Periinfarction block was originally described by First et al and has been used to include certain intraventricular conduction defects other than left and right bundle branch block associated with myocardial infarction. There is considerable disagreement as to the genesis of the conduction defect. Other terms, such as "intrainfarction block" and "postinfarction block" have been proposed to imply that the block may not originate at the periphery of the necrotic area. Grant suggested that the delay in conduction in one of the divisions of the left bundle branch is responsible. Indeed, the findings in many reported cases of periinfarction block are consistent with those of the hemiblocks. Involvement of the more distal part of the Purkinje fibers or interruption of the normal muscle-to-muscle conduction (parietal block) probably account for the others.

The vectorcardiographic findings considered as typical of periinfarction block consist of abnormal initial **QRS** vectors diagnostic of myocardial infarction and slowly inscribed terminal vectors which are directed opposite to the initial forces. The duration of the terminal slowing is 0.03 sec or longer. The changes are best seen in the planar projection in which the abnormal initial forces are most clearly displayed. The duration of the QRS loop may or may not exceed the usual "normal limits."

Periinfarction block may be differentiated from bundle branch block by the direction of the slowly inscribed terminal **QRS** vectors. In left bundle branch block they are directed to the left and posteriorly; in right bundle branch block, rightward and anteriorly. In periinfarction block they are variable but always opposite to the initial vectors. However, frequently, the distinction is difficult. This is particularly true in anterolateral myocardial infarction with periinfarction block. The terminal vectors are oriented to the left and posteriorly and resemble closely those of left bundle branch block.

MYOCARDIAL INJURY AND ISCHEMIA

When the myocardial damage is of lesser degree and not accompanied by necrosis, the changes of the **QRS** vectors described above for the various types of myocardial infarction will not be observed. The abnormalities are confined instead, to the **ST** and **T** vectors resulting in an injury or ischemic pattern.

Myocardial Injury (Figs. 11.21, 11.34, 11.35)

Under normal conditions, the various areas of the ventricular myocardium are in an equal state of polarization during diastole and no potential difference is manifested. After the completion of depolarization, the potential will again return to zero. Therefore, the QRSsÊ loop is inscribed as a closed loop. In a significant number of normal subjects the QRSsÊ loop does not close and a small **ST** vector* is present. This is attributed to the early onset of repolarization in some region of the myocardium before the depolarization process has completed. The magnitude of the **ST** vector is, however, small and usually less than 0.1 mV but exceptions do occur especially in younger subjects. The direction is anterior, inferior, and to the left.

The origin of the abnormal **ST** vector in myocardial injury has been attributed to either the presence of a current of injury or a blocking of depolarization. According to the "current of injury" theory, some believe that the injured muscle is only partially polarized during electrical diastole. Its potential becomes less positive (or more negative) in comparison to that of the uninjured myocardium. A vector representing the potential difference between the injured and uninjured tissue at this

---

* As described previously, the **ST** vector is defined by a straight line joining the origin and terminus of the QRSsÊ loop, with the latter representing the positive end.

M.C. 191116

Frontal   R. Sagittal   Transverse

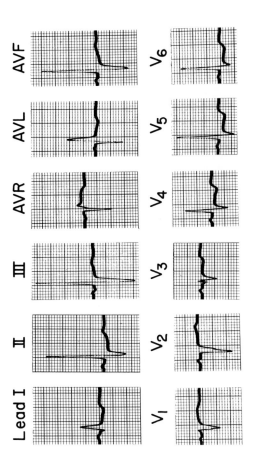

Fig. 11.33. Anterolateral myocardial infarction with periinfarction block. The infarct was proved at autopsy. In the vectorcardiogram the transverse and sagittal planes demonstrate a decrease of the anterior QRS forces. The frontal plane QRS loop is inscribed counterclockwise and its maximum vector is directed at about 70°. The initial deflection and efferent limb are oriented inferiorly, at first slightly to the right and then to the left. The late portion of the QRS loop is slowly inscribed and the terminal deflection is 180° discordant to the early portion of the QRS loop. The wide angle between the initial and terminal vectors is also well demonstrated in the right sagittal plane and is consistent with periinfarction block. In the electrocardiogram there is a QR deflection in leads I and aVL with slight prolongation of the QRS interval. A q wave is also present in leads V_2 and V_3.

time would thus be directed away from the former and toward the latter. At the completion of depolarization, the potential difference no longer exists between the various parts of the myocardium, and the magnitude of this vector becomes zero. It may also be said that, in effect, during the depolarization process another vector of the same magnitude but opposite polarity has neutralized the vector representing the current of injury existing before the onset of depolarization. The direction of this vector is away from the uninjured and toward the injured muscle.

The proponents of the "blocking of depolarization" theory believe that although the injured muscle is repolarized normally, its depolarization is incomplete. Its potential at the end of depolarization is relatively more positive than that of the uninjured. A vector representing the potential difference at this time would be directed toward the injured and away from the uninjured tissue. Therefore, according to either theory, it can be said that when a portion of the myocardium is injured, a vector force (**ST** vector) is uncovered during depolarization which is directed toward the area of injury (Fig. 11.34). In fact, it is very likely that both mechanisms are involved and their effects are additive.

Since the **ST** vector points away from the uninjured muscle and toward the injured area, a subepicardial myocardial injury of the anterior wall would result in an **ST** vector directed anteriorly. Conversely, a subendocardial injury of the same region would produce an **ST** vector directed toward the left ventricular cavity, that is, posteriorly. By the same token, involvement of the subepicardial muscle of the inferior wall would be associated with an inferiorly directed **ST** vector, and the direction will be reversed if the subendocardium is injured. The **ST** vectors associated with involvement of the other areas will not be individually described as they can readily be derived with the same principle (Fig. 11.35). As a rule, the abnormal vector is demonstrated most clearly in the plane which is more or less parallel to the spatial vector.

In the acute stage of a transmural myocardial infarction, the associated injury potential results in an **ST** vector which is similar to that of the subepicardial injury of the region. The magnitude of the **ST** vector decreases as the infarction approaches its subacute phase.

In the conventional electrocardiogram, leads facing the injured wall record ST segment elevation if the subepicardial layer is involved and ST depression if the subendocardial layer is involved. In the former case, the **ST** vector is projected on the positive side of the lead axes and in the latter, the negative side. Thus, for example, the ST segment is elevated in the precordial leads in anterior wall subepicardial injury and depressed in subendocardial injury. The changes expected in injury of other areas can similarly be derived by using the same reasoning.

Myocardial Ischemia (Figs. 11.36 and 11.37)

Ischemia of the myocardium impairs its recovery process. When a portion of the ventricular wall is so affected, the normal sequence of ventricular repolarization will be disturbed and the resultant potential altered. Consequently, abnormalities are manifested in the **T** vectors.

Although the pathophysiology responsible for the various types of T-vector changes associated with myocardial ischemia is still poorly understood, the descrip-

A.

Subendocardial injury

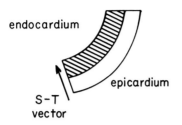

Subepicardial injury

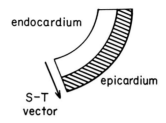

B.

Subendocardial injury of anterior wall

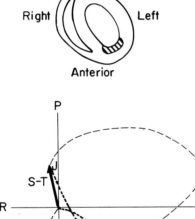

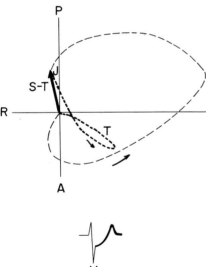

Subepicardial injury of anterior wall

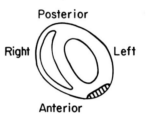

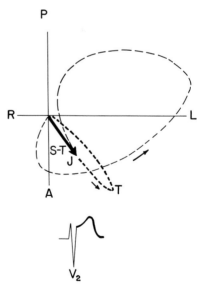

Fig. 11.34. Myocardial injury. (A) Diagrams give the direction of the **ST** vector in subendocardial and subepicardial injury. (B) The transverse plane vectorcardiogram (not including the P loop) and the QRS-T complex in lead V_2 in anterior wall subendocardial and subepicardial injury.

MYOCARDIAL INJURY

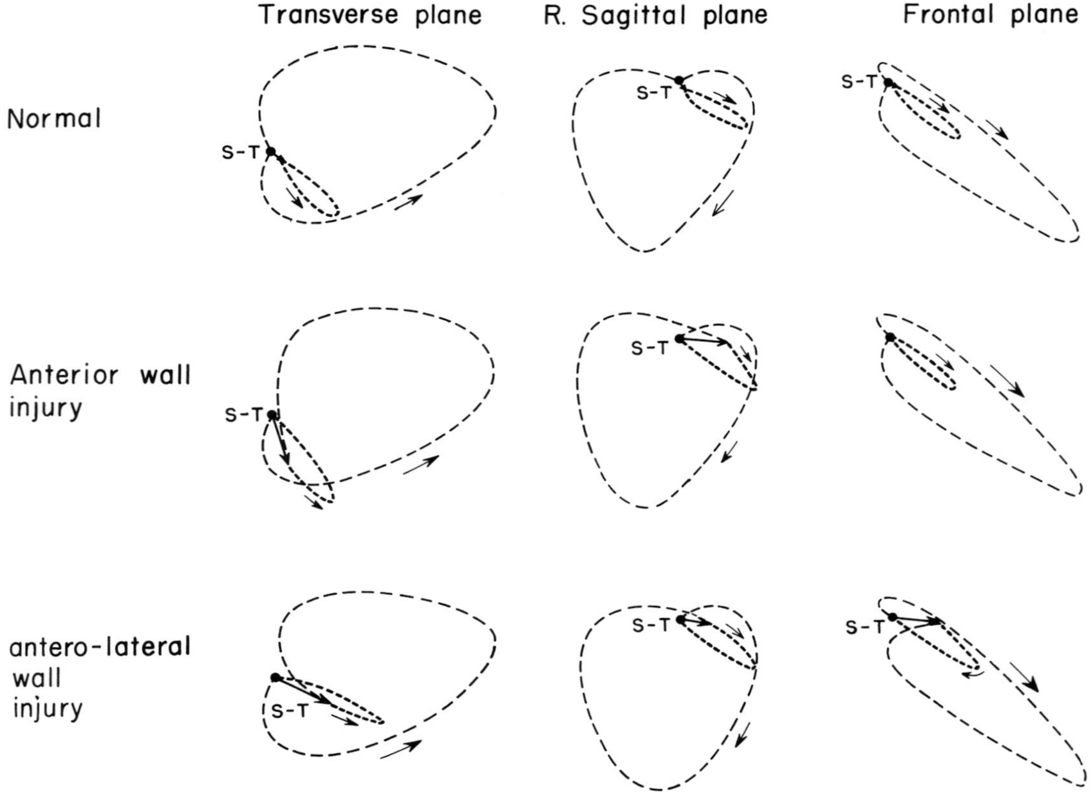

Transverse plane   R. Sagittal plane   Frontal plane

Normal

Anterior wall injury

antero-lateral wall injury

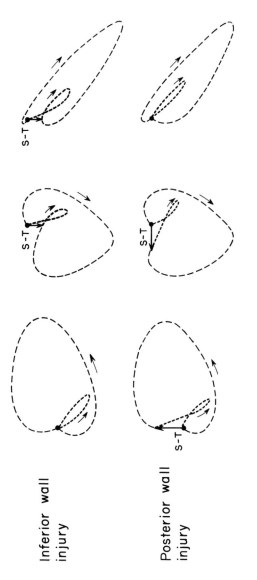

Fig. 11.35. Myocardial injury. Schematic diagrams depicting the direction of the **ST** vector in normal subject and transmural or subepicardial injury of various locations.

A. Subendocardial ischemia   Subepicardial ischemia

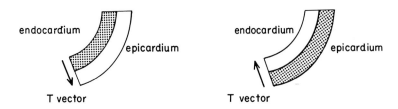

B. Subendocardial ischemia   Subepicardial ischemia
of anterior wall   of anterior wall

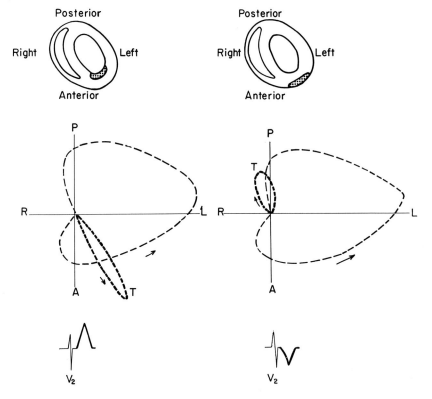

Fig. 11.36. Myocardial ischemia. (A) Diagrams give the direction of the **T** vector in subendocardial and subepicardial ischemia. (B) The changes of the transverse plane T loop and the T wave in lead V₂ in anterior wall subendocardial and subepicardial ischemia.

tion given below is based mainly on the theory suggested by Sodi-Pallares, which appears to be a reasonable explanation in most instances.

Normally, the ventricular repolarization proceeds from the epicardium toward the endocardium. A reduction of blood supply to an area of the subendocardium would further delay the onset of its recovery. When it finally begins to repolarize, its potential is no longer opposed by the forces originated from the other portions of

MYOCARDIAL ISCHEMIA

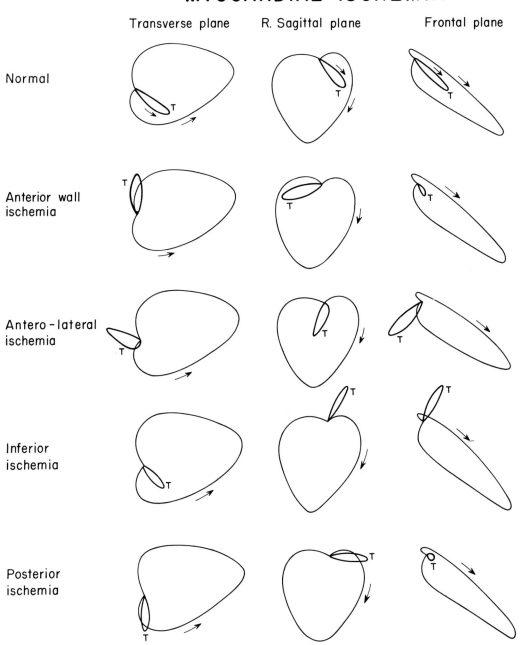

Fig. 11.37.   Myocardiol ischemia. Schematic diagrams depicting the direction of the T loop in normal subject and transmural or subepicardial ischemia of various locations. The direction of inscription of the T loop in myocardial ischemia varies as well as the configuration which may be narrow or abnormally wide.

the myocardium and becomes abnormally prominent. Since the direction of the spread of the process remains essentially the same, the orientation of the T vectors is unchanged. Therefore, for instance, subendocardial ischemia of the anterior wall is associated with abnormally large T vectors directed anteriorly and that of the inferior wall, with abnormally large T vectors directed inferiorly.

When there is ischemia of the subepicardial layer, the delay of the onset of recovery of this region may reverse the normal direction of ventricular repolarization. The process now proceeds from the endocardium toward the epicardium. Consequently, the direction of the T vectors is also reversed. Therefore, subepicardial ischema of the anterior wall will be accompanied by T vectors directed posteriorly and that of the inferior wall by T vectors directed superiorly.

Transmural ischemia apparently has an effect similar to that of the subepicardial ischemia. The T vectors are also directed away from the site of the lesion. Similar changes are observed in the acute and subacute stages of a transmural myocardial infarction and may persist for a variable, sometimes indefinite, period after the onset of the infarction.

In addition to the alteration of its orientation and magnitude, the TsÊ loop in myocardial ischemia is characteristically inscribed at a uniform speed. This is in contrast to the consistent slow inscription of the outgoing limb of the normal loop which is indicated by the close spacing of the dashes. The direction of inscription is often, but not always, reversed. In many instances the TsÊ loop becomes abnormally wide with its length-to-width ratio less than 2.6 to 1 (Figs. 11.7 and 11.12). (The length-to-width ratio of the spatial T loop may be approximately determined by using the longest maximum T vector among the three planes against the largest width among the three planes.)

In the conventional electrocardiogram, tall T waves are recorded in leads facing the ventricular wall containing the zone of subendocardial ischemia as the T vectors are directed toward the positive side of the lead axes. Inverted T waves are recorded in these same leads if ischemia involves the subepicardium since the T vectors now project on the negative side of the lead axes. For example, subendocardial ischemia of the anterior wall is associated with tall T waves in the precordial leads and subepicardial ischemia of the same region, with T-wave inversion in these leads. The loss of the normal slow inscription of the outgoing limb of the TsÊ loop correlates with the loss of the gradual slope of the first half of the T wave seen in the normal T wave. Consequently, the T wave in myocardial ischemia becomes symmetrical in appearance. The electrocardiographic counterpart of the abnormally wide TsÊ loop is difficult to recognize from the routine scalar leads. Simultaneous recording of multiple leads is required (see Reference 4).

REFERENCES

1. Burch GE, Horan LG, Ziskind J, Cronvich JA: A correlative study of postmortem, electrocardiographic, and spatial vectorcardiographic data in myocardial infarction. Circulation 18:325, 1958
2. Benchimol A, Desser KB, Massey BJ: Coexisting left anterior hemiblock and inferior wall myocardial infarction. Vectorcardiographic features. Am J Cardiol 29:7, 1972
3. Cabrera E, Rocha JC, Flores G: El vectorcardiograma de los infartos miocardios con trastornos de conduccion intraventricular. Arch Inst Cardiol Mexico 29:625, 1959

4. Chou TC, Helm RA, Lach R: The significance of a wide TsÊ loop. Circulation 30:400, 1964

5. DePasquale N, Burch GE: The spatial vectorcardiogram in left bundle branch block and myocardial infarction, with autopsy studies. Am J Med 29:633, 1960

6. Doucet P, Walsh TJ, Massie E: A vectorcardiographic study of right bundle branch block with the Frank lead system. Clinical correlation in myocardial infarction. Am J Cardiol 16:342, 1965

7. Doucet P, Walsh TJ, Massie E: A vectorcardiographic and electrocardiographic study of left bundle branch block with myocardial infarction. Am J Cardiol 17:171, 1966

8. First SR, Bayley RH, Bedford DR: Peri-infarction block; electrocardiographic abnormality occasionally resembling bundle branch block and local ventricular block of other types. Circulation 2:31, 1950

9. Grant RP: Peri-infarction block. Prog Cardiovasc Dis 2:237, 1959

10. Gunnar RM, Pietras RJ, Blackaller J, Dadmun SE, Szanto PB, Tobin JR Jr: Correlation of vectorcardiographic criteria for myocardial infarction with autopsy findings. Circulation 35:158, 1967

11. Gunnar RM, Winslow EBJ, Cabin GI, Pietras RJ, Boswell J, Szanto PB: Autopsy correlation of vectorcardiographic criteria for the diagnosis of myocardial infarction. Proc XI Int Vectorcardiography Symp. Amsterdam and London, North-Holland, 1970, p 333

12. Hoffman I, Taymor RC, Gootnick A: Vectorcardiographic residua of inferior infarction. Seventy-eight cases studied with the Frank system. Circulation 29:562, 1964

13. Hoffman I, Taymor RC, Morris MH, Kittell I: Quantitative criteria for the diagnosis of dorsal infarction using the Frank vectorcardiogram. Am Heart J 70:295, 1965

14. Hugenholtz PG, Ryan TJ, Woerner T, Levine HD: Recognition of anterior wall infarction in patients with left ventricular hypertrophy. A study of the Frank vectorcardiogram. Circulation 27:386, 1963

15. Hugenholtz PG, Whipple GH, Levine HD: A clinical appraisal of the vectorcardiogram in myocardial infarction. I. The cube system. Circulation 24:808, 1961

16. Hugenholtz PG, Forkner CE Jr, Levine HD: A clinical appraisal of the vectorcardiogram in myocardial infarction. II. The Frank system. Circulation 24:825, 1961

17. Libanoff AJ, Boiteau GM, Allenstein BJ: Diaphragmatic myocardial infarction with peri-infarction block. Studies of the electrocardiogram and vectorcardiogram. Am J Cardiol 12:772, 1963

18. Massie E, Walsh TJ: Clinical Vectorcardiography and Electrocardiography. Chicago, Year Book, 1960, pp 255–339

19. Mathur VS, Levine HD: Vectorcardiographic differentiation between right ventricular hypertrophy and posterobasal myocardial infarction. Am J Cardiol 17:131, 1966

20. Mayer JW, Castellanos A Jr, Lemberg L: The spatial vectorcardiogram in peri-infarction block. Am J Cardiol 11:613, 1963

21. McConahay DR, McCallister BD, Hallermann FJ, Smith RE: Comparative quantitative analysis of the electrocardiogram and the vectorcardiogram. Correlations with the coronary arteriogram. Circulation 42:245, 1970

22. Neuman J, Blackaller J, Tobin JR Jr, Szanto PB, Gunnar RM: The spatial vectorcardiogram in left bundle branch block. Am J Cardiol 16:352, 1965

23. Richman HG, Yokoi M, Gleason D, Nishijima K, Simonson E: Reliability of the vectorcardiographic diagnosis of myocardial infarction. Proc XI Int Vectorcardiography Symp. Amsterdam and London, North-Holland, 1970, p 343

24. Sodi-Pallares D, Calder RM: New Bases of Electrocardiography. St. Louis, Mosby, 1956, pp 531–533

25. Walsh TJ, Tiongson PM, Stoddard EA, Massie E: The vectorcardiographic QRSsÊ-loop findings in inferoposterior myocardial infarction. Am Heart J 63:516, 1962

26. Wolff L, Wolff R, Samartzis MD, Mazzoleni A, Soffe AM, Reiner L, Matsuoka S:

Vectorcardiographic diagnosis. A correlation with autopsy findings in 167 cases. Circulation 23:861, 1961

27. Young E, Williams C: The frontal plane vectorcardiogram in old inferior myocardial infarction. Criteria for diagnosis and electrocardiographic correlation. Circulation 37:604 1968

28. Young E, Levine HD, Vokonas PS, Kemp HG, Williams RA, Gorlin R: The frontal plane vectorcardiogram in old inferior myocardial infarction. II. Mid-to-late QRS changes. Circulation 42:1143, 1970

12

Atrial Enlargement

Normal atrial depolarization begins at the sinoatrial node and spreads radially first through the right atrial and then the left atrial musculature. Therefore, the initial vectors of the PsÊ loop represent the potential from the right atrium and the terminal vectors that of the left atrium. The midportion of the PsÊ loop represents the combined forces from both atria and the interatrial septum. Anatomically, the right atrium is located anteriorly, and the left atrium, posteriorly. The right atrial vectors are directed inferiorly, leftward and anteriorly, and the left atrial vectors are directed inferiorly, leftward and posteriorly. Therefore, in right atrial enlargement the initial anterior vectors increase in magnitude and the PsÊ loop is displaced anteriorly. In left atrial enlargement the late posterior forces are increased and the loop is displaced posteriorly. In biatrial enlargement both the initial anterior and the late posterior components of the loop become prominent.

Right Atrial Enlargement (Figs. 12.1-12.3)

The spatial P loop in right atrial enlargement is directed inferiorly, slightly to the left and most of the loop is located anteriorly. The magnitude of the loop and its maximum spatial vector is abnormally large. The duration of the P loop is usually within normal limits. The loop has a relatively smooth contour. The atrial **T** vector is often quite large and points in a direction opposite to that of the maximum **P** vector. (The atrial **T** vector is represented by a vector drawn from the beginning of the PsÊ loop, E, to the end of the loop, O,) Therefore, the spatial P loop often remains widely opened.

Transverse plane. In the transverse plane projection the P loop is directed leftward with most of the loop area located anteriorly. The direction of inscription usually remains counterclockwise as in the normal individual. The maximum **P** vector is directed anteriorly and to the left and its magnitude often, but not necessarily always, exceeds the normal upper limit of 0.1 mV. The anterior displacement of the enlarged P loop explains the prominent P wave seen in the right

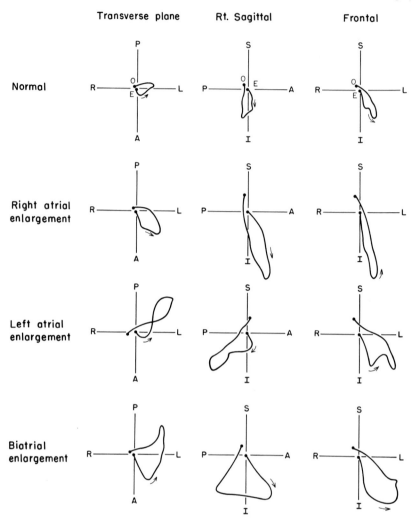

Fig. 12.1. Schematic diagrams comparing the normal P loop with the P loop in right atrial, left atrial, and biatrial enlargement.

precordial leads of the conventional electrocardiogram. The atrial **T** vector is small in this projection.

Right sagittal plane. In the right sagittal plane most of the P loop is located anteriorly and inferiorly, and the maximum **P** vector is similarly oriented. The magnitude of the maximum **P** vector exceeds the upper limit of normal (0.18 mV). The loop is inscribed clockwise as in the normal person. The loop usually ends superiorly and slightly posteriorly to its origin with an abnormally large atrial **T** vector.

Frontal plane. In the frontal plane projection the P loop is directed inferiorly and slightly to the left. Although the direction of the maximum **P** vector is still within the normal range (15° to 90°), the vector tends to be vertical in position and approaches 90°. However, only rarely does it exceed 90°. The loop is usually inscribed counterclockwise, but a figure-of-eight pattern is also encountered with the distal portion of the loop being inscribed clockwise. The magnitude of the maximum vector is greater than the normal upper limit of 0.2 mV. In many instances the loop appears to be quite narrow. The atrial **T** vector is usually quite large and is directed superiorly and slightly to the right being opposite to the direction of the maximum **P** vector.

The pattern of "P pulmonale" in the conventional electrocardiogram is related to the abnormally large and more or less vertical P loop. The magnitude of the projections of the **P** vectors on the lead axes of leads II, III, and aVF is increased. Since the duration of the P loop is normal, the P wave is therefore tall but not wide. It should be pointed out that a long narrow P loop is not necessarily always associated with a tall and *narrow* P wave in the scalar electrocardiogram. If the duration of the P loop is increased, the P wave will be wide. The abnormally large atrial **T** vector directed superiorly has its counterpart in the downward displacement of the PR segment in the inferior leads.

Left Atrial Enlargement (Figs. 12.1, 12.4 and 12.5)

In left atrial enlargement the PsÊ loop is directed inferiorly, leftward, and mostly posteriorly. The magnitude of the loop and its maximum spatial vector is increased but usually not to the degree seen in right atrial enlargement. The duration of the PsÊ loop may or may not be increased. The loop is often quite irregular in contour. The atrial **T** vector may or may not be abnormally large and is directed opposite to the maximum spatial **P** vector.

Transverse plane. In the transverse plane projection the P loop is directed to the left with most of the loop area located posteriorly. Either the loop is inscribed counterclockwise, or it presents a figure-of-eight pattern. In the latter instance the proximal portion is inscribed counterclockwise and the distal portion clockwise. The maximum **P** vector is directed to the left and posteriorly, and its magnitude exceeds the normal upper limit of 0.1 mV. The atrial **T** vector, if visible, is directed rightward and anteriorly. The large posteriorly oriented P loop explains the wide and deep negative terminal deflection of the P wave often seen in lead V₁ of the conventional electrocardiogram.

Right sagittal plane. In the right sagittal plane most of the P loop is located inferiorly and posteriorly. The direction of inscription is usually clockwise even though a figure-of-eight pattern is also seen. The magnitude of the maximum **P** vector may or may not exceed the normal upper limit of 0.18 mV. The atrial **T** vector is directed superiorly and usually anteriorly.

Frontal plane. In the frontal plane projection the P loop is oriented inferiorly and to the left. Although the direction of the maximum **P** vector is still within the normal range, it is usually less vertical than that of the normal person or patient with right atrial enlargement. The loop is inscribed counterclockwise. In one group of left atrial enlargement, mostly that caused by mitral valvular disease, the P loop tends to

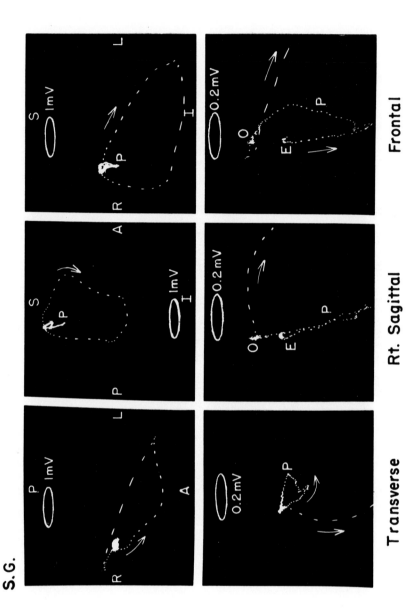

S.G.

Transverse   **Rt. Sagittal**   **Frontal**

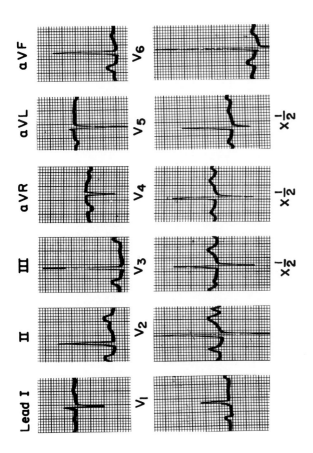

Fig. 12.2. Right atrial enlargement in a 19-year-old patient with tetralogy of Fallot. In the bottom panel of the vectorcardiogram the enlarged P loop and the beginning of QRS loop are recorded.

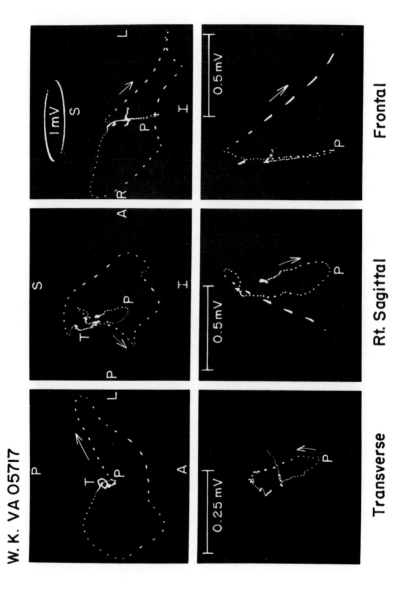

W. K. VA 05717

Transverse   Rt. Sagittal   Frontal

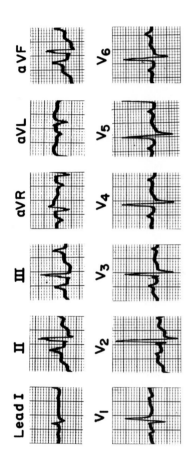

Fig. 12.3. Right atrial enlargement in a 65-year-old man with chronic cor pulmonale.

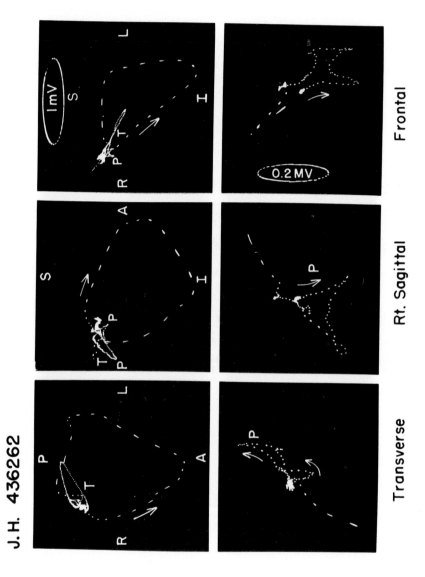

J.H. 436262

Frontal

Rt. Sagittal

Transverse

262

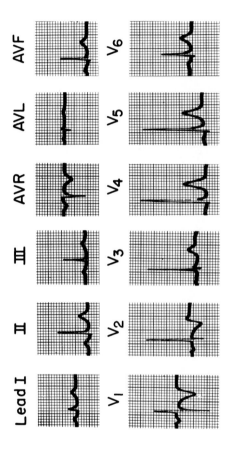

Fig. 12.4. Left atrial enlargment in a 56-year-old man with mitral stenosis. The relatively large anterior component of the P loop in the right sagittal plane suggests that right atrial enlargement may also be present.

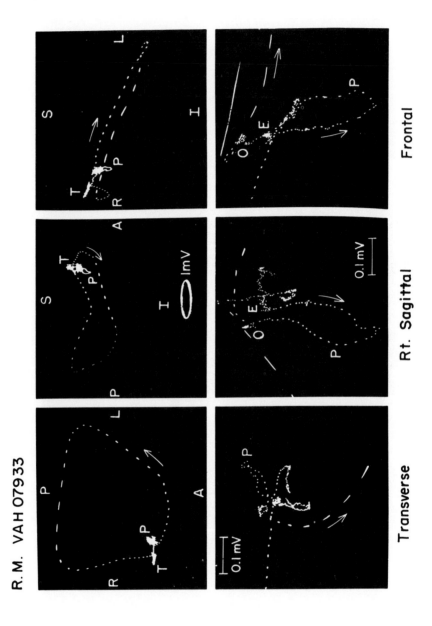

R.M. VAH 07933

Frontal

Rt. Sagittal

Transverse

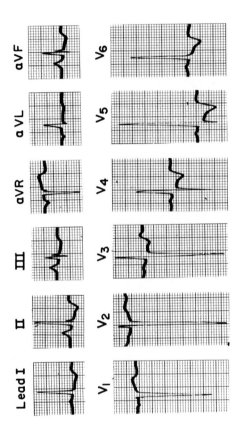

Fig. 12.5. Left atrial enlargement in a 47-year-old man with hypertensive cardiovascular disease.

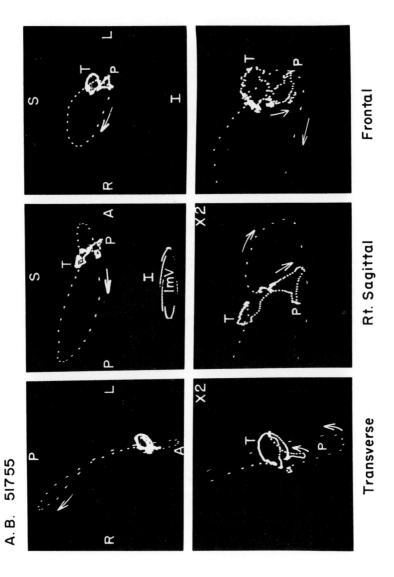

A. B. 5I755

Frontal

Rt. Sagittal

Transverse

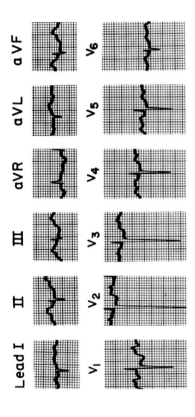

Fig. 12.6. Biatrial enlargement in a 35-year-old woman with mitral stenosis and chronic lung disease.

be more irregular in contour and bifid in appearance with the terminal part of the loop directed more leftward and upward. The duration of the loop is often increased. The magnitude of the maximum **P** vector, however, usually remains within the normal limits in this projection. The conventional electrocardiogram displays the "P mitrale" pattern with a broad and notched P wave seen usually in leads I and II. When the left atrial enlargement is caused by hypertensive cardiovascular or aortic valvular disease, the P loop may often be relatively smooth and elongated with an increase of the magnitude of its maximum vector. The duration of the loop may or may not increase. The P wave in the limb leads of the electrocardiogram therefore could resemble closely the pattern of "P pulmonale."

Biatrial Enlargement (Figs. 12.1 and 12.6)

The increase of both the right and left atrial potential in biatrial enlargement augments both the early anterior and the late posterior forces. Therefore, the enlarged PsÊ loop has a large anterior as well as a large posterior component. These characteristic changes are best demonstrated in the transverse and sagittal planes. The transverse plane P loop may be inscribed counterclockwise or may present a figure-of-eight pattern. A large triangular loop in the sagittal plane is quite typical of this condition. The loop is inscribed clockwise in this projection and two "maximum" vectors of almost equal magnitude can usually be identified, one directed anteriorly and one posteriorly. The direction of inscription of the loop remains normal (clockwise) in this projection and also in the frontal plane (counterclockwise).

In the conventional electrocardiogram lead V_1 records a P wave with an initial tall upright deflection followed by a large negative terminal component and represents the counterpart of the changes seen in the transverse plane projection. The limb leads, especially leads II, III, and aVF, usually display a tall and broad P wave which is the equivalent of the increase in the magnitude and duration of the P loop in the frontal plane.

REFERENCES

1. Chou TC, Helm RA: The pseudo P pulmonale. Circulation 32:96, 1965
2. Scheuer J, Kahn M, Bleifer S, Donoso E, Grishman A: The atrial vectorcardiogram in health and disease. Am Heart J 60:33, 1960
3. Sano T, Hellerstein, HK, Vayda E: P vector loop in health and disease as studied by the technique of electrical dissection of the vectorcardiogram (differential vectorcardiography). Am Heart J 53:854, 1957

13

Pulmonary Emphysema, Pulmonary Embolism

PULMONARY EMPHYSEMA

Pulmonary Emphysema (Figs. 13.1-13.3)

Pulmonary emphysema, with or without cor pulmonale, often presents rather characteristic vectorcardiographic and electrocardiographic patterns by which the condition may be recognized. Although the exact mechanism is not entirely understood, several factors have been suggested to account for the changes. The lung is a relatively poor electrical conductor. Emphysema further increases the resistance to the transmission of the cardiac potential toward the body surface and alters the characteristics of the lead vectors. The low position of the diaphragm is accompanied by a more vertical heart. There is also some clockwise rotation of the heart along its longitudinal axis, the importance of which is, however, debatable. In the following paragraphs the discussion is limited to the findings seen in patients without clinical evidence of cor pulmonale. It should be mentioned that a slight or even moderate degree of cor pulmonale may often be present but cannot be detected clinically.

The main feature of the vectorcardiographic changes in pulmonary emphysema is the posterior displacement of the QRSsÊ loop; the magnitude of the spatial loop is reduced. There is no evidence of a conduction delay, and the duration of the QRSsÊ loop remains normal. The **ST** vector, if present, is small. The TsÊ loop is directed more inferiorly. There is an increase in the average magnitude of the PsÊ loop. The loop also becomes more vertical in position.

Transverse plane. In the transverse plane projection the entire QRS loop is rotated in a counterclockwise direction so that the main body of the loop is oriented more posteriorly and medially than the normal QRS loop (Fig. 13.1). The initial deflection is written anteriorly and either to the right or more commonly, to the left. (In the normal person the right anterior direction is the most common.) The direction of inscription of the loop is counterclockwise. The terminal deflection is

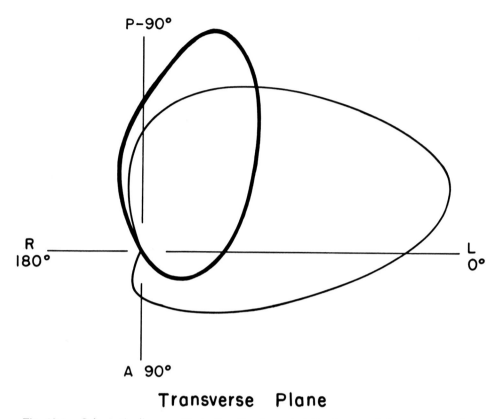

Transverse Plane

Fig. 13.1. Schematic diagram illustrating the characteristic changes of the transverse plane QRS loop in pulmonary emphysema as compared with that of the normal individual. The normal loop is drawn with a thin line and the emphysema loop with a heavy line. Note the smaller magnitude and the posterior rotation of the QRS loop in pulmonary emphysema.

directed posteriorly and slightly to the right. Occasionally, there is a rather marked rightward displacement of the terminal deflection, and the area of the QRS loop located in the right posterior quadrant becomes abnormally large and exceeds the normal upper limit, which is about 20 percent of the total QRS area. In such an instance it is probable that right ventricular hypertrophy is present. The maximum **QRS** vector is reduced in amplitude. It is directed to the left but more posteriorly than that of the average normal person. The 0.02-sec instantaneous vector may sometimes be oriented posterior to the 0° to 180° axis in patients without coronary artery disease. Therefore, a false-positive diagnosis of anterior myocardial infarction may be made. The T loop is usually normal in its orientation, magnitude, and direction of inscription. The abnormalities of the PsÊ loop are not well displayed in this projection.

The posterior orientation of the QRS loop corresponds to the "clockwise rotation" seen in the precordial leads of the conventional electrocardiogram. Most of the loop area is now on the negative side of the lead axis of V_1 through V_4 resulting in a leftward shift of the transitional zone, and a predominantly upright QRS deflection is not recorded until lead V_5 or V_6 is reached. The small r wave seen in the right and midprecordial leads is related to the small initial anterior QRS forces. An S wave is often present in the left precordial leads because of the terminal rightward forces. However, the magnitude of the S wave is usually small in the absence of cor pulmonale. The T wave in the precordial leads is usually normal. There is no significant change seen in the precordial P wave.

Right sagittal plane. The posterior rotation of the QRS loop is also well displayed in the right sagittal projection. The magnitude of the early anterior forces is reduced, and the loop is inscribed clockwise. Most of the loop area is located in the inferoposterior quadrant. The maximum **QRS** vector is directed more posteriorly, but its magnitude in this projection usually remains normal. This is because although the maximum spatial vector is smaller, its direction is now more parallel to the sagittal plane. Posterior displacement of the 0.02-sec **QRS** vector beyond 90° is sometimes observed. The T loop reveals no significant changes. The magnitude of the P loop is often increased. The loop may be oriented slightly anteriorly or posteriorly but is essentially vertical in position. Its direction of inscription remains clockwise.

Frontal plane. In the frontal plane projection the QRS loop usually appears to be quite small and is attributed to both a reduction in the magnitude of the spatial loop and its posterior orientation, so that the loop is more or less perpendicular to the frontal plane. The loop may be inscribed either clockwise or counterclockwise. The maximum **QRS** vector is usually more inferior (i.e., more vertical) than that of the normal individual. In some patients there is a relatively large area of the loop located to the right, and abnormally large late superior forces are also occasionally seen, especially when the loop is inscribed counterclockwise. The average T loop is displaced more inferiorly. Its magnitude is within the normal range. The magnitude of the maximum **P** vector is increased, and the P loop is essentially vertical in position and approaches and sometimes exceeds 90°. The loop is inscribed counterclockwise and is often quite narrow.

The reduction in the size of the QRS loop in the frontal plane projection explains the overall low voltage of the QRS complex in the limb leads of the scalar electrocardiogram. Because of the more vertical direction of the maximum **QRS** vector the voltage of the QRS complex in lead I is especially small. The presence of the late rightward and superior **QRS** vectors in certain patients is equivalent to the $S_1S_2S_3$ pattern in the limb leads, as these vectors project on the negative side of the lead axis of leads I, II, and III. The P and T waves in lead I are also small because of the vertical position of the P and T loops. The increase in the magnitude of the P loop and its vertical orientation correlate with the tall P wave in the inferior leads, the P pulmonale.

PULMONARY EMBOLISM (Figs. 13.4A and B)

In pulmonary embolism the vectorcardiographic and electrocardiographic changes depend in a large measure on the size of the embolus and the time of the recording in relation to the onset of the acute event. Characteristically, the abnormalities are transient in nature but the rapidity of the changes varies. In

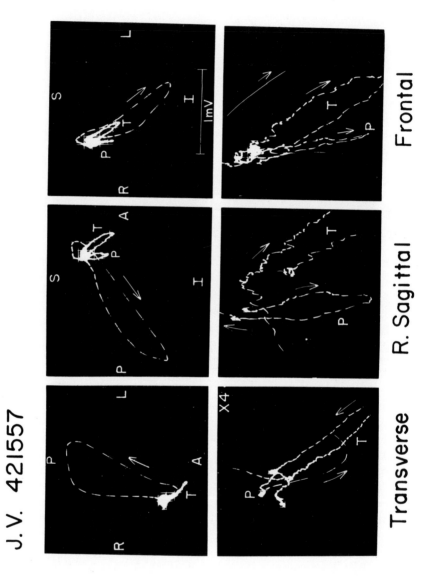

J.V. 421557

Transverse   R. Sagittal   Frontal

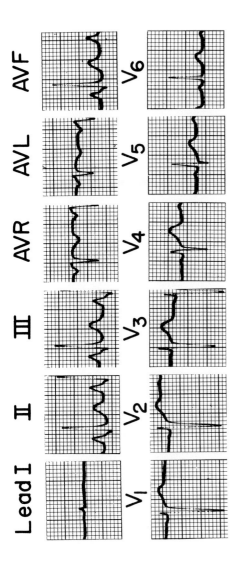

Fig. 13.2. Pulmonary emphysema in a 54-year-old man. In the transverse plane of the vectorcardiogram there is a rather marked posterior rotation of the QRS loop and its maximum **QRS** vector. The 0.02-sec **QRS** vector is also oriented posteriorly. These findings correlate with the poor progression of the R wave in the right and midprecordial leads in the conventional electrocardiogram. The transitional zone is between leads V_4 and V_5. The relatively vertical orientation of the P, QRS, and T loops in the frontal plane explains the low voltage of all the complexes in lead I. The increase in the magnitude of the maximum **P** vector correlates with the P-pulmonale pattern in the electrocardiogram. (Each dash in the vectorcardiogram represents 2.5 msec.)

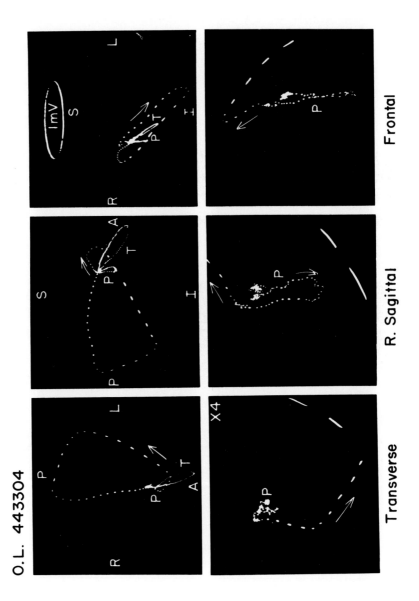

O.L. 443304

Frontal

R. Sagittal

Transverse

274

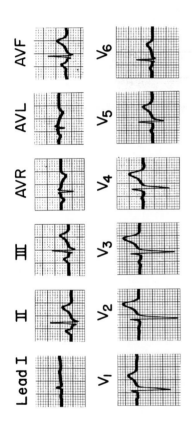

Fig. 13.3. Pulmonary emphysema in a 57-year-old man. In the lower panel of the vectorcardiogram only the enlargement of the P loop and of the beginning of the QRS loop is shown. Note the typical posterior rotation of the QRS loop in the transverse plane and the long narrow vertical P loop in the frontal plane. The apparent disproportionally small QRS and T waves in lead I of the electrocardiogram in relation to the frontal plane QRS and T loops occur because the lead vector of lead I is not horizontal but is tilted somewhat superiorly and leftward and therefore subtends wider angles with the **QRS** and **T** vectors.

275

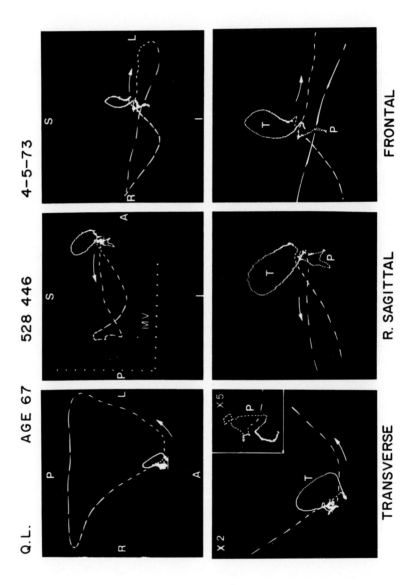

Q.L.　　AGE 67　　528 446　　4-5-73

TRANSVERSE　　R. SAGITTAL　　FRONTAL

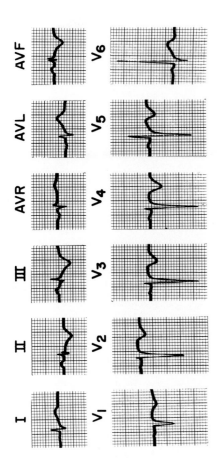

Fig. 13.4. (A) Pulmonary embolism. The tracings were recorded from a 67-year-old woman several hours after the onset of chest pain. The clinical findings and lung scan supported the diagnosis of pulmonary embolism. Both the vectorcardiogram and electrocardiogram are quite typical for acute right heart strain as described in the text. Note the direction of the initial **QRS** vectors, the prominent terminal appendage, and the direction of the T loop for comparison with Fig. 13.4B.

277

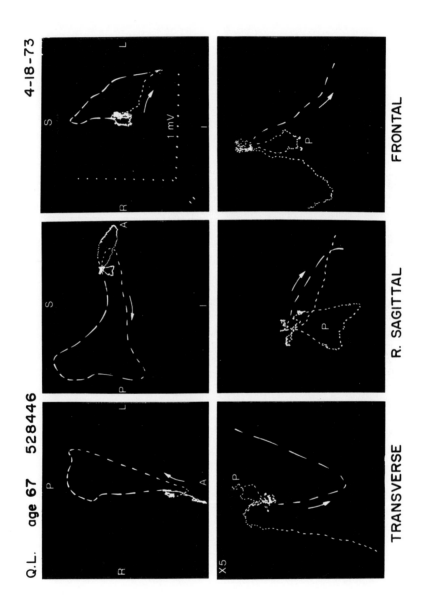

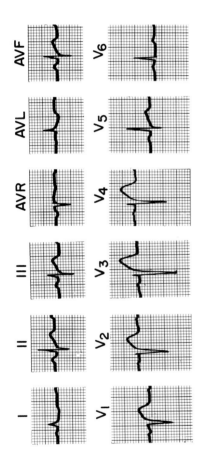

Fig. 13.4. (B) (See Fig. 13.4A) The tracings were recorded from the same patient 2 weeks later. Note the more anterior and inferior direction of the initial QRS forces and the disappearance of the terminal appendage. The QRS loop is now inscribed clockwise in the right sagittal plane and counterclockwise in the frontal plane. The T loop is oriented anteriorly, rightward, and inferiorly. Although the vectorcardiogram and electrocardiogram are still abnormal, they are no longer suggestive of acute right heart strain.

clinical practice the so-called typical findings are observed only in a small percentage of patients. Furthermore, other organic heart diseases often coexist and modify or mask the alterations caused by pulmonary embolism.

The sudden increase of the pulmonary vascular resistance results in an acute dilatation of the right ventricle and right atrium. A clockwise rotation of the heart along its longitudinal axis and right ventricular conduction delay probably occur and are believed to be the major causes for the QRS changes. Myocardial hypoxemia secondary to the sudden reduction of cardiac output and relative coronary insufficiency is probably responsible for some of the repolarization abnormalities.

In the vectorcardiogram the major changes involve the initial and terminal QRS forces. The early **QRS** vectors are displaced superiorly, leftward, and posteriorly. The late vectors are displaced rightward, posteriorly, and usually superiorly. These late forces are often quite prominent and form a terminal appendage. In the majority of cases there is no evidence of a conduction delay. Occasionally, slow inscription of the terminal portion of the loop is present resembling that of right bundle branch block. The spatial T loop is displaced posteriorly, superiorly, and usually leftward. The PsÊ loop may become more vertical and increase in magnitude.

Transverse plane. In the transverse plane the entire QRS loop is rotated posteriorly. It is inscribed counterclockwise. The initial deflection is inscribed to the left and slightly anteriorly. The main body of the loop is more posterior than normal. The late part of the afferent limb and the terminal deflection form an acute angle pointing rightward and posteriorly. It is in this projection the terminal appendage appears most prominent. The magnitude of the maximum **QRS** vector is not increased, but its direction is more posterior than normal. The 0.02-sec **QRS** vector may be directed posteriorly in the absence of coronary artery disease. It is apparent that the changes of the QRS loop in this plane are not unlike those of pulmonary emphysema with chronic cor pulmonale. In our limited experience the "pointed" terminal appendage is more common in acute cor pulmonale. However, it is to be emphasized that the transient nature of these changes is most important for the recognition of acute pulmonary embolism.

The transverse plane T loop is directed posteriorly and usually leftward. It may be inscribed clockwise in this projection.

The posterior displacement of the initial deflection and efferent limb of the QRS loop correlates with the leftward displacement of the transitional zone with slow progression of the R wave in the right and mid precordial leads in the conventional electrocardiogram. The rightward and posteriorly directed terminal appendage explains the relatively deep S wave in the left precordial leads. If the terminal appendage is approaching the 0 to 180° axis, it may project on the positive side of the lead axis of V_1 and lead V_1 may then record an RsR' complex. The T-wave inversion in the right and sometimes mid precordial leads is related to the posterior and leftward orientation of the T loop.

Right sagittal plane. In the right sagittal plane the superior and posterior displacement of the early **QRS** vectors often results in a counterclockwise or figure-of-eight inscription of the QRS loop. The T loop is directed superiorly and posteriorly. It is often inscribed counterclockwise.

Frontal plane.   In the frontal plane projection the initial deflection of the QRS loop is written to the left and either horizontally or slightly superiorly. The duration of the initial superior forces, unlike that in inferior myocardial infarction, usually does not exceed 0.025 sec. The loop is inscribed either clockwise or in a figure-of-eight pattern. The terminal appendage is directed rightward and usually superiorly. The T loop is displaced superiorly and leftward.

The well known S_1Q_3 pattern in the conventional electrocardiogram in pulmonary embolism has its counterpart in the superior displacement of the initial deflection (Q_3) and the rightward orientation of the terminal QRS forces (S_1). As the superior displacement of the early forces is of lesser degree than that observed in inferior myocardial infarction, abnormal Q wave is seldom recorded in lead II although it may be present in lead aVF. T-wave inversion in the inferior leads (II, III, and aVF) is related to the superior orientation of the T loop.

REFERENCES

1. Criep LH, Siberlatt M: The effect of bronchial asthma on the heart, with special reference to the spatial vectorcardiogram. J Allergy 31:191, 1960
2. Karlen WS, Wolff L; The vectorcardiogram in pulmonary embolism. II. Am Heart J 51:839, 1956
3. Spodick DH, Hauger-Klevene JH, Tyler JM, Muench H, Dorr CA: The electrocardiogram in pulmonary emphysema. Relationship of characteristic electrocardiographic findings to severity of disease as measured by degree of airway obstruction. Am Rev Resp Dis 88:14, 1963
4. Wasserburger RH, Kelly JR, Rasmussen HK, Juhl JH: The electrocardiographic pentalogy of pulmonary emphysema. A correlation of roentgenographic findings and pulmonary function studies. Circulation 20:831, 1959
5. Wolff R: Observations on the vectorcardiographic changes in experimental and clinical pulmonary embolism, in Sasahara AA, Stein M (eds): Pulmonary Embolic Disease. New York and London, Grune & Stratton, 1965, pp 199–205

14

Wolff-Parkinson-White Syndrome

WOLFF-PARKINSON-WHITE SYNDROME

The syndrome of short P-R interval with abnormal QRS complex was first recognized as a distinct clinical entity by Wolff, Parkinson, and White, in 1930. It has also been called the *anomalous atrioventricular excitation syndrome, ventricular preexcitation syndrome*, and the *bundle of Kent syndrome*. The characteristic electrocardiographic findings include:

1. A P-R interval of 0.12 sec or less with normal P wave;
2. Abnormally wide QRS complex with a duration of 0.10 sec or more;
3. The presence of an initial slurring of the QRS complex, the delta wave;
4. Secondary ST- and T-wave changes; and
5. The frequent association of paroxysmal rapid heart action.

The widening of the QRS complex is at the expense of the P-R interval and the sum of the duration of the P-R interval, and the QRS complex remains normal. The arrhythmias are practically all supraventricular in origin with paroxysmal atrial tachycardia being most common. Atrial fibrillation and atrial flutter are less frequent.

The syndrome is most likely congenital in origin and affects individuals of all ages. Although the vast majority of the patients have no associated heart disease, the condition is observed frequently in the presence of certain congenital cardiac malformations, especially the Ebstein's anomaly. Patients with primary myocardial disease and hypertrophic subaortic stenosis also have a higher incidence of the Wolff-Parkinson-White (WPW) syndrome than the general population. The possibility that the syndrome is acquired has been proposed, but the evidence is so far rather meager. It has been observed after myocardial infarction and during cardiac catherization. Patients with thyrotoxicosis also have higher incidence of the syndrome.

It is generally agreed that premature excitation of a portion of the ventricular musculature is responsible for the electrocardiographic alterations seen in this

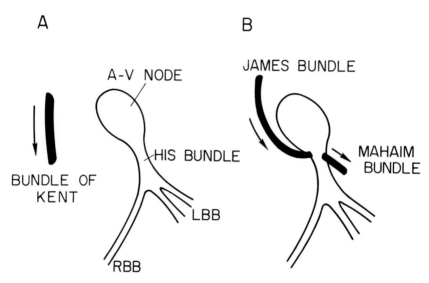

Fig. 14.1. Schematic diagrams illustrating the mechanisms proposed to explain the Wolff-Parkinson-White syndrome.

syndrome. The wide QRS complex, in fact, represents a "fusion beat." The electrical potential from the area of preexcitation inscribes the delta wave which shortens the P-R interval, and the remaining part of the QRS complex originates from the activation of the rest of the ventricles through the usual pathway. However, there is a considerable difference of opinion as to the mechanism by which the preexcitation is brought about. The most generally accepted explanation of the classical WPW syndrome assumes the presence of a lateral AV bypass or the bundle of Kent which allows the atrial impulse to bypass the AV node and activates part of the ventricle prematurely (Fig. 14.1A). Indeed, recently epicardial mapping during open-heart surgery has demonstrated such an area of ventricular preexcitation along the AV groove at the right lateral border or posterobasal region of the heart. A lateral accessory bundle has also been identified anatomically in about 50 percent of the patients with the WPW syndrome in whom a careful histologic examination has been performed. However, it is questionable whether the bundle of Kent theory is applicable in all instances. An alternative mechanism has been proposed which is based on the bypass fibers described by James and Mahaim (Fig. 14.1B). The pathway of James is a paranodal tract which bypasses the upper and central AV node where the normal AV conduction delay occurs to connect with the lower third of the node or directly with the bundle of His. The P-R interval is therefore shortened when the impulse is conducted through the James fibers. The bypass fibers of Mahaim may serve as a short direct connection between the lower AV node or the His bundle and the ventricular septum. Excitation through these fibers will result in preexcitation of the ventricular septum resulting in a delta wave. Such a combination of connections has been demonstrated anatomically in a patient with this syndrome.

    The syndrome is often intermittent, and the configuration of the WPW complex may vary from beat to beat. Occasionally the P-R interval may be within the normal limits or the QRS duration is less than 0.10 sec. Rosenbaum has classified the cases of WPW syndrome into two types. Type A includes those in which the delta wave is upright in all of the precordial leads. In type B the delta wave is predominantly downward in lead V_1 but is upright in the left precordial leads. In type A WPW complex the area of preexcitation is believed to be located in the posterobasal portion of the left ventricle; in type B, at the lateral border of the right ventricle near the AV groove. In both instances, the spread of the depolarization wave in the area of preexcitation appears to proceed from the epicardium to the endocardium. Variant forms of the WPW syndrome have also been described. In the Lown-Ganong-Levine (LGL) syndrome the P-R interval is shortened, but the QRS complex is normal. The accelerated AV conduction may be the result of AV nodal bypass through the James fibers. In other patients the P-R interval is normal but a delta wave is present. Under this circumstance the atrial impulse may travel through the AV node in the normal fashion but the abnormal ventricular excitation occurs because of the presence of Mahaim fibers.

Vectorcardiographic Findings

The atrial depolarization is not altered in the WPW syndrome. The PsÊ loop is therefore normal. The shortening of the P-R interval is usually difficult to recognize in the vectorcardiogram. The electronic beam remains stationary during the period of the P-R segment and its duration is thus difficult to ascertain. Occasionally, the QRSsÊ loop may follow the PsÊ loop directly without any interruption.

The changes in the QRSsÊ loop are most characteristic, and the diagnosis is based primarily on the slowly inscribed initial portion of the loop representing the delta vectors—the delta deflection. The duration of the delta deflection usually ranges from 0.02 to 0.07 sec. The course of the remaining portion of the QRSsÊ loop is also altered. The magnitude of the maximum spatial **QRS** vector may be abnormally large in the absence of ventricular hypertrophy. The total duration of the QRS loop is increased. Secondary TsÊ loop changes are often observed. Depending on the direction of the delta deflection in the transverse plane projection, the vectorcardiogram in the WPW syndrome may likewise be classified into two types, types A and B. They are equivalent to the electrocardiographic classification proposed by Rosenbaum.

Type A WPW Syndrome (Figs. 14.2–14.5)

Transverse plane. In type A WPW syndrome, as stated previously, the ventricular preexcitation probably begins at the epicardium of the posterobasal region of the left ventricle and spreads anteriorly. Therefore, the vectors representing the potential of the abnormal depolarization process are oriented similarly. In the transverse plane the general direction of the delta deflection is anterior, either to the left or slightly to the right. Most of its component vectors are anterior to 25°. The entire QRS loop is also displaced anteriorly with the maximum **QRS** vector located in the left anterior quadrant. The direction of inscription of the loop is usually counterclockwise, although a figure-of-eight pattern is occasionally seen.

The direction and magnitude of the T loop and its maximum vector vary a great deal and may or may not be within the normal range. An anterior and rightward orientation of the maximum **T** vector is, however, rare. The direction of inscription of the T loop is usually clockwise which is abnormal.

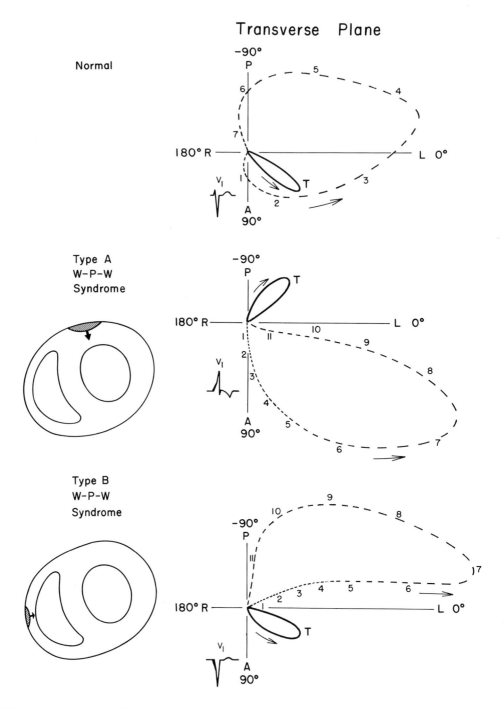

Fig. 14.2. Schematic diagrams illustrating the area of preexcitation and the direction of its representative vector in type A and B Wolff-Parkinson-White syndrome. Their transverse plane vectorcardiograms are compared with that of the normal individual. The scalar QRS-T complexes in lead V_1 are also shown.

The anterior orientation of the delta deflection and the remainder of the QRS loop in type A WPW syndrome is the counterpart of the upward inscription of the delta wave and the rest of the QRS complex seen in all of the precordial leads of the conventional electrocardiogram. Since the orientation of the T loop is variable, the T wave may therefore be either upright or inverted and either concordant or discordant to the QRS complex. The equivalent of the abnormal sense of rotation of the T loop is difficult to recognize in the routine scalar leads.

Right sagittal plane. In the right sagittal projection the anterior orientation of the slowly inscribed delta deflection is also demonstrated. It may be directed superiorly or inferiorly. The QRS loop is usually inscribed clockwise with the great majority of the loop area located anteriorly. The T loop is usually directed inferiorly and is inscribed counterclockwise.

Frontal plane. In the frontal plane projection the orientation of the delta deflection varies a great deal but usually is to the left, either superiorly or inferiorly. The direction of the inscription of the QRS loop may be either clockwise or counterclockwise, or the loop may present a figure-of-eight pattern. Most of the loop area is located to the left. When the delta deflection is directed superiorly and the loop is inscribed clockwise, an erroneous diagnosis of inferior wall myocardial infarction may be made if the initial conduction abnormalities are not realized. The direction of the T loop scatters rather widely but is inferior in most of the cases. It may rotate either clockwise or counterclockwise.

In the limb leads of the conventional electrocardiogram the delta wave may be either upright or downward in any given lead and is related to the variable orientation of the delta deflection in the vectorcardiogram. The T wave is usually upright in the inferior leads since the T loop is directed inferiorly in most instances.

Type B WPW Syndrome (Figs. 14.2, 14.6 and 14.7)

Transverse plane. In type B WPW syndrome the ventricular preexcitation probably begins at the epicardium of the basal portion of the right ventricle at its lateral border, and the impulse spreads in a generally right-to-left direction. The delta deflection is therefore oriented to the left, usually posteriorly, but sometimes slightly anteriorly. Most of the component vectors of the delta deflection are posterior to 25°. The rotation of the QRS loop is quite variable. The majority of the loop area is located to the left with the maximum QRS vector oriented in a direction similar to that of the delta deflection.

The direction of the T loop and its maximum vector is widely scattered. The T loop may be located in any one of the four quadrants. In contrast to type A WPW syndrome, the transverse plane T loop in type B is usually inscribed counter-clockwise.

The predominantly downward inscription of the delta wave in the precordial lead V_1 of the conventional electrocardiogram is related to the leftward and essentially posterior orientation of the delta deflection. Most of the component delta vectors are projected on the negative side of the lead axis of lead V_1. The delta wave, as well as the rest of the QRS complex, is upright in the left precordial leads since the vectors project on the positive side of the lead axis of these leads. The variable

E.B. VCG 1341 age 43

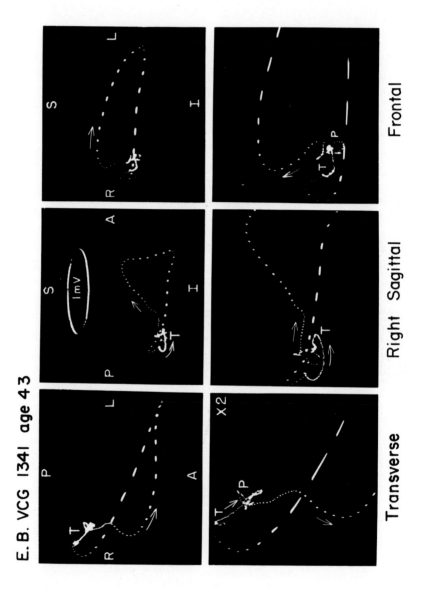

Frontal   Right Sagittal   Transverse

288

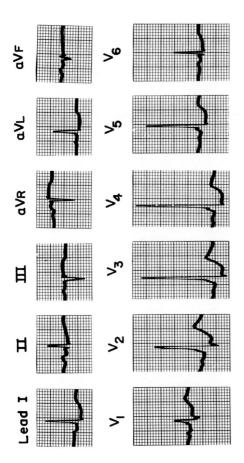

Fig. 14.3. Type A Wolff-Parkinson-White syndrome. The vectorcardiogram and electrocardiogram were recorded from a 43-year-old man who has a history of repeated episodes of tachycardia. Examination shows no other evidence of heart disease. Note most of the slowly inscribed initial portion of the QRS loop, the delta deflection, is directed anteriorly and superiorly. There is an abnormal ST vector, the direction of which is opposite to that of the delta deflection. The T loop is small and is inscribed clockwise in the transverse plane and counterclockwise in the right sagittal plane.

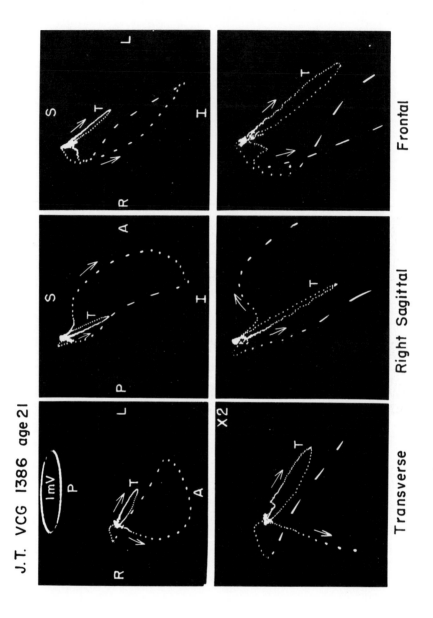

J.T. VCG 1386 age 21

Transverse   Right Sagittal   Frontal

290

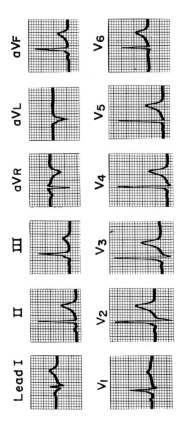

Fig. 14.4. Type A Wolff-Parkinson-White syndrome in a 21-year-old otherwise normal woman. The duration of the delta deflection is 0.028 sec. Although the magnitude and direction of the T loop is normal in all the planar projections, its direction of inscription is the reverse of the normal in the transverse and sagittal planes.

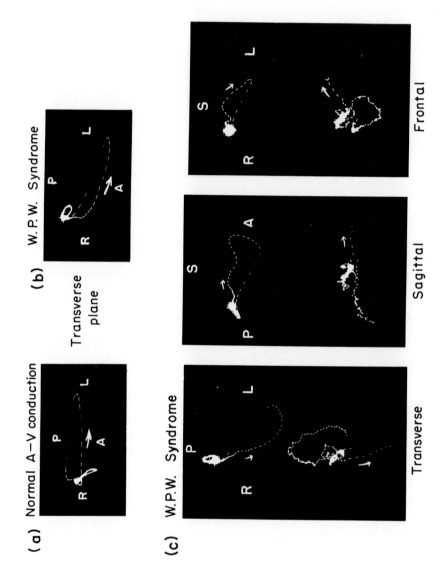

(a) Normal A–V conduction

(b) W.P.W. Syndrome

Transverse plane

(c) W.P.W. Syndrome

Transverse   Sagittal   Frontal

292

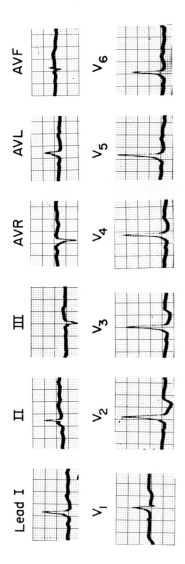

Fig. 14.5. Intermittent type A Wolff-Parkinson-White syndrome with normal P-R interval: (a) and (b) transverse plane vectorcardiogram recorded within a period of a few minitues. (a) Normal AV conduction, and (b) Type A WPW syndrome. (c) Vectorcardiogram and electrocardiogram recorded on the same patient a few days later. The P-R interval is normal (0.15 sec). Note that the transverse plane vectorcardiogram is different from that in (b).

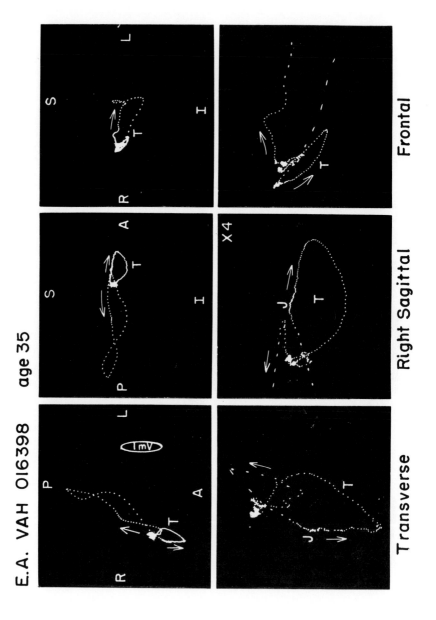

E.A. VAH OI6398   age 35

Frontal

Right Sagittal

Transverse

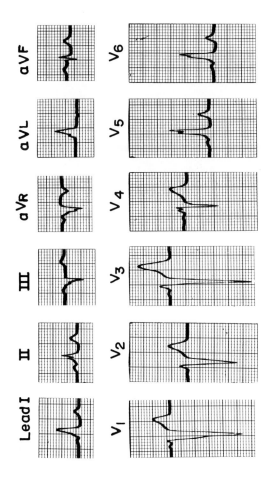

Fig. 14.6. Type B Wolff-Parkinson-White syndrome in a 35-year-old healthy man. Note most of the delta deflection is oriented to the left, posteriorly and more or less horizontally. The direction of the **ST** vector is opposite to that of the delta deflection. The T loop is inscribed counterclockwise in the transverse plane and clockwise in the right sagittal plane.

295

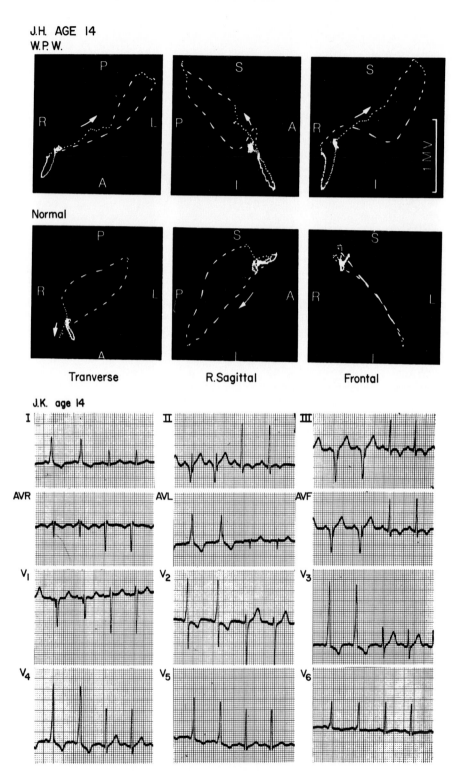

Fig. 14.7. Intermittent type B Wolff-Parkinson-White syndrome. The patient is a 14-year-old boy with no clinical evidence of heart disease. Note the leftward, posterior and superior orientation of the delta deflection during the WPW syndrome. During normal AV conduction the T loop is directed superiorly. The cause of the repolarization abnormalities is unknown.

orientation of the T loop is seen in the precordial leads as a T wave of different polarities. The T wave may be either concordant or discordant to the QRS complex

Right sagittal plane.   The orientation of the delta deflection is widely scattered in this projection. The remaining portion of the QRS loop likewise does not present any specific pattern. The direction of the T loop is also variable, but it is usually inscribed clockwise.

Frontal plane.   In the frontal plane projection the delta deflection and the rest of the QRS loop are oriented to the left, either superiorly or inferiorly. The loop may be inscribed clockwise, counterclockwise, or present a figure-of-eight pattern. The orientation of the T loop is variable, and its direction of inscription is usually counterclockwise.

In the conventional electrocardiogram lead I records an upward delta wave and QRS complex since the vectors are directed leftward. The inferior leads may reveal either upward or downward complexes. When the delta deflection is directed superiorly, a wide Q wave is recorded in the inferior leads and may lead to the erroneous diagnosis of inferior myocardial infarction.

REFERENCES

1. Bleifer S, Kahn M, Grishman A, Donoso E: Wolff-Parkinson-White syndrome. A vectorcardiographic electrocardiographic and clinical study. Am J Cardiol 4:321, 1959
2. Boineau JP, Moore EN: Evidence for propagation of activation across an accessory atrioventricular connection in types A and B pre-excitation. Circulation 41:375, 1970
3. Burch GE, DePasquale NP: Electrocardiographic and vectorcardiographic detection of heart disease in the presence of the pre-excitation syndrome (Wolff-Parkinson-White syndrome). Ann Intern Med 54:387, 1961
4. Burchell HB, Frye RL, Anderson MW, McGoon DC: Atrioventricular and ventriculoatrial excitation in Wolff-Parkinson-White syndrome (type B). Temporary ablation at surgery. Circulation 36:663, 1967
5. Chung K-Y, Walsh TJ, Massie E: Wolff-Parkinson-White syndrome. Am Heart J 69:116, 1965
6. Durrer D, Roos JP: Epicardial excitation of the ventricles in a patient with Wolff-Parkinson-White syndrome (type B). Circulation 35:15, 1967
7. Durrer D, Schuilenburg RM, Wellens HJJ: Preexcitation revisited. Am J Cardiol 25:690, 1970
8. Ferrer MI: New concepts relating to the preexcitation syndrome. JAMA 01:162, 1967
9. Hecht HH (moderator), Kennamer R, Prinzmetal M, Rosenbaum FF, SodiPallares D, Wolff L, Brooks C, Pick A, Rijlant P, Robb JS: Anomalous atrioventricular excitation: panel discussion. Ann NY Acad Sci 65:826, 1956–1957
10. Lister JW, Worthington FX Jr, Gentsch TO, Swenson JA, Nathan DA, Gosselin AJ: Preexcitation and tachycardias in Wolff-Parkinson-White syndrome, type B. A case report. Circulation 45:1081, 1972
11. Preston TA, Kirsh MM: Permanent pacing of the left atrium for treatment of WPW tachycardia. Circulation 42:1073, 1970
12. Wolff L, Richman JL: The diagnosis of myocardial infarction in patients with anomalous atrioventricular excitation (Wolff-Parkinson-White syndrome). Am Heart J 45:545, 1953

SECTION II

Pediatric Aspects

INTRODUCTION

One of our purposes in Section II is to describe and evaluate for the internist the contribution of vectorcardiography to the diagnosis of heart disease in the pediatric age group. It is mandatory to appreciate that the evolution of the vectorcardiogram in the normal growing child is a dynamic process characterized primarily by slow regression of right ventricular dominance and concomitant progression of left ventricular dominance. This appreciation will allow separation of the normal from the abnormal ventricular hypertrophy. In our experience, analysis of vectorcardiograms has been helpful in supplementive evaluation and understanding of scalar electrocardiograms associated with specific congenital heart diseases. In many instances, analysis of the vector loops has alerted the clinician to features which may be unusual or incompatible with the working clinical diagnosis.

The evolution of medical and surgical management of congenital heart disease has resulted in the development of a cadre of patients who have reached adolescence or early adult life. Another of our purposes is to identify vectorcardiographic abnormalities which are present in many of these patients who have had excellent symptomatic improvement from surgical correction of the congenital cardiac anomaly.

Attempts to correlate the abnormal hemodynamic load in the heart with the changes in the vectorcardiogram have also been helpful. Since these changes result in varying combinations of cardiac chamber hypertrophy and dilatation, we will make free reference to the vectorcardiographic analysis of the various types of ventricular enlargement described in earlier sections of this text. We will amplify these analyses when specific diseases produce unusual changes in the younger age group.

TRANSVERSE   RT. SAGITTAL   FRONTAL

AGE

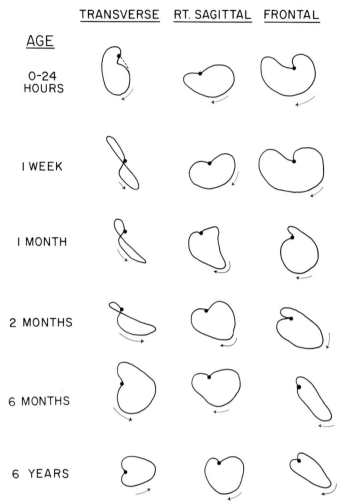

0-24
HOURS

I WEEK

I MONTH

2 MONTHS

6 MONTHS

6 YEARS

Fig. A.1. Schematic diagrams to illustrate the evolution of the QRS loop in the normal full-term infant and child. In the first 24 hr of life, right ventricular dominance is expressed by rightward and anterior forces with a clockwise transverse loop. The initial forces in about half of normal babies are leftward and anterior in the transverse plane (shown by the dotted line). A gradual and progressive increase in leftward and posterior forces and decrease in rightward and anterior forces is associated with the development of normal left ventricular dominance and regression of the normal right ventricular forces of the neonate.

EVOLUTION OF THE NORMAL VECTORCARDIOGRAM

The Full Term Infant (Figs. A.1–A.6)

In the fetus at term the vascular resistance of the pulmonary circulation is higher than that in the systemic circulation. Thus, the intrauterine work of the heart results in nearly equal right and left ventricular mass. The ratio of the weight of the right ventricle to that of the left ventricle in the normal full-term infant is approximately 1.1 to 1.3. Immediately after birth, dramatic changes occur in the circulation. Systemic vascular resistance rises when the placental circulation is eliminated and pulmonary vascular resistance falls when the lungs expand. These profound changes do not occur instantaneously, but are effected over a period of hours or days.

These anatomic and hemodynamic changes are reflected in the QRS loop of the normal neonate (Figs. A.1 to A.3). The normal right ventricular dominance is expressed by rightward and anterior forces with a clockwise inscription of the

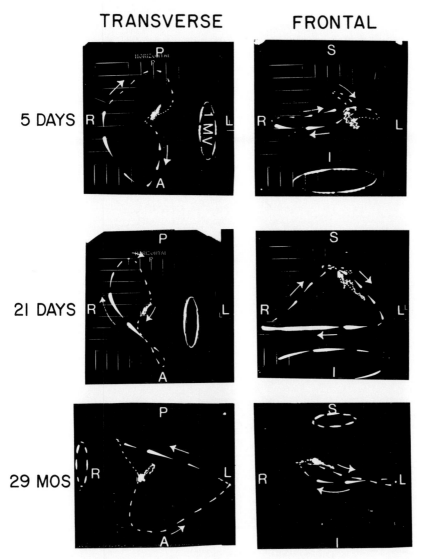

Fig. A.2. Vectorcardiograms in the same normal child at age 5 days, 21 days, and 29 months, which illustrate right ventricular dominance at age 5 days and evolution of progressive left ventricular forces to normal at age 29 months. Ellipse in each vectorcardiographic reproduction indicates a 1-mV signal. Corresponding electrocardiograms are shown in Fig. A.3.

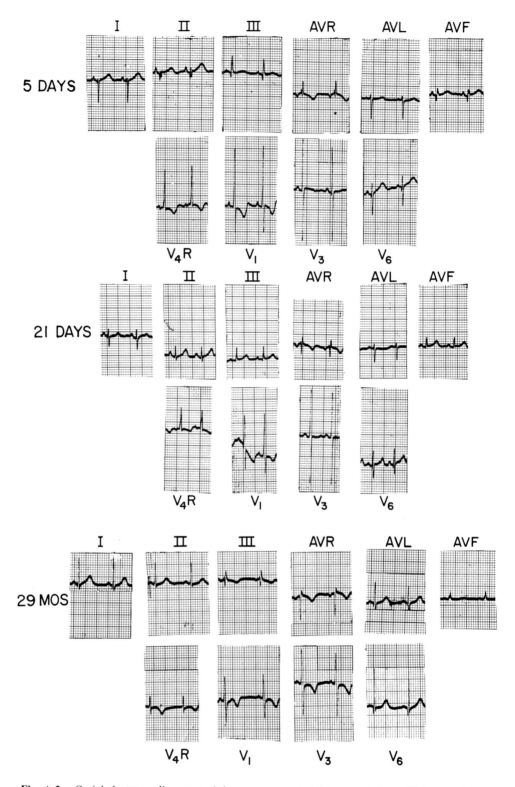

Fig. A.3. Serial electrocardiograms of the same normal child at age 5 days, 21 days, and 29 months. These tracings demonstrate the normal progression from right axis deviation and right ventricular dominance to normal axis deviation and left ventricular dominance. The corresponding vectorcardiograms are shown in Fig. A.2.

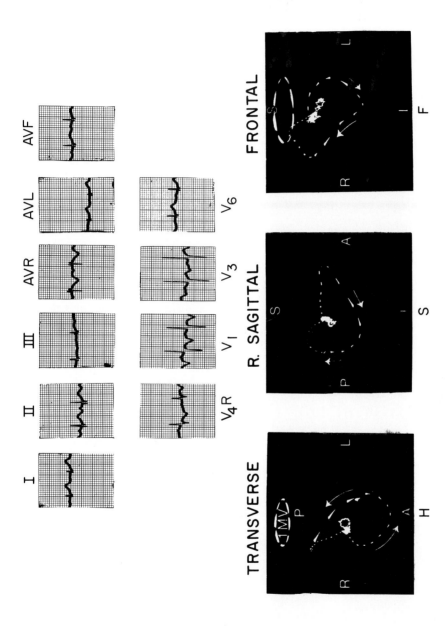

Fig. A.4. Electrocardiogram and vectorcardiogram of normal 21-month-old baby.

transverse loop. However, in about half of normal neonates in the first day of life, the initial forces in the transverse plane are leftward and anterior. During the first few months of life, there is a gradual and progressive decrease in rightward and anterior forces with a concomitant increase in posterior and leftward forces. During this time, but especially in the first months of life, the loop in the transverse plane is variable and may become narrow and counterclockwise, narrow and clockwise, or show a figure-of-eight configuration. Eventually, and usually by the age of 2 months, the transverse loop is open, counterclockwise, and directed to the left and anteriorly. Left ventricular dominance is usual by the age of 6 months so that the transverse loop is leftward and inscribed in a counterclockwise manner. The precordial leads of the scalar electrocardiogram reflect these changes. The right precordial leads show a monophasic R wave or an R/S ratio greater than 1 with an rS complex in V in early life. This lack of right-to-left progression of the precordial R wave is characteristic in the normal infant and differs significantly from the normal adult pattern (Figs. A.4 to A.6).

The Premature Infant (Figs. A.7–A.8)

The circulatory changes in the premature infant after birth may differ significantly from that of the full-term baby, in that the fall of pulmonary vascular

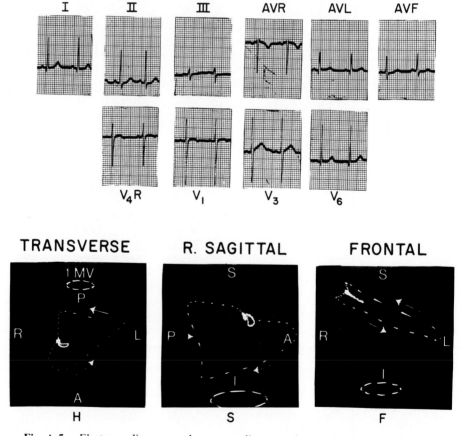

Fig. A.5. Electrocardiogram and vectorcardiogram of normal 6-year-old child.

resistance is frequently more rapid in these immature babies (Figs. A.7 and A.8). Also, the significant right ventricular dominance which develops in late intrauterine life may not have occurred in the very premature babies. These hemodynamic changes are reflected in the vectorcardiogram of the normal premature infant. At birth, the QRS voltage is low, and the transverse loop is frequently inscribed counterclockwise with prominent leftward forces. These dominant leftward forces progress to the normal "adult" pattern without signs of right ventricular dominance. The precordial leads of the scalar electrocardiogram reflect these findings and show an R/S ratio equal to or less than 1 in V_1, and a well-defined qR complex in V_6. However, there is marked variability especially in the first week of life. In some premature babies the QRS loop is indistinguishable from that found in the full-term baby which is characterized by right ventricular dominance.

RIGHT VENTRICULAR VOLUME OVERLOAD

Left-to-right shunting of blood with resultant volume overload of the right ventricle may occur with normal pulmonary arterial pressures or with varying degrees of pulmonary hypertension and increased pulmonary vascular resistance.

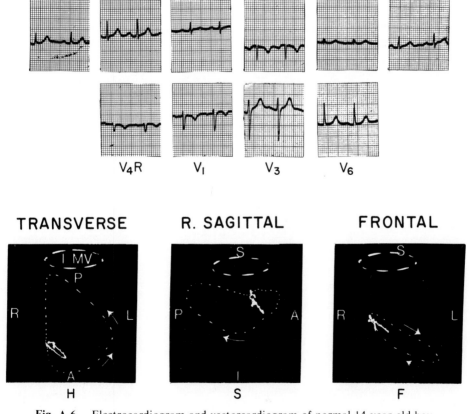

Fig. A.6. Electrocardiogram and vectorcardiogram of normal 14-year-old boy.

PREMATURE INFANT

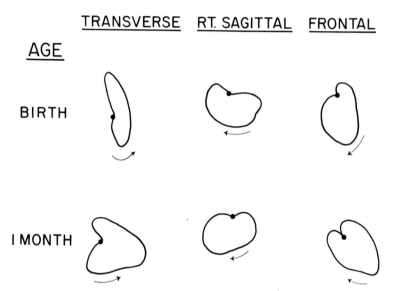

TRANSVERSE   RT. SAGITTAL   FRONTAL

AGE

BIRTH

I MONTH

Fig. A.7. Schematic drawing to illustrate evolution of the QRS loop in a premature infant who was otherwise normal (Compare with full-term infant shown in Fig. A.1). Prominent leftward forces with a counterclockwise transverse loop is present at birth and this may progress to the normal "adult" pattern at age 1 month. However, in some premature infants the QRS loop simulates that seen in the full-term baby (Fig. A.1) which is characterized by right ventricular dominance.

Atrial septal defects of the ostium secundum and ostium primum types and partial anomalous pulmonary venous return are classic examples of right ventricular volume overload with normal pulmonary arterial pressures and resistances. These conditions contrast with total anomalous venous return and with complete atrioventricular canal which are frequently associated with significant elevation of pulmonary vascular resistance. Pulmonary valvular incompetence resulting in right ventricular volume overload in childhood is most frequently encountered after surgical relief of right ventricular outflow obstruction or after many years of extreme elevation of pulmonary vascular resistance. These conditions are discussed under systolic overload of the right ventricle. Tricuspid incompetence resulting in right ventricular volume overload is uncommon in the pediatric age group, although this is seen occasionally with Ebstein's malformation, in neonates with normal hearts and after right ventriculotomy.

Atrial Septal Defects

In atrial septal defect, with or without partial anomalous venous return, the left-to-right shunting of blood results in volume overload of the right ventricle which becomes dilated and hypertrophied. In the majority of the cases investigators believe that the hypertrophy involves primarily the outflow tract of the right ventricle. When pulmonary hypertension is present, there is additional pressure overload of the right ventricle and right ventricular hypertrophy will be more severe and generalized. The vectorcardiogram and electrocardiogram are usually quite useful in establishing the diagnosis, and they are especially valuable for the differentiation between the ostium secundum and the ostium primum type of the defect.

Ostium Secundum Defect (Figs. A.9-A.11)

In a small percentage of the patients the PsÊ loop is suggestive of right atrial enlargement. The magnitude of the maximum **P** vector is increased and the loop is displaced anteriorly. The QRSsÊ loop is abnormal in the great majority of cases. The most consistent finding is the rightward and anterior displacement of the late portion of the loop. Most of the spatial loop is located inferiorly. The duration of the QRSsÊ loop may be increased and may occasionally exceed 0.12 sec. Slow inscription of the terminal deflection indicating a conduction delay may or may not

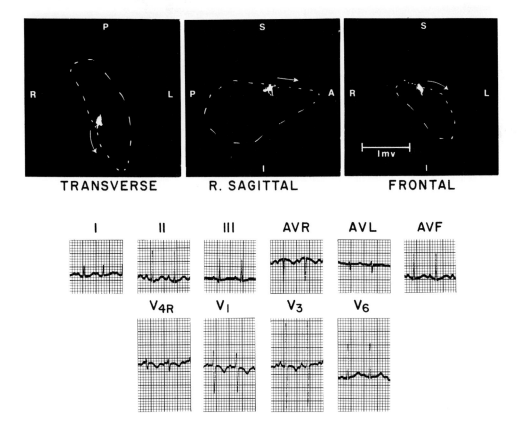

Fig. A.8. Premature infant. He weighed 2100 gm. and was 6 weeks old at the time these vectorcardiograms and electrocardiograms were obtained. His cardiovascular system was normal clinically. Left ventricular dominance with a counterclockwise transverse loop and prominent leftward forces contrast with the right ventricular dominance of the normal full-term infant (compare with Fig. A.2).

Atrial Septal Defect

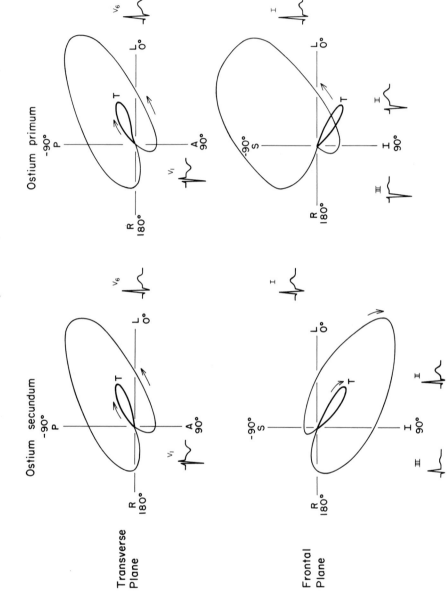

Fig. A.9. Schematic diagrams illustrating the changes in the transverse and frontal plane QRS and T loops in the ostium secundum and ostium primum types of atrial septal defect.

be observed. The TsÊ loop is usually directed to the left and may be anterior or posterior, inferior or superior, and is more or less opposite to the terminal **QRS** vectors. The **ST** vector, if present, is usually small.

Transverse Plane. In the transverse plane projection the configuration of the QRS loop varies, depending primarily on the degree of the anterior and rightward displacement of the loop and the length of the segment involved. Most commonly, the alteration is limited to the terminal deflection and the later portion of the afferent limb. An appendage-like protrusion is seen in the right posterior or right anterior quadrant. The direction of inscription of the loop remains counterclockwise. Thus, the changes are essentially those observed in type C right ventricular hypertrophy described in Chapter 7 of Section I. When the displacement of the afferent limb is marked, a figure-of-eight or clockwise loop will be seen which is consistent with type A right ventricular hypertrophy. However, in either case, abnormal terminal slowing of the inscription of the loop may also be present to suggest a right ventricular conduction defect. When the configuration of the QRS loop is correlated with the hemodynamic data, a counterclockwise loop is usually observed in patients whose pulmonary arterial pressure is relatively normal, and a clockwise loop in patients with moderate or severe degree of pulmonary hypertension. Exceptions, however, do occur.

The T loop is usually directed to the left, either anteriorly or, more commonly, posteriorly. The direction of inscription of the loop is clockwise in the great majority of patients.

The anterior and rightward displacement of the late **QRS** vectors is manifested in lead V_1 of the conventional electrocardiogram as a secondary R wave (R'). These vectors now project on the positive side of the lead axis of V_1. An RSR' (or rSr', RSr', rSR') complex is, therefore, the most common and typical pattern seen in atrial septal defect. The width of the R' varies and depends on the presence or absence of terminal conduction delay. The magnitude of the R' correlates with the degree of displacement of the terminal vectors and in the absence of marked conduction delay often, but not necessarily, reflects the severity of the right ventricular hypertrophy. The RSR' pattern may be recorded in lead V_1 with either a counterclockwise or a clockwise loop. It is usually difficult to predict the direction of inscription of the loop from the scalar lead unless multiple precordial leads are taken simultaneously. An S wave is recorded in the left precordial leads and is the equivalent of the R in lead V_1. The T wave is usually inverted in lead V_1 and upright in leads V_5 and V_6, as the T loop is directed to the left and usually is posterior to 25°.

Right sagittal plane. In the right sagittal projection most of the QRS loop is oriented inferiorly, either anteriorly or posteriorly. The loop is usually inscribed clockwise or presents a figure-of-eight pattern. A counterclockwise inscription of the loop is occasionally observed. A terminal conduction delay may or may not be present. The orientation of the T loop varies, but the direction of inscription is quite consistently counterclockwise.

Frontal plane. The QRS loop in the frontal plane projection is most helpful in the differentiation of the ostium secundum from the ostium primum type of defect. In the secundum type most of the loop is located inferiorly and the maximum **QRS**

J. R. age 19 ♂

Transverse   Sagittal   Frontal

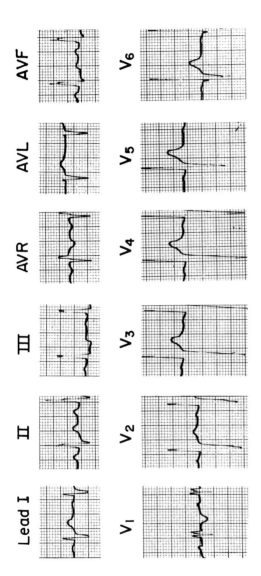

Fig. A.10. Atrial septal defect, secundum type. The patient is 19 years old and the diagnosis was confirmed at surgery. The pulmonary arterial pressure was normal. In the vectorcardiogram the transverse and frontal plane QRS loops reveal abnormally large rightward terminal vectors. Some terminal conduction delay is present. The loop is inscribed counterclockwise in the transverse plane and clockwise in the frontal plane. Note the counterclockwise T loop in the right sagittal plane. The electrocardiogram presents the typical RSR pattern in lead V_1. (In this illustration each dash in the vectorcardiogram represents 2.5 msec instead of the usual 2.0 msec.)

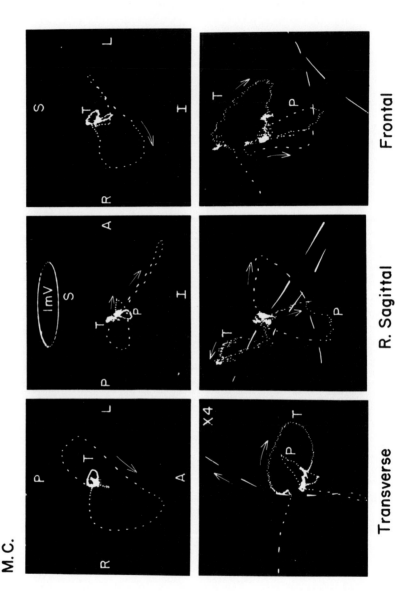

M.C.

Transverse

R. Sagittal

Frontal

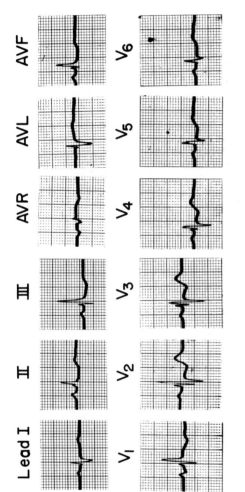

Fig. A.11. Atrial septal defect, secundum type. The vectorcardiogram and electrocardiogram were recorded from a 56-year-old woman. The diagnosis of secundum type of atrial septal defect was proved at surgery. Her pulmonary arterial pressure was 60/15 mm Hg. In the vectorcardiogram the transverse plane QRS loop is inscribed clockwise. There is no evidence of a terminal conduction delay. The vectorcardiographic findings are consistent with type A right ventricular hypertrophy.

vector is below the 0 to 180° axis. The loop is inscribed clockwise even though a figure-of-eight pattern is occasionally seen. It is often abnormally wide owing to the rightward displacement of the afferent limb and the terminal deflection. The T loop is usually directed to the left and is more commonly inferior. It is inscribed clockwise.

In the conventional electrocardiogram an S wave is recorded in lead I because of the increased terminal rightward forces. It may be wide if terminal conduction delay is present. The T wave in lead I is upright as the T loop is oriented to the left. Since most of the loop area and the maximum **QRS** vector are oriented inferiorly, the inferior leads (leads II, III, and aVF) display predominantly upright deflections.

Ostium Primum Defect (Figs. A.9 and A.12).

The vectorcardiogram in ostium primum defect differs from that of the secundum type mainly in that the spatial QRS loop is directed superiorly. In the transverse plane projection the findings are rather similar, since pulmonary arterial pressures and resistances are usually normal. In the sagittal plane the superiorly oriented QRS loop may be inscribed clockwise or counterclockwise or presents a figure-of-eight pattern. The T loop is usually directed inferiorly, either anteriorly or posteriorly. The direction of inscription is usually counterclockwise.

In the frontal plane the changes in the QRS loop are quite characteristic. It is displaced superiorly with the majority of the loop and the maximum **QRS** vector located above the 0° to 180° axis. The direction of inscription of the loop is counterclockwise. The T loop is oriented to the left and inferiorly and may be inscribed either clockwise or counterclockwise. In the conventional electrocardiogram lead I displays an RS complex similar to that in the secundum defect. However, because of the superior orientation of the QRS loop and the maximum **QRS** vector, the inferior leads display a predominantly downward (rS) deflection.

These vectorcardiographic findings occur in more than 95 percent of ostium primum defects, but are not specific for this disease. About 15 percent of isolated simple ventricular septal defects have a counterclockwise and largely superior loop in the frontal plane and the differentiation of this condition from ostium primum defects generally depends on the interpretation of left ventriculograms. These vectorcardiographic findings are also present in tricuspid atresia, in some instances of complete transposition of the great arteries, double outlet right ventricle, ventricular inversion (L-transposition), single ventricle, patent ductus arteriosus, coarctation of the aorta and occasionally in valvular pulmonic stenosis.

The genesis of the vectorcardiographic and electrocardiographic patterns in ostium primum defects has been attributed to the presence of a left ventricular conduction defect. Durrer and associates have demonstrated in surgical patients early excitation of the posterobasal region of the left ventricle. They believe that the prominent leftward and superior forces are originated from the lateral and anterior parts of the left ventricle, being no longer opposed by the potential from the posterobasal wall which was depolarized prematurely.

Common Atrioventricular Canal (Fig. A.13)

The major hemodynamic abnormalities of this complicated defect are large left-to-right shunt at both ventricular and atrial levels, atrioventricular valve incompet-

P.A. 434119

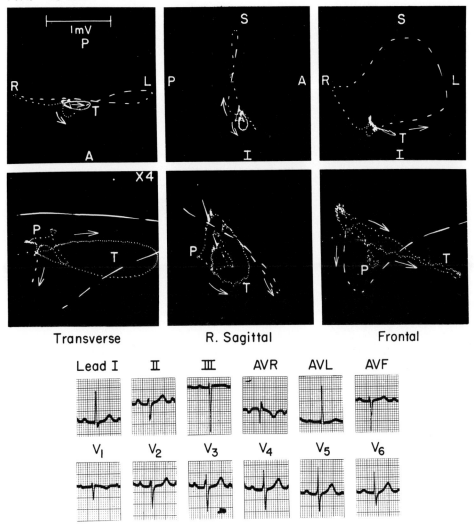

Transverse   R. Sagittal   Frontal

Lead I   II   III   AVR   AVL   AVF

V_1 V_2 V_3 V_4 V_5 V_6

Fig. A.12. Atrial septal defect, primum type. The vectorcardiogram and electrocardiogram were recorded from a 22-year-old woman, and the diagnosis of a primum defect was confirmed at surgery. The pulmonary arterial pressure was normal. In the transverse plane of the vectorcardiogram a large rightward terminal deflection is present. However, an R is not recorded in lead V_1 of the electrocardiogram. This may be explained by the fact that the terminal deflection is more or less perpendicular to the lead axis of V_1. Note the characteristic superior orientation of the QRS loop in the right sagittal and frontal planes; the loop is inscribed counterclockwise in the latter projection. There is no evidence of a terminal conduction delay.

315

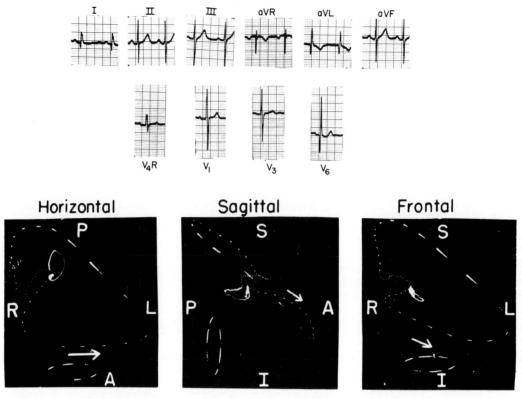

Fig. A.13. Common atrioventricular canal with large left-to-right shunt and elevated pulmonary vascular resistance. The large QRS voltages in the transverse plane with very prominent anterior and leftward forces are attributed to biventricular hypertrophy. The frontal QRS loop is counterclockwise and a major part of loop is superior in the frontal and right sagittal planes. Terminal slowing is present. The electrocardiogram shows a prolonged P-R interval. The positive T waves in V_4R and V_1 are caused by right ventricular hypertrophy. Ellipse in each vectorcardiogram is a 1-mV signal.

ence and left ventricular right atrial shunts. Peak pulmonary arterial pressures reach systemic levels early in life, but left-to-right shunts dominate because pulmonary vascular resistance is less than systemic. With progress of the disease and extreme elevation of pulmonary vascular resistance, bidirectional shunting occurs with resultant hypoxemia.

The vectorcardiograms are similar to those described under ostium primum defect, but with the additional finding of significant right ventricular hypertrophy. This is associated with the classic superiorly oriented, counterclockwise frontal QRS loop. Signs of left ventricular hypertrophy may be superimposed, but these are not always striking even in the presence of significant mitral regurgitation or persistence of a torrential pulmonary blood flow.

RIGHT VENTRICULAR PRESSURE OVERLOAD

Valvular Pulmonic Stenosis

The severity of obstruction to right ventricular outflow can usually be estimated by analysis of the vectorcardiographic changes. This applies particularly to patients with *severe obstruction* (right ventricular peak systolic pressures greater than 100 mm Hg), who generally show signs of type A right ventricular hypertrophy (Chapter 7, Section I). In patients with *moderate obstruction* (right ventricular peak systolic pressures between 50 to 100 mm Hg), type B or C right ventricular hypertrophy are usually present. This implies that with increasing right ventricular peak systolic pressure the QRS loop in the transverse plane becomes progressively more anterior and rightward. However, there are many exceptions to the above generalities. In about one-fifth of patients with severe obstruction, the QRS loop in the transverse plane is inscribed in a counterclockwise direction but rightward forces remain prominent. Also, many patients with moderate obstructions have a clockwise transverse loop of type A right ventricular hypertrophy. Ellison and Restieaux consider that the increase in right maximum spatial voltage is more reliable in assessing the degree of severity of pulmonic stenosis.

Concomitant signs of right atrial enlargement are present in some patients with severe obstruction (Chapter 12, Section I). The T loop is normal in most children, being directed leftward inferiorly and slightly anteriorly. An upright T wave in the right precordial leads of the scalar electrocardiogram is found frequently in children with right ventricular hypertrophy, which is associated with an anterior T loop.

The vectorcardiogram is variable in patients with *mild obstruction* (peak right ventricular systolic pressure of less than 50 mm Hg). Generally rightward and anterior forces are prominent, but the normal counterclockwise inscription is maintained in the transverse plane. However, a significant number of patients have vectorcardiographic signs simulating those seen in ostium secundum atrial septal defect with abnormally large rightward terminal vectors and a rSR' pattern in the right precordial electrocardiographic leads.

Regression of signs of right ventricular hypertrophy *after surgery* occur slowly even after adequate valvotomy. Some patients with type A right ventricular hypertrophy show a decrease in rightward and anterior forces and the direction of inscription of the QRS loop in the transverse plane becomes counterclockwise. Although vectorcardiographic signs of right ventricular hypertrophy may regress completely, some patients retain signs of significant hypertrophy even though the gradient across the pulmonic valve has almost been abolished.

A minority of patients with isolated valvular pulmonic stenosis require infundibulectomy in addition to valvotomy because of associated infundibular obstruction. These patients frequently develop signs of complete right bundle branch block postoperatively. These postoperative signs are described under tetralogy of Fallot.

Pulmonary Arterial Branch Stenosis (Fig. 7.5)

The vectorcardiographic signs of isolated pulmonary arterial branch stenosis depend on the severity of obstruction and therefore closely simulate those described above under valvular pulmonic stenosis. Since pulmonary arterial branch stenosis is frequently associated with other congenital anomalies, the vectorcardiographic signs depend on the dominating lesion. The most common associated abnormalities include patent ductus arteriosus (as seen in congenital rubella), pulmonary valvular stenosis, tetralogy of Fallot, ostium secundum atrial septal defect, and supravalvular aortic stenosis. When the associated anomaly results in right ventricular hypertrophy, signs of superimposed pulmonary arterial branch stenosis are not detectable by the vectorcardiogram. However, an associated large patent ductus arteriosus may result in signs of biventricular hypertrophy. Frequently these patients have left ventricular dominance, and signs of mild right ventricular hypertrophy are masked. The syndrome of combined pulmonary arterial branch stenosis and supravalvular aortic stenosis usually results in biventricular hypertrophy, but the vectorcardiogram may show signs of isolated right ventricular hypertrophy even in the presence of severe supraaortic obstruction.

Tetralogy of Fallot (Figs. 7.4, A.14–A.16)

A specific combination of ventricular septal defect and pulmonic stenosis comprises the tetralogy of Fallot. The ventricular septal defect is large and the pulmonic stenosis is severe, so that both ventricles have near equal peak systolic pressures. The shunt across the ventricular septum is bidirectional or exclusively from right to left. These hemodynamics result in marked right ventricular hypertrophy. The left ventricle is either normal or small because of decreased pulmonary blood flow which results in diminution of venous return to the left ventricle. Ventricular septal defect with pulmonic stenosis and exclusive left-to-right shunt, the so called pink tetralogy is discussed under ventricular septal defect.

Type A right ventricular hypertrophy is the classic vectorcardiographic finding in patients with severe cyanotic tetralogy of Fallot prior to surgery. These signs are found in all age groups including infants. The transverse QRS loop is clockwise and displaced anteriorly and to the right (see Fig. 7.4). The initial forces may be directed normally or leftward and anteriorly. Patients with less severe right ventricular outflow obstruction and larger pulmonary blood flow may still retain signs of type A right ventricular hypertrophy. However, others in this group show a counterclockwise transverse QRS loop of type B right ventricular hypertrophy. The frontal plane loop is usually inscribed clockwise and is oriented inferiorly with an abnormally large rightward force. In rare instances a counterclockwise superior frontal loop is present. In these patients, the differential diagnosis of tetralogy of Fallot from endocardial cushion defect with pulmonic stenosis usually depends on the findings at left ventriculography. After palliative shunt operations pulmonary blood flow is increased so that venous return to the left ventricle is enhanced. This results in varying degrees of left ventricular enlargement. If the palliative shunt is small, there is little effect on the vectorcardiogram, and signs of type A right ventricular hypertrophy persist. However, large shunts with torrential pulmonary blood flow may occur after surgery especially with the Potts operation (side-to-side anastomosis of the descending thoracic aorta and left pulmonary artery) or the Waterston shunt (side-to-side anastomosis of the ascending aorta to the right pulmonary artery). In these patients signs of varying degrees of left ventricular hypertrophy are superimposed on those of right ventricular hypertrophy so that a significant portion of the QRS loop is displaced to the left (Fig. A.15). Rarely, pulmonary vascular disease develops after many years of large pulmonary blood flow which results in a loss of left ventricular forces and return of isolated right ventricular hypertrophy.

Striking vectorcardiographic changes are usual after complete surgical repair. Postoperative complete right bundle branch block is usual (Fig. A.16), although not invariable and has been attributed to trauma of the right branch of the bundle of His during repair of the ventricular septal defect. The location of the right bundle along the posteroinferior aspect of infracristal ventricular septal defects has been confirmed by several authors. Right ventriculotomy and infundibular resection also contribute to the development of complete right bundle branch block. Ellison and Restieaux in-

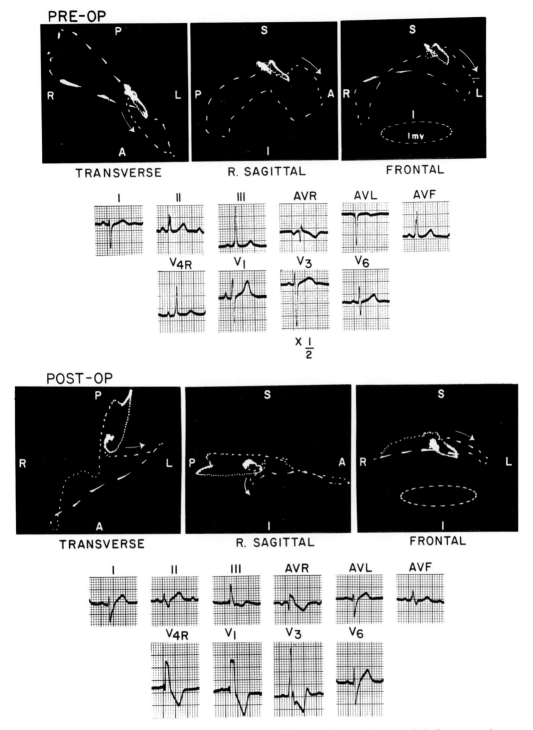

Fig. A.14. Tetralogy of Fallot. This 7-year-old boy was intensely cyanotic before operation. The preoperative vectorcardiograms and electrocardiograms show right ventricular hypertrophy. In the transverse plane, the QRS loop presents a figure-of-eight pattern with an initial counterclockwise inscription. The late portion of the loop is rightward, posterior, and clockwise. The positive T waves in the right precordium are also characteristic of right ventricular hypertrophy. Postoperative complete right bundle branch block is present.

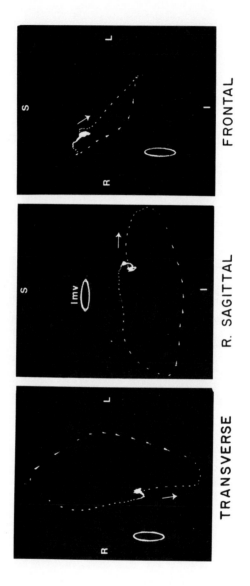

TRANSVERSE   R. SAGITTAL   FRONTAL

320

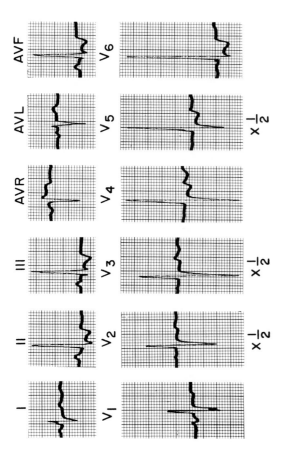

Fig. A.15. Tetralogy of Fallot. This 20-year-old man had a large Potts anastomosis performed during infancy which resulted in a torrential pulmonary blood flow and marked left ventricular hypertrophy. The QRS voltage is increased in all planes with a counterclockwise leftward and largely posterior transverse loop. The anterior forces are also increased and suggest associated right ventricular hypertrophy.

321

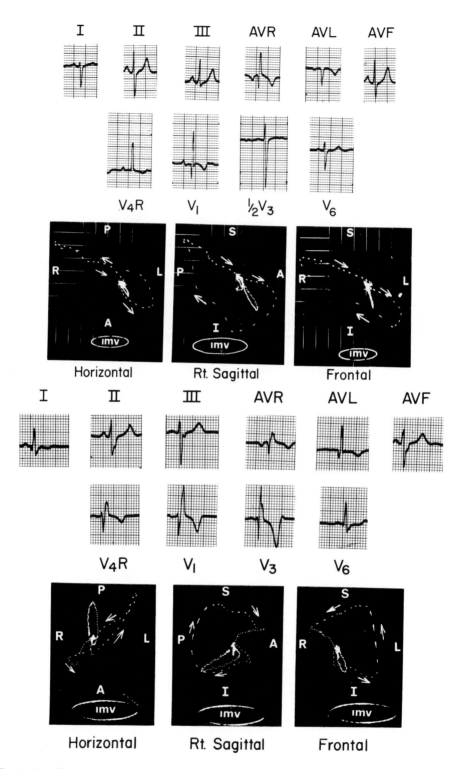

Fig. A.16. Tetralogy of Fallot. *Preoperatively,* right ventricular hypertrophy was present with prominent anterior and leftward initial QRS forces with late rightward and posterior forces. The frontal loop is clockwise. *Postoperatively,* the frontal QRS loop is counterclockwise with a superior orientation, indicating the presence of left anterior hemiblock. Complete right bundle branch block is also present.

dicated that an adequate surgical repair which resulted in peak right ventricular systolic pressure below 50 mm Hg was associated with a return of the right maximum spatial voltage to normal even though the intraventricular conduction delay resulted in bizarre vectorcardiographic loops.

Left anterior hemiblock may also be induced by surgical therapy of tetralogy of Fallot (Fig. A.16), and these findings are superimposed on those of complete right bundle branch block. About 10 percent of our patients who underwent surgical correction of Fallot's tetralogy developed this bifascicular block after operation. This complication has been attributed to selective injury of the anterior fascicles of the left bundle branch during repair of the ventricular septal defect. To date, none of our patients with postsurgical left anterior hemiblock and right bundle branch block have developed complete heart block, although the long-term prognosis is guarded.

Pulmonary Atresia with Intact Ventricular Septum

In the common form of this disease, the right ventricular cavity is small or minute, is encroached upon by hypertrophied muscular trabeculae and the right ventricular wall is thick. Less frequently, the right ventricular cavity is normal or dilated and the wall hypertrophied. In the latter group, signs of severe right ventricular hypertrophy are usual and indistinguishable from severe isolated valvular pulmonic stenosis. Patients with small right ventricular cavities frequently show left ventricular dominance for age with decreased right ventricular forces. These babies usually show a counterclockwise transverse QRS loop with a clockwise, inferior frontal loop. The latter findings may help differentiate this disease from tricuspid atresia since the latter frequently shows a counterclockwise superiorly oriented frontal QRS loop. However, there are many variations in the frontal loop pattern so that this finding is not diagnostic.

Eisenmenger Situation

The term *Eisenmenger situation* is used to describe a combination of severe pulmonary hypertension with reversed or bidirectional shunt through a ventricular septal defect, an atrial septal defect, patent ductus arteriosus, or other communications between the aorta and lesser circulation. This implies that the principal physiologic abnormality is extreme elevation of pulmonary vascular resistance. Generally the vectorcardiographic expression of this hemodynamic abnormality is in the form of type A right ventricular hypertrophy with right atrial enlargement. This is seen especially with ventricular septal defects. However, this generalization does not apply to all patients with the Eisenmenger situation. The electrocardiographic differentiation of obstructive from hyperkinetic pulmonary hypertension is difficult in ostium secundum atrial septal defect, although many of these patients show type A right ventricular hypertrophy (Fig. A.11). Complete right bundle branch block may occur and may mask the signs of significant right ventricular hypertrophy. In others, the vectorcardiographic signs of marked right ventricular hypertrophy may not be obvious so that the transverse QRS loop retains a counterclockwise orientation with large rightward terminal vectors and a clockwise frontal plane loop. Patients with endocardial cushion defect and marked elevation of pulmonary vascular resistance retain the abnormal superior counterclockwise frontal QRS loop with signs of either type A or B right ventricular hypertrophy. When the Eisenmen

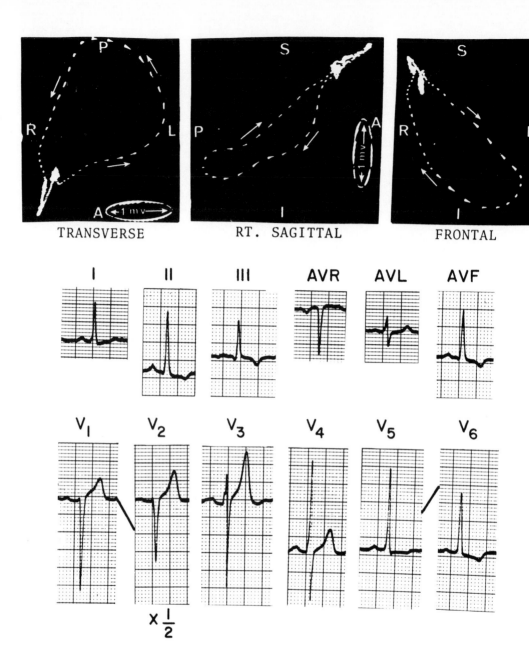

TRANSVERSE   RT. SAGITTAL   FRONTAL

I   II   III   AVR   AVL   AVF

V_1 V_2 V_3 V_4 V_5 V_6

$\times \frac{1}{2}$

Fig. A.17. Congenital aortic stenosis is 19-year-old man with a gradient of 110 mm Hg at rest. At operation his tricuspid aortic valve was calcified and was replaced with a prosthetic valve. These vectorcardiograms and electrocardiograms which were obtained preoperatively show left ventricular hypertrophy. In the transverse plane the major portion of the large magnitude QRS loop is leftward and posterior with a counterclockwise inscription. The T loops are discordant to the QRS loops.

ger situation complicates aortic runoff (e.g., patent ductus arteriosus), isolated type A right ventricular hypertrophy is usual, but some show signs of biventricular hypertrophy.

LEFT VENTRICULAR SYSTOLIC OVERLOAD

Obstruction to left ventricular outflow in children and adolescents is usually caused by congenital abnormalities in the region of the aortic valve, coarctation of the aorta, or primary myocardial disease. Varying degrees of left ventricular hypertrophy are present when the obstruction is moderate or severe. The vectorcardiogram is of value to help assess the degree of severity and may suggest the site of obstruction.

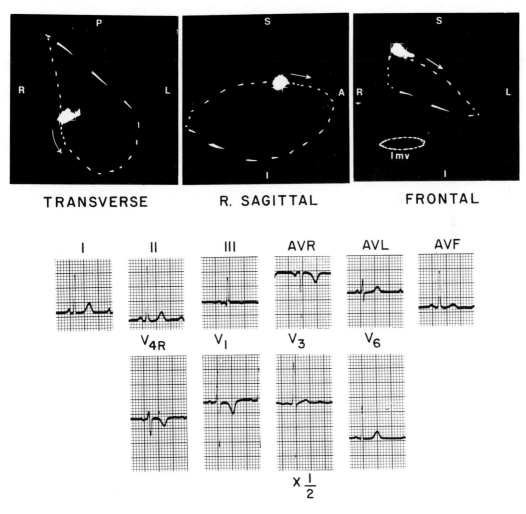

Fig. A.18. Severe aortic stenosis in a 6-year-old boy who had repeated syncopal episodes. Peak systolic gradient 110 mm Hg. across aortic valve. These preoperative vectorcardiograms and electrocardiograms do not suggest that the obstruction is severe.

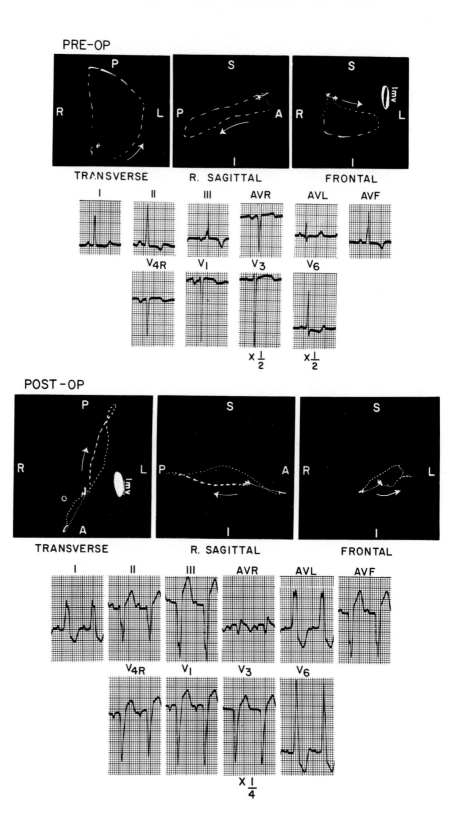

PRE-OP

TRANSVERSE   R. SAGITTAL   FRONTAL

I   II   III   AVR   AVL   AVF

V_{4R} V_1 V_3 V_6

$x\frac{1}{2}$ $x\frac{1}{2}$

POST-OP

TRANSVERSE   R. SAGITTAL   FRONTAL

I   II   III   AVR   AVL   AVF

V_{4R} V_1 V_3 V_6

$X\frac{1}{4}$

Aortic Valvular and Subvalvular Stenosis (Figs. A.17–A.19)

In the transverse plane the initial anterior QRS forces tend to be decreased and generally are directed leftward and anteriorly. However, this is not universal and in about one-third of patients the initial forces are normally directed anteriorly and rightward. The QRS loop is usually counterclockwise and a figure-of-eight pattern is less common. The major forces are directed leftward and posterior and generally they are more posterior with increasing severity. Terminal rightward forces are usually absent although Ellison and Restieaux found this sign in 10 percent of their patients with isolated aortic stenosis. The P loop is usually normal. The T loop is concordant if the obstruction is mild and discordant in severe cases, but this separation is not clear cut since many patients with severe disease have concordant T loops. Generally, a change of the T loop wave from concordant to discordant indicates progression of the disease. In the frontal plane the QRS loop is usually clockwise leftward and inferior. A counterclockwise superior orientation of the loop is unusual.

Estimation of severity of aortic stenosis and progression of the degree of obstruction is not easily assessed in children and many investigators have analyzed the vectorcardiogram to develop an accurate noninvasive method to estimate the gradient produced by the obstruction. The symptoms of dizziness and classic angina pectoris may be difficult to elucidate in a child, and the physical signs of left ventricular outflow obstruction may be unreliable to assess severity. Therefore, great reliance is frequently placed on the scalar electrocardiogram to indicate severity of disease by noting increased left ventricular voltage and inverted left precordial T waves. It is noteworthy that in 13 percent of the patients studied by Fowler and associates, the scalar electrocardiogram suggested mild disease when the gradient exceeded 70 mm Hg. Hugenholtz and Gamboa and Ellison and Restieaux found a close relationship between the magnitude of spatial voltages directed to the left and the left ventricular peak systolic pressure. The mean value of the maximal spatial voltages to the left increased from 2.2 mV when the stenosis was trivial to more than 4 mV in severe disease. These signs were much more accurate than the 12-lead scalar electrocardiogram. These authors use an increase in maximal spatial voltage to the left as an indication for cardiac catheterization and repeat catheterization is avoided if there is no further increase in voltage. They have also developed regression equations to estimate left ventricular pressure from voltage criteria. Fowler and his associates used the sum of maximum voltage of the QRS loop in the frontal and transverse planes as well as the QRS-T angle in these planes to estimate the severity of the disease. From this information, they developed regression equations and a nomogram to estimate the gradient across the aortic valve. This data contrasts with

---

Fig. A.19. Severe aortic stenosis in 9-year-old boy. Preoperatively, left ventricular hypertrophy is evident because the left maximal spatial QRS voltages are large and are directed leftward and posteriorly. Valvotomy of the tricuspid stenotic valve did not reduce the gradient since marked subvalvular muscular hypertrophy was also present. The latter required resection of part of the hypertrophied interventricular septum in the outflow portion of the left ventricle. This resulted in postoperative left bundle branch block.

the experience of Reeve and associates, who found no significant relationship between the maximal spatial vectors and the peak left ventricular systolic pressure. In this study there was a considerable overlap of the maximal spatial vectors in the normal controls and those with aortic valve disease, although the values tended to be higher in the latter group.

It appears that further confirmatory evidence is still necessary for determining the vectorcardiographic criteria of severity of aortic stenosis. Although the qualitative changes of the loop inscriptions posteriorly and leftward are of value, quantitative data relating the voltage with the severity of obstruction are still controversial.

After operation and successful reduction of left ventricular pressure, abnormal vectorcardiographic findings frequently persist. Although there may be some improvement, the vectorcardiogram has been disappointing in assessing severity postoperatively. The diminished initial forces remain unchanged, large leftward and posterior voltages may persist and sometimes the discordant T loops remain. In rare instances, subvalvular resection of part of the interventricular septum may be necessary to alleviate the gradient which may result in the development of complete left bundle branch block (Fig. A.19).

Supravalvular Aortic Stenosis and Coarctation of the Aorta (Fig. A.20)

Classically the vectorcardiogram in supraclavicular aortic stenosis and coarction of the aorta (Fig. A.20) is normal or shows signs of left ventricular hypertrophy. However, in some patients with coarctation of the aorta the scalar electrocardiogram may suggest signs of right ventricular enlargement because of right axis deviation and signs of right ventricular hypertrophy or incomplete right bundle branch block. Evaluation of our patients with supravalvular aortic stenosis and with coarctation of the aorta showed distinctive vectorcardiographic patterns. The most characteristic finding in isolated supravalvular aortic stenosis was the displacement of the transverse QRS loop rightward and posteriorly with the maximum vector directed to the right of $-90°$. About half of the patients with coarctation of the aorta had similar transverse loops. These findings were reflected in the scalar electrocardiogram by deep S waves in the left precordial leads. The initial forces in the transverse plane were either normal or directed leftward. The association of leftward initial forces and rightward terminal vectors was a distinctive finding, especially in supravalvular aortic stenosis. Of interest is that 10 percent of the patients with uncomplicated aortic valvular stenosis studied by Ellison and Restieaux had transverse loops directed rightward and posteriorly.

The mechanisms of these signs are of interest. None of our patients with supravalvular aortic stenosis or coarctation of the aorta had associated right-sided disease, such as pulmonary arterial branch stenosis, and the right ventricular pressures were within normal limits. We postulated that the rightward and posterior transverse loop described above was caused by hypertrophy of the posterobasal portion of the left ventricle or was a manifestation of left posterior hemiblock. The significance of these observations is that the scalar electrocardiogram and vectorcardiogram may be misinterpreted as indicating right ventricular hypertrophy.

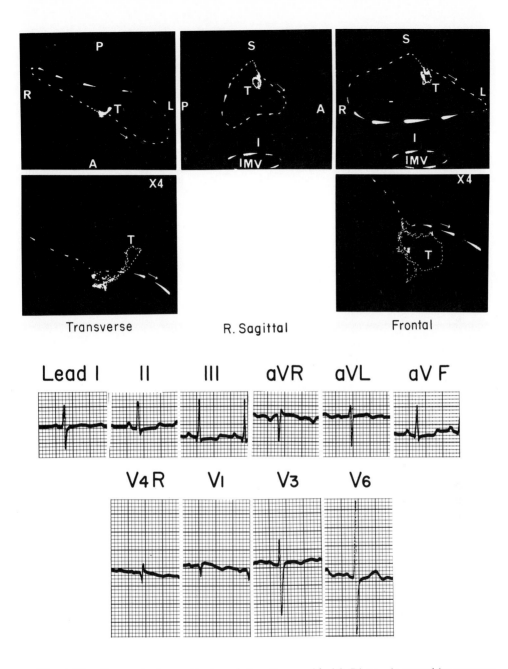

Fig. A.20. Supravalvular aortic stenosis in a 5-year-old girl. Diagnosis proved by aortography and by demonstrating a 21-mm Hg gradient across the obstruction. In the transverse plane the initial QRS forces are leftward and anterior and the terminal vector is rightward and posterior. The latter finding is associated with a deep S wave in V_6. The frontal QRS loop is clockwise and inferior. These vectorcardiographic findings could be attributed to posterobasal left ventricular hypertrophy or left posterior hemiblock.

329

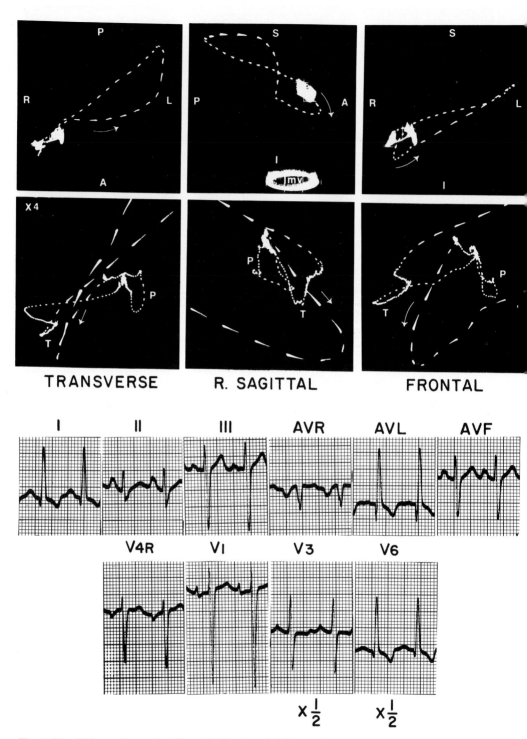

Fig. A.21. Triscuspid atresia with underdeveloped right ventricle. This 15-year-old boy had a Blalock-Taussig anastomosis in infancy. In the transverse plane the large QRS loop is leftward and posterior. The frontal QRS loop is counterclockwise and superior. The large P loops suggest right atrial enlargement.

LEFT VENTRICULAR VOLUME OVERLOAD

In children, the conditions which most frequently result in left ventricular volume overload are patent ductus arteriosus, aortic incompetence, mitral incompetence, and tricuspid atresia with underdeveloped right ventricle. The signs of left ventricular enlargement are variable but definite with severe lesions. The loop in the transverse plane is frequently wide, counterclockwise and is directed primarily leftward and posteriorly with a large maximum QRS vector. Less frequently, the posterior loop is narrow or inscribed in a figure-of-eight. When hypertrophy is marked, the ST vector is abnormally large and the T loop discordant. In the frontal plane the initial QRS forces are directed mainly to the right either inferiorly or superiorly. The maximum vector is to the left and inferiorly except in most cases of tricupsid atresia in which it is directed superiorly. The loop inscription is extremely variable being counterclockwise, clockwise, or as a figure-of-eight.

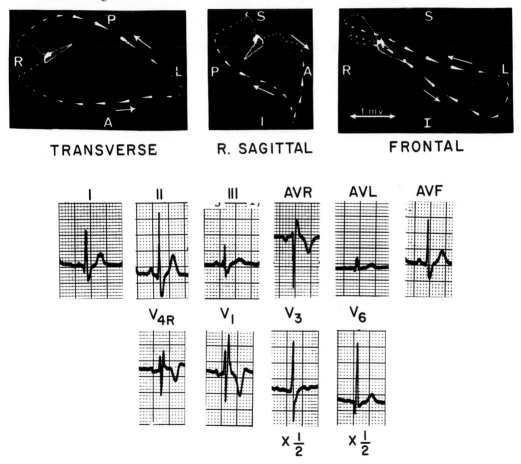

TRANSVERSE   R. SAGITTAL   FRONTAL

Fig. A.22. Ventricular septal defect of moderate size. This 6-year-old boy had a large pulmonary blood flow, but the pulmonary arterial resistance was normal. The transverse QRS loop is inscribed normally, but the voltage is large indicating left ventricular hypertrophy. The rightward and slowly inscribed terminal QRS vector corresponds to the secondary R waves in the right precordium and these signs are caused by a right ventricular conduction defect.

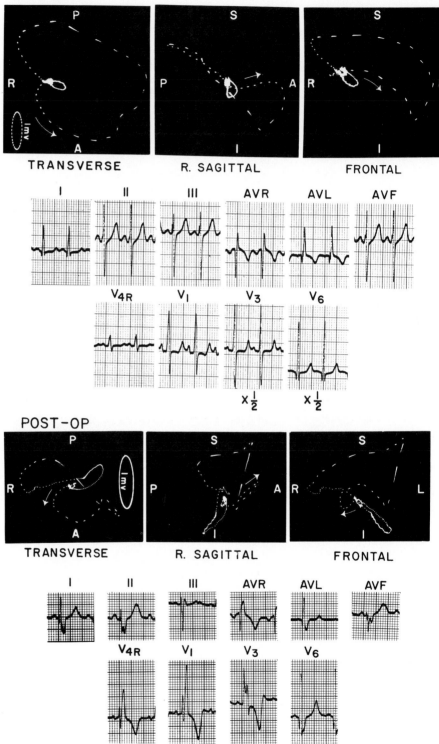

Tricuspid atresia. There are certain distinctive features in tricuspid atresia (Fig. A.21). The P loop is large and is directed primarily leftward, anteriorly and inferiorly, suggesting right atrial enlargement. Some investigators have suggested that right atrial enlargement is more pronounced if the atrial septal defect is small. Davachi and associates found isolated right atrial enlargement more frequently if tricuspid atresia was associated with subpulmonic stenosis. However, signs of biatrial enlargement are common. Ellison and Restieaux found significant right atrial enlargement in younger patients and biatrial hypertrophy was common in older patients.

The frontal plane QRS loop in tricuspid atresia usually shows counterclockwise superior orientation and only rarely is the axis at 0° or inferiorly. The abnormal left axis deviation could be explained by the unusually early origin of the left bundle. The QRS loop in the transverse plane is as described above. Ellison and Restieaux indicate that a more anteriorly directed transverse loop with significant rightward terminal forces suggests an associated large ventricular septal defect and a larger right ventricular cavity than usually encountered.

VOLUME OVERLOAD OF BOTH VENTRICLES WITH OR WITHOUT PRESSURE OVERLOAD

Ventricular Septal Defect (Figs. A.22-A.26)

Ventricular septal defects present varying hemodynamic effects which are determined primarily by the size of the defect and the ratio of pulmonary resistance to systemic vascular resistance. In patients with small defects, the shunt is trivial, pulmonary vascular resistance is normal, and the vectorcardiogram is normal. When the defect is moderate, the left-to-right shunt is significant but pulmonary vascular resistance is usually normal. These patients generally show progressive increase of left ventricular voltage and signs of biventricular involvement (Fig. A.22). In the transverse plane, the QRS loop is usually open, inscribed counterclockwise with prominent anterior and posterior forces. In patients with large defects, significant left-to-right shunts, and increased pulmonary arterial pressure and resistance, the transverse QRS loop may still be counterclockwise, but there is a tendency toward a figure-of-eight or clockwise inscription as right ventricular pressures approach systemic levels. The initial forces are increased in magnitude, generally directed rightward and anteriorly and less frequently leftward and anteriorly. The large initial forces have been attributed to septal hypertrophy and to diastolic overload of the left ventricle. These contrast with the small initial forces seen in many patients with

Fig. A.23. Large isolated infracristal ventricular septal defect in a 3-year-old boy. The left-to-right shunt was torrential before operation and the pulmonary vascular resistance was moderately elevated. The preoperative transverse vectorcardiogram indicates the presence of biventricular enlargement because of the wide counterclockwise QRS loop with a large anterior and leftward efferent limb and an afferent limb which later becomes posterior and rightward. The frontal QRS loop is counterclockwise and mostly superior. The postoperative vectorcardiogram shows that the major portion of the frontal loop is counterclockwise but is more superior than preoperatively. Also right bundle branch block developed after operation.

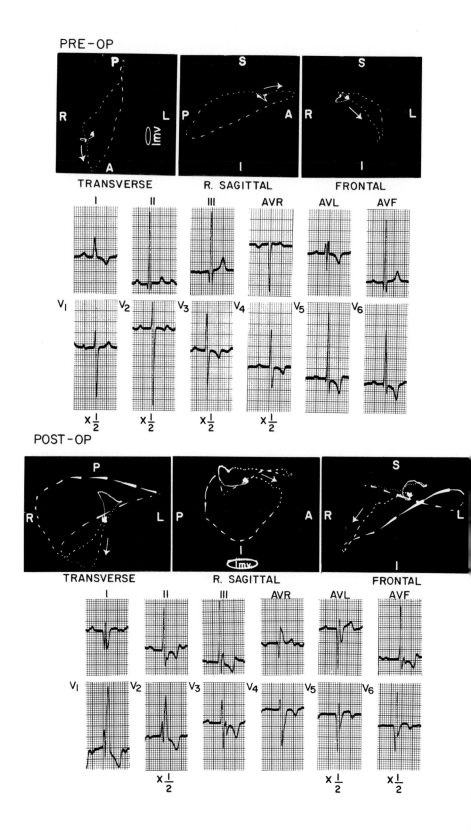

PRE-OP

TRANSVERSE R. SAGITTAL FRONTAL

POST-OP

TRANSVERSE R. SAGITTAL FRONTAL

aortic stenosis. As right ventricular pressure rises, the terminal QRS forces become prominent and are generally directed rightward, posteriorly, and superiorly. Occasionally, the terminal forces are anterior and inferior. In the majority, the frontal QRS loop is inscribed clockwise or is a figure-of-eight and is directed inferiorly and leftward. Generally, there is no significant change in the frontal loop with moderate rises in right ventricular pressure. Vectorcardiographic signs of ventricular septal defects with the Eisenmenger complex have been described earlier in this chapter.

About 16 percent of patients with isolated ventricular septal defect have a counterclockwise superior frontal loop (Fig. A.23). This finding is not related to the hemodynamic abnormality and may be found in small, moderate, or large defects. In these patients, clear differentiation of isolated ventricular septal defect from an endocardial cushion defect depends on the findings at left ventriculography.

The vectorcardiographic signs produced by ventricular septal defect and pulmonic stenosis with persistent left to right shunt depend on the severity of obstruction. If right ventricular pressure is only slightly or moderately elevated, the vectorcardiographic findings are nonspecific and show signs of biventricular hypertrophy. As right ventricular pressure approaches systemic levels, right ventricular forces become more prominent, or may be dominant. The vectorcardiographic signs in these patients are also nonspecific. They may simulate those described under large ventricular septal defect or in some instances may show signs of isolated type A right ventricular hypertrophy.

The signs produced by ventricular septal defect and aortic valve incompetence depend on the severity of the lesion, especially the degree of aortic regurgitation. These patients show signs of marked left ventricular hypertrophy when the lesion is severe (Fig. A.24) with large counterclockwise, leftward and posterior transverse QRS loops. Surgical treatment of the patient shown in Figure A.24 required aortic valve replacement and was complicated by myocardial infarction.

Some infants with isolated large ventricular septal defects are treated by palliative pulmonary artery banding. The effect of this operation is to reduce pulmonary blood flow, but there is resultant marked right ventricular hypertrophy, usually type A (Fig. A.25). Surgical closure of isolated ventricular septal defects also results in characteristic vectorcardiographic signs. Complete right bundle branch is common (Figs. A.23, A.25, A.26) and has been attributed to the right ventriculotomy or to surgical trauma to the right bundle as it courses along the posteroinferior aspect of infracristal ventricular defects. Of interest is that complete right bundle branch block may occur without right ventriculotomy when the ventricular defect is closed via a right atriotomy and the tricuspid valve. Six percent of our patients who underwent surgical closure of a ventricular septal defect developed left anterior hemiblock and complete right bundle branch block (Fig. A.26). Left

---

Fig. A.24. Ventricular septal defect with severe aortic incompetence due to an unsupported aortic cusp. The left-to-right shunt in this 14-year-old boy was moderate. Marked left ventricular hypertrophy is present preoperatively with the large magnitude counterclockwise transverse loop being directed leftward and posteriorly. The frontal loop is counterclockwise and inferior. This patient required aortic valve replacement. Postoperatively he developed an anterolateral myocardial infarction with the major portion of the transverse loop being inscribed in a clockwise manner.

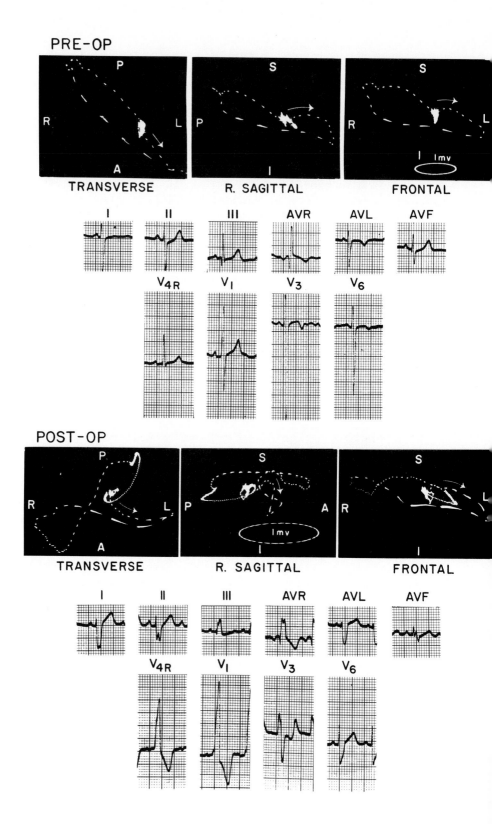

anterior hemiblock was attributed to selective injury of the anterior fascicles of the left bundle. To date none of these patients have developed complete heart block, but the long-term prognosis remains guarded.

Complete Transposition of the Great Arteries (Fig. A.27)

The vectorcardiogram can be useful in assessing the hemodynamic effects on the ventricles in arterial transposition (d loop). Babies with arterial transposition, intact ventricular septum, and relatively low-peak pressures in the posterior (left) ventricle have signs of isolated right ventricular hypertrophy, usually type A. In the transverse plane, the QRS loop is inscribed in a clockwise manner and is directed anteriorly and rightward. The frontal plane QRS loop is generally clockwise, inferior, and rightward. Dominance of the right ventricle is understandable since it supports the systemic circulation. Diminution of left ventricular forces is striking and occurs despite increased pulmonary blood flow and volume overloading of the left ventricle.

Arterial transposition with nearly equal peak systolic pressures in both ventricles. This defect is usually associated with other lesions, such as large ventricular septal defect, pulmonic stenosis, severe pulmonary vascular disease, large patent ductus arteriosus, or surgical pulmonary arterial banding (Fig. A.27). When arterial transposition is associated with a large ventricular septal defect, the QRS loop in the transverse plane is written in a counterclockwise manner or figure-of-eight configuration. The frontal plane loop is counterclockwise in about half of these patients. Thus, in patients with arterial transposition, a clockwise, anterior, rightward and open loop in the transverse plane suggests an intact ventricular septum, whereas a counterclockwise or figure-of-eight transverse loop suggests posterior ventricular hypertension, usually associated with a ventricular septal defect. Although it is agreed that the vectorcardiogram is superior to the scalar electrocardiogram in detecting combined ventricular hypertrophy in arterial transposition, it is still not clear whether all instances of elevated left ventricular pressures are reflected in the vectorcardiogram. Ellison and Restieaux found that they could make a fairly reliable assessment of left ventricular pressure because generally, a clockwise transverse QRS loop was associated with a left ventricular pressure less than two-thirds of that in the right ventricle. A counterclockwise transverse loop indicated that the left ventricular pressure was more than two-thirds of the right ventricular pressure. Mair and associates found that in patients with nearly equal peak systolic pressures in both ventricles, the vectorcardiogram was not helpful in separating patients with large pulmonary flow from those with relatively diminished pulmonary flow (as in pulmonary stenosis, severe pulmonary vascular disease, or pulmonary arterial bands). These authors found that progression of pulmonary vascular disease could not be detected reliably by serial vectorcardiograms.

Fig. A.25.   Large ventricular septal defect. This boy required pulmonary arterial banding at the age of 3 months. His preoperative vectorcardiogram and electrocardiogram were obtained at age 6 years prior to pulmonary artery debanding and closure of the ventricular septal defect. At that time signs of marked right ventricular hypertrophy were present. Postoperatively, he developed complete right bundle branch block.

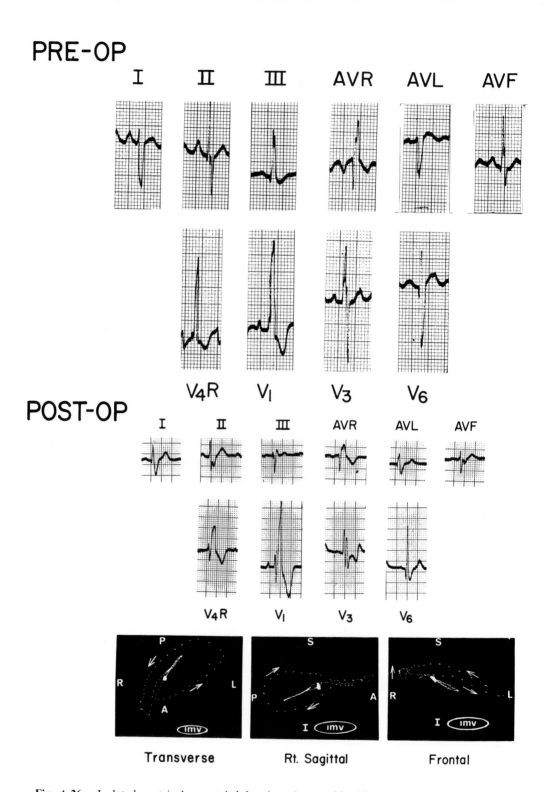

Fig. A.26. Isolated ventricular septal defect in a 3-year-old with preoperative pulmonary artery pressure of 80/21 mm Hg., and a pulmonary-systemic flow ratio of 2:8:1. Preoperative electrocardiogram shows right axis deviation and right ventricular hypertrophy. Postoperative electrocardiogram and vectorcardiogram indicate a change of frontal plane axis to the left, a counterclockwise, mostly superior, frontal loop and advanced right bundle branch block.

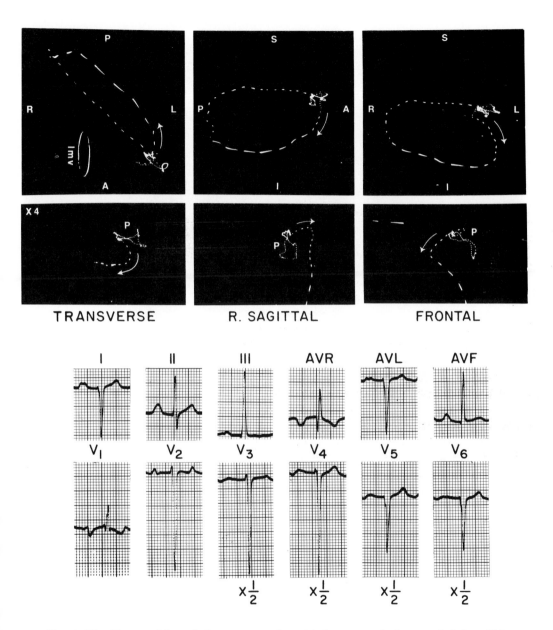

Fig. A.27. Transposition of the great arteries with large ventricular septal defect. This patient underwent pulmonary arterial banding and atrial septectomy during infancy. This vectorcardiogram and electrocardiogram were obtained at age 21 years and show signs of right ventricular hypertrophy and biatrial enlargement. The voltage of the QRS loops is increased. The initial forces in the transverse plane are clockwise, leftward, and anterior but the major portion of this loop is rightward, posterior, and counterclockwise. The large frontal loop is clockwise, inferior, and to the right.

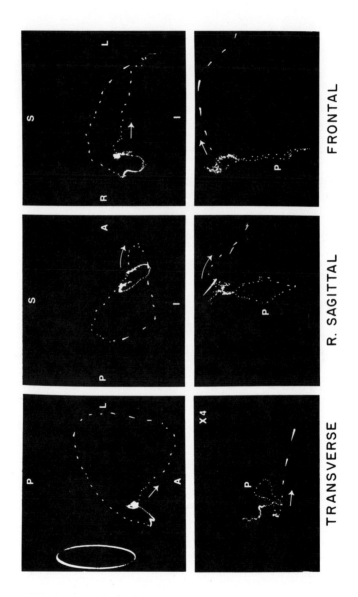

FRONTAL

R. SAGITTAL

TRANSVERSE

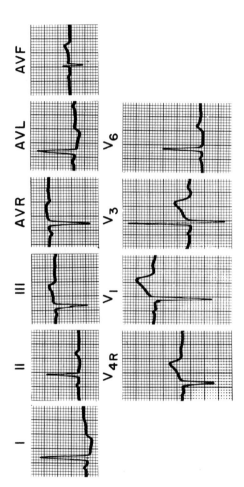

Fig. A.28. Corrected transposition of the great arteries in a 13-year-old girl without other associated intracardiac defects at cardiac catheterization. The initial QRS forces are characteristic and are directed leftward and anteriorly.

341

Complete transposition of the great arteries with right ventricular hypoplasia.
This defect is associated with reduced rightward QRS forces, and a posteriorly
directed counterclockwise transverse loop.

Corrected Transposition of the Great Arteries (Figs. A.28, A.29).

This condition is also known as ventricular inversion or L-transposition.
Systemic venous blood passes through a bicuspid atrioventricular valve into a "right-
sided" ventricle which is structurally similar to that of the normal left ventricle. The
venous blood is ejected into the lungs and returns to the left atrium, which empties
through a tricuspid valve into a ventricle which is structurally similar to the right
ventricle. The ascending aorta is more leftward and the pulmonary artery more
posterior. Physiologically, blood flow is normal since systemic venous blood is
oxygenated and arterialized blood ejected in the normal manner. However, associated lesions are common, especially ventricular septal defect, pulmonic stenosis, and
incompetence of the left atrioventricular valve. Since ventricular inversion is present,
the early depolarization of the ventricular septum is from right to left. Thus, the
characteristic initial QRS forces in corrected transposition are leftward and either
posteriorly or anteriorly as best seen in the transverse loop (Fig. A.28). This also
explains the q wave in the right precordial leads and the absence of an initial q in V_5
and V_6 of the scalar electrocardiogram. The initial **QRS** vector may also be superior.
The remainder of the QRS loop depends on the presence and severity of the
associated lesions. Elevated anterior ventricular pressure owing to pulmonic stenosis
or extreme elevation of pulmonary vascular resistance is associated with a clockwise
or figure-of-eight inscription of the transverse QRS loop with prominent rightward
forces. Large leftward and posterior forces suggest posterior ventricular enlargement
which is frequently caused by left atrioventricular valve incompetence. Conduction
abnormalities are common including complete heart block (Fig. A.29).

Single Ventricle (Fig. A.30)

Usually the single ventricle has the morphology of a left ventricle and the right
ventricle is rudimentary. The pulmonary artery arises from the single ventricle and
the aorta from the rudimentary chamber. Transposition of the great vessels is usual
and these patients are further subdivided according to inversion or noninversion of
the ventricles. With ventricular inversion, the rudimentary right ventricle is located
superiorly and leftward, and the aorta arises anteriorly and to the left of the
pulmonary artery (l loop). In noninverted ventricles, the rudimentary right ventricle
is anterior superior and to the right, and the aorta arises anterior and to the right of
the pulmonary trunk (d loop).

There is confusion in the literature concerning the vectorcardiographic findings
in these patients because anatomic classification may not be clear. Generally, in
single ventricle with l loop, the initial QRS forces are leftward, anterior (sometimes
posterior), and superior with the major part of the transverse QRS loop being
rightward and anterior. Single ventricle with d loop (noninversion) usually shows a
pattern of severe left ventricular hypertrophy. The initial forces are to the right and
inferior with marked leftward and posterior shift of the QRS loop.

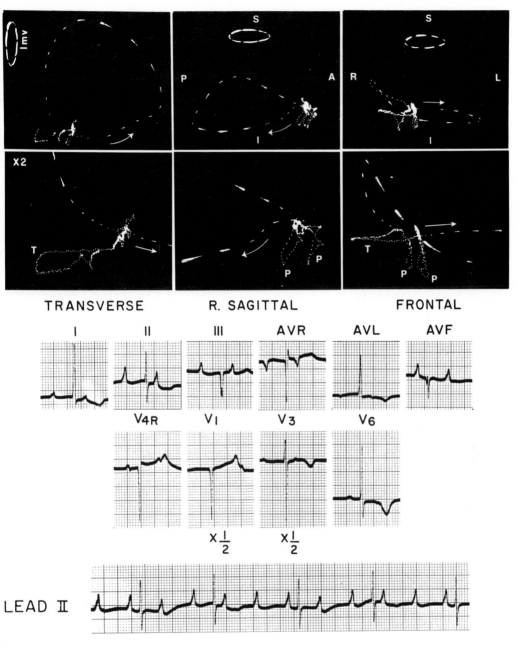

TRANSVERSE   **R. SAGITTAL**   **FRONTAL**

I   II   III   AVR   AVL   AVF

V4R   V1   V3   V6

$x\frac{1}{2}$ $x\frac{1}{2}$

LEAD II

Fig. A.29. Corrected transposition of the great arteries. This 2-year-old boy developed Stokes-Adams attacks because of complete heart block shown in the strip of lead 2 of the electrocardiogram and by the two P loops for each QRS T loop. The initial QRS forces are characteristically leftward, anterior, and inferior. At cardiac catheterization associated cardiac anomalies were not detected.

343

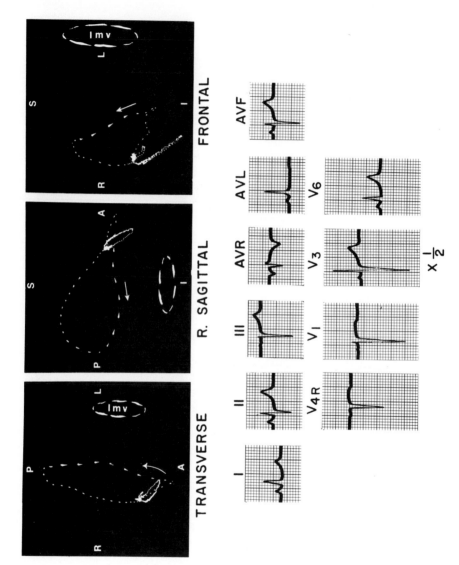

Fig. A.30. Single ventricle with d loop (noninversion) and pulmonic stenosis. The QRS loop shows the pattern of left ventricular hypertrophy. In the transverse plane the QRS loop is displaced leftward and posteriorly and the frontal loop is counterclockwise and superior.

MISCELLANEOUS DISEASES

Ebstein's Anomaly (Figs. A.31, A.32)

The classic electrocardiogram in Ebstein's anomaly consists of prolongation of the PR interval, right atrial enlargement, right bundle branch block which is sometimes atypical, and Wolff-Parkinson White syndrome (especially type B). The vectorcardiogram frequently shows low voltage and an increased QRS duration which is attributed to right bundle branch block manifested as delayed conduction especially in the terminal portion of the QRS loop. In the transverse plane, the QRS loop is leftward and posterior being inscribed in a counterclockwise or figure-of-eight configuration. The frontal loop is inferior, clockwise, or in the form of a figure-of-eight. The P waves are frequently large and suggest right atrial enlargement. The vectorcardiographic signs of Wolff-Parkinson White syndrome are described in Chapter 14.

Anomalous Origin of the Left Coronary Artery from the Pulmonary Artery (Fig. A.33)

Perfusion of the left ventricular myocardium varies in this condition and depends primarily on the collateral coronary circulation and the volume of blood flow from the left coronary artery to the pulmonary artery. Frequently, this anomaly leads to anterolateral myocardial infarction in infancy. Loss of leftward anterior

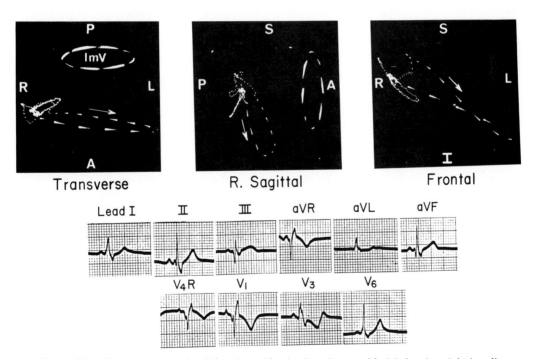

Fig. A.31. Ebstein's anomaly of the tricuspid valve in a 7-year-old girl showing right bundle branch block and type B Wolff-Parkinson-White syndrome. She also had episodes of paroxysmal supraventricular tachycardia.

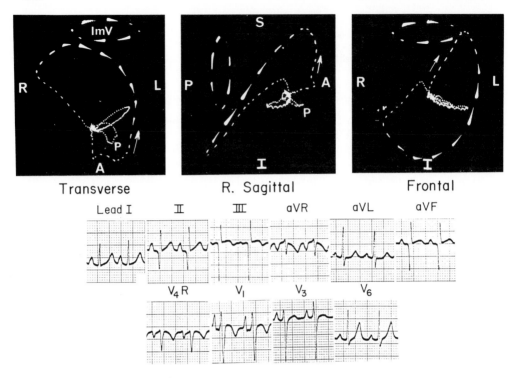

Fig. A.32. Ebstein's anomaly of the tricuspid valve proved by cardiac catheterization in a 1-year-old boy. The large P loop is directed leftward, anteriorly and inferiorly indicating right atrial enlargement. The QRS loop resembles that seen in diaphragmatic (inferior) myocardial infarction. In the right sagittal plane, the initial forces are displaced superiorly and anteriorly and the loop is counterclockwise. In the frontal plane, the initial forces are abnormally superior and leftward and the whole loop is inscribed clockwise.

forces result in an abnormal transverse QRS loop which is inscribed clockwise, rightward and posteriorly. The frontal loop is frequently superiorly oriented with a counterclockwise inscription. The T loops are also abnormal and are directed rightward anteriorly and inferiorly. Recovery of some leftward QRS forces occurs in patients who survive infancy. In these patients, some leftward anterior forces return so that the transverse loop may become counterclockwise or show a figure-of-eight pattern.

Cardiac Malposition (Fig. A.34)

Dextrocardia with total situs inversus is frequently associated with a normally functioning heart without intracardiac defects. However, patients with isolated dextrocardia or isolated levocardia almost invariably have associated complex cardiac anomalies. The most frequently encountered defects include ventricular inversion (L transposition), single ventricle, and atrioventricular valvular anomalies. Since the anatomic assessment of these anomalies depend on localizing atrial situs, the relative position of the ventricles and the presence or virtual absence of the ventricular septum, vectorcardiography is of help in arriving at a correct diagnosis.

Generally, atrial and visceral situs are similar so that a normal tracheobronchial tree bifurcation and normally situated stomach bubble on the chest x-ray suggests normal atrial position. The vectorcardiogram confirms these findings so that a leftward, anterior, and inferior P loop is associated with normally situated atria. In dextrocardia with situs inversus, the P loop is rightward anterior and inferior.

Analysis of the initial QRS forces is of help in localizing the ventricles. The presence of l transposition (ventricular inversion) is associated with leftward initial forces. In d loop with noninversion, the initial forces are to the right. Generally,

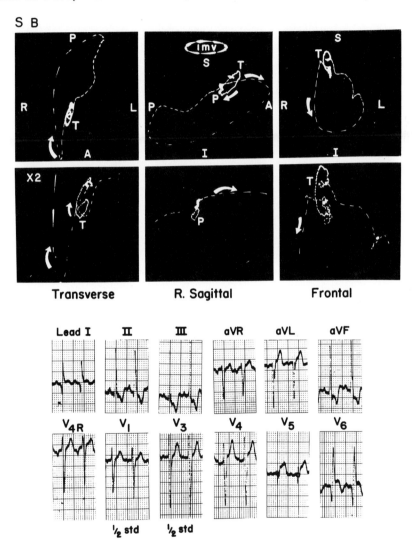

Fig. A.33. Aberrant origin of the left coronary artery from the pulmonary artery in a baby who succumbed in cardiac failure at age 4 months. Diagnosis confirmed at autopsy. Vectorcardiogram and electrocardiogram show signs of anterolateral myocardial infarction. In the transverse plane, initial QRS forces are normal, but the efferent limb which is inscribed clockwise is displaced rightward and posteriorly. This results in the deep wide Q waves in the left precordium.

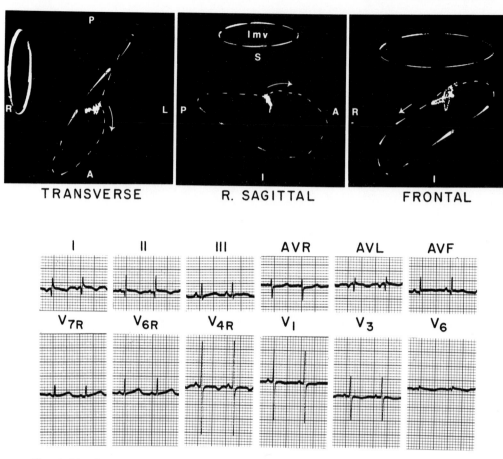

TRANSVERSE   R. SAGITTAL   FRONTAL

Fig. A.34. Dextrocardia with total situs inversus. Associated cardiac defects were not demonstrable. This vectorcardiogram and electrocardiogram are mirror image of normal in this newborn child.

accurate diagnosis in specific patients depends on all available noninvasive and invasive methods because of the complexity of these anomalies.

Glycogen Storage Disease (Type 2) (Fig. A.35)

Vectorcardiographic abnormalities produced by primary myocardial diseases have been described elsewhere. However, type 2 glycogen storage disease has specific findings. This disease is characterized by an increase in cardiac, hepatic, and skeletal muscle glycogen and a decrease in alpha glucosidase. The condition is lethal in symptomatic patients, usually within the first few years of life. The common vectorcardiographic finding is marked increase in left ventricular forces. The transverse QRS loop is counterclockwise, leftward and posterior. In a minority of patients associated right ventricular enlargement is manifested by late prominent rightward forces. Large initial forces are directed normally to the right and anterior, and are associated with large septal Q waves. Frequently, the P-R interval is short and the early part of the QRS is inscribed slowly so that the loop superficially resembles that seen in the Wolff-Parkinson-White syndrome. The P loops may indicate biatrial enlargement and the T loops may be discordant. Investigators have suggested that glycogen is an efficient electrical conductor. Rapid conduction through the atria would result in a short P-R interval and the increased voltage has been explained on large forces generated by glycogen.

SOME SPECIFIC PEDIATRIC PROBLEMS

Counterclockwise Superior Frontal QRS Loop

Endocardial cushion defect. Left axis deviation with a counterclockwise superiorly oriented frontal QRS loop is rare in normal children and generally

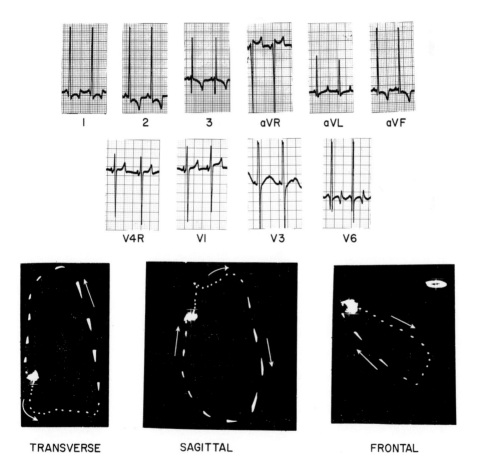

Fig. A.35. Glycogen storage disease type II. The diagnosis was proved biochemically, by electron microscopy and at autopsy. A 1-mV signal is shown at the top right of frontal vectorcardiogram. There is marked increase in voltage of all QRS loops with signs of massive left ventricular hypertrophy. The P-R interval is short. The abnormal T waves were attributed to left ventricular hypertrophy. However, the patient was receiving digitalis at the time of the tracing.

suggests the presence of an endocardial cushion defect. However, this finding is not specific for this anomaly and may be found in a variety of congenital cardiac defects. Before describing these anomalies, it is advantageous to point out that more than 95 percent of all forms of endocardial cushion defect show a counterclockwise superior frontal loop, and this sign is useful to distinguish cushion defects from ostium secundum atrial septal defects. The presence of a counterclockwise superior frontal loop in endocardial cushion defect does not depend on the associated hemodynamics, and it is found with small or large left-to-right shunts, normal or increased pulmonary vascular resistance, and with varying degees of mitral or tricuspid incompetence. Furthermore, this finding persists after successful repair of the defect, even after regression of signs of biventricular hypertrophy. The types of endocardial cushion defect associated with this abnormal frontal loop include ostium primum defects, atrioventricular canal, and common atrium. In rare instances, isolated clefts of the anterior mitral leaflet are associated with abnormal left axis deviation, and these patients may represent forme fruste types of endocardial cushion defects.

Ostium secundum atrial septal defects.   These abnormalities with or without partial anomalous venous return are usually associated with right axis deviation. However, 3 percent of these patients with uncomplicated defects show abnormal left axis deviation. Superior counterclockwise frontal loops can also develop in rare instances after surgical closure of a secundum atrial septal defect in patients who had right axis deviation before operation.

Ventricular Septal Defects.   Neufeld and associates described isolated ventricular septal defects of the atrioventricular canal type and these patients have abnormal left axis deviation. However, 16 percent of simple *ventricular septal defects* have a counterclockwise superiorly oriented frontal loop. Ellison and Restieaux suggest that it may be possible to separate simple ventricular defects from endocardial cushion defects by timing the superior orientation of the frontal loop. In simple ventricular septal defects, the frontal loop does not become superior until an average of 40 msec from the onset of the QRS, whereas in endocardial cushion defect the frontal loop is superior earlier.

Origin of both great vessels from the right ventricle.   This condition (also known as double-outlet right ventricle) is invariably associated with a ventricular septal defect through which left ventricular blood is ejected into the aorta. Although the frontal plane axis is variable, Neufeld and associates found a significant number of patients with superior counterclockwise frontal QRS loop especially when the ventricular defect was infracristal and pulmonic stenosis was absent. The abnormal frontal loop was attributed to the posterior displacement of the conduction tissue by the ventricular defect.

Left ventricular outflow obstruction.   This defect caused by the various forms of aortic stenosis or coarctation of the aorta is only rarely associated with a counterclockwise superior frontal loop in children. Also, increasing severity of obstruction is not associated with a progressive leftward displacement in frontal axis. Reports indicate that occasionally patients with coarctation of the aorta and those with aortic stenosis and insufficiency also have a counterclockwise superior frontal loop.

Pulmonary stenosis.   This condition is usually associated with a rightward, inferior, and clockwise frontal loop. However, a small number of patients with isolated pulmonic stenosis do have a counterclockwise superior frontal loop. This abnormality did not reflect the severity of obstruction and was seen in mild or severe disease.

Tetralogy of Fallot.   There are many reports of a counterclockwise superior frontal loop in tetralogy of Fallot. This finding was not associated with severity of the lesion nor were other defects present with the Fallot's tetralogy. Generally, these patients require left ventriculography to exclude an associated endocardial cushion defect.

Ebstein's anomaly.   Ebstein's anomaly may be associated with a counterclockwise superior frontal loop. This is also found in some patients with Ebstein's malformation and type B Wolff-Parkinson-White syndrome.

Tricuspid atresia with underdeveloped right ventricle.   This diagnosis is usually considered in cyanotic patients with counterclockwise superior frontal loops. However, this abnormal frontal loop also occurs in *transposition of the great arteries*. In these patients, the presence of a counterclockwise superior frontal loop does not correlate with the associated anatomic or hemodynamic changes. It is found in transposition with intact ventricular septum, ventricular septal defect, ventricular septal defect with pulmonic stenosis and with pulmonary vascular disease. Patients with *single ventricle* and noninversion (d loop) frequently show a counterclockwise superior frontal loop and contrast with those who have an l loop when the frontal plane is generally inscribed inferiorly and clockwise.

INITIAL QRS FORCES

In normal children the QRS forces (Q loop) are directed anteriorly and usually rightward and superiorly. There are many clinical situations in which the initial vector is unusual in that it is directed primarily leftward, resulting in virtual absence of Q waves in V_5 and V_6. This sign is present on the first day of life in half of normal full-term babies (Fig. A.1) and is attributed to the right ventricular dominance of the normal neonate. The evolution of normal left ventricular dominance results in normal anterior rightward and superior initial forces by the age of 1 month. This course of events contrasts with those seen in premature babies who frequently have a rightward and anterior initial vector from birth (Fig. A.7).

Right ventricular hypertrophy.   The initial QRS forces in patients with congenital cardiac defects which result in right ventricular hypertrophy may be directed primarily leftward. Generally, this occurs when the hypertrophy is marked and the normal anterior rightward initial forces persist when the hypertrophy is mild or moderate. However, there is a significant overlap in these two groups so that the initial forces in some patients with severe right ventricular hypertrophy may still be directed rightward.

Left ventricular hypertrophy. The initial QRS forces in left ventricular hypertrophy are also variable. Leftward, anterior, and superior displacement of the initial vector is common and has been attributed to possible septal fibrosis. The leftward, posterior, and large voltage of the remainder of the loop clearly separates these patients from those with right ventricular hypertrophy. Large normally directed initial forces (rightward and anteriorly) are associated with deep Q waves in the left precordium and are seen in left ventricular enlargement with a hypertrophied interventricular septum.

The magnitude and direction of the initial QRS forces are not diagnostic for specific lesions which result in either left or right ventricular hypertrophy. However, certain congenital cardiovascular lesions are frequently associated with abnormal initial QRS forces.

Corrected transposition. This condition (also known as ventricular inversion or l loop) is associated with the initial forces being directed leftward, and either posteriorly or slightly anteriorly. The abnormal orientation of these initial forces is attributed to early depolarization of the ventricular septum from right to left because of ventricular inversion.

Single ventricle with l loop. Single ventricle (double-inlet left ventricle) with l loop is also associated with leftward, anterior (sometimes posterior), and superior initial forces.

Aortic stenosis and aortic coarctation. Most patients with supravalvular aortic stenosis and many with coarctation of the aorta have leftward and anterior initial QRS forces associated with rightward terminal vectors. These findings have been attributed to posterobasal left ventricular hypertrophy or to left posterior hemiblock.

Cardiac malposition. In patients with cardiac malposition, the initial QRS forces are directed leftward in the presence of ventricular inversion.

Wolff-Parkinson-White syndrome and left bundle branch block. The details of the initial QRS forces in Wolff-Parkinson-White syndrome and left bundle branch block have been given in Chapters 8 and 14. Left bundle branch block is rare in children but may be seen in patients with primary myocardial disease or after surgical incision of the left side of the interventricular septum in the outflow portion of the ventricle (Fig. A.19).

COMPLETE RIGHT BUNDLE BRANCH BLOCK

In the pediatric age group, complete right bundle branch block is seen most frequently after surgery which involves right ventriculotomy with or without closure of a ventricular septal defect. This has been attributed to surgical trauma to the right bundle as it courses along the posteroinferior aspect of infracristal ventricular defects. Closure of ventricular septal defects through the right atrium and tricuspid valve may also be complicated by right bundle branch block so that incision of the free wall of the right ventricle is not essential for the production of this sign. However, we have observed complete right bundle branch block after incision of the right ventricle for relief of isolated infundibular pulmonic stenosis with intact ventricular septum.

In children, complete right bundle branch block is rare in ostium secundum atrial septal defects, whereas this finding is more common in adults. *Ebstein's anomaly* is frequently associated with an unusual type of complete right bundle branch block and with low-voltage QRS complexes. Complete right bundle branch block is known to occur in about 15 percent of adults with chronic rheumatic heart disease. We have seen this abnormality in two children with first episode acute rheumatic fever and mild-to-moderate carditis. It is not known whether complete right bundle branch block was present in these patients prior to the onset of acute rheumatic fever. It is also known that complete right bundle branch block may occur rarely in children who are considered to have normal cardiovascular systems. We have not encountered complete right bundle branch block in children with chronic cor pulmonale.

REFERENCES

1. Abramson, H Burton CR: The spatial vectorcardiogram in proven atrial septal defect. Br Heart J 24:103, 1962

2. Besterman E: Atrial septal defect with pulmonary hypertension. Br Heart J 23:587, 1961.

3. Burch GE, DePasquale N: The Anomalous left coronary artery. an experiment of nature. Am J Med 37:159, 1964

4. Burch GE, DePasquale N: The spatial vectorcardiogram in proved congenital atrial septal defect. Am Heart J 58:319, 1959

5. Cabrera E, Gaxiola A: Diagnostic contribution of the vectorcardiogram in hemodynamic overloading of the heart. Am Heart J 60:296, 1960

6. Caylor GG, Ongley P, Nadas AS: Relation of systolic pressure in the right ventricle to the electrocardiogram. A study of patients with pulmonary stenosis and intact ventricular septum. N Engl J Med 258:979, 1958

7. Coelho E, DePaiva E, DePadua F, Nunes A, Amram S, Bordalo E Sa, Luis S: Tetralogy of Fallot. Angiocardiographic, electrocardiographic, vectorcardiographic and hemodynamic studies of the Fallot-type complex. Am J Cardiol. 7:538, 1961

8. Daoud G, Kaplan S, Benzing G, Gallaher ME: Auscultatory findings of pure infundibular stenosis. Am J Dis Child 108:73, 1964

9. Davachi F, Lucas Jr, RV Moller JH: The Electrocardiogram and vectorcardiogram in tricuspid atresia. Correlation with pathologic anatomy. Am J Cardiol 25:18, 1970

10. Downing Jr, JW, Kaplan S, Bove KE: Postsurgical left anterior hemiblock and right bundle-branch block. Br Heart J 34:263, 1972

11. Durrer D, Roos JP, van Dam RT: The genesis of the electrocardiogram of patients with ostium primum defects (ventral atrial septal defects). Am Heart J 71:642, 1966

12. DuShane JW, Weidman WH, Brandenburg RO, Kirklin JW: Differentiation of interatrial communications by clinical methods: ostium secundum, ostium primum,

common atrium, and total anomalous pulmonary venous connection. Circulation 21:363, 1960

13. Elliott LP, Schiebler GL: A roentgenologic-electrocardiographic approach to cyanotic forms of heart disease. Pediatr Clin North Am 18:1133, 1971

14. Ellison RG, Restieaux NJ: Vectorcardiography in congenital heart disease: a method for estimating severity, Philadelphia, WB Saunders Company, 1972

15. Feldt RH, DuShane JW, Titus JL: The anatomy of the atrioventricular conduction system in ventricular septal defect and tetralogy of Fallot: correlations with the electrocardiogram and vectorcardiogram. Circulation 34:774, 1966

16. Fowler RS, Shams A, Keith JD: The vectorcardiogram in aortic stenosis in childhood, in I Hoffman (ed): Vectorcardiography 2. Philadelphia, Lippincott, 1971, p 568

17. Gamboa R, Gersony WM, Nadas AS: The Electrocardiogram in tricuspid atresia and pulmonary atresia with intact ventricular septum. Circulation 34:24, 1966

18. Gaum WE, Chou T-C, Kaplan S: The vectorcardiogram and electrocardiogram in supravalvular aortic stenosis and coarctation of the aorta. Am Heart J 84:620, 1972

19. Gessner IH, Elliott LP, Schiebler GL, Van Mierop LHS, Miller B Lynn: The Vectorcardiogram in double inlet left ventricle, with or without ventricular inversion, in Hoffman I (ed): Vectorcardiography 2. Philadelphia, Lippincott, 1971 p 624

20. Grant RP: The syndrome of dextroversion of the heart. Circulation 18:25, 1958

21. Guller B, DuShane JW, Titus JL: The atrioventricular conduction system in two cases of tricuspid atresia. Circulation 40:217, 1969

22. Hamby RI, Hoffman I, Glassman E: The T loop in right ventricular hypertrophy. Dis Chest 55:105, 1969

23. Hugenholtz PG, Gamboa R: Effect of chronically increased ventricular pressure on electrical forces of the heart. Circulation 31:511, 1964

24. James FW, Kaplan S: The Normal electrocardiogram in the infant and child, in Fisch C (ed): Cardiovascular Clinics, vol. 5, no 3. Philadelphia, FA Davis, 1973, p 295

25. Kahn M, Bleifer SB, Grishman A, Donoso E: The vectorcardiogram and electrocardiogram before and after valvulotomy for pulmonic stenosis. Am Heart J 58:327, 1959

26. Kaplan S: Atrial septal defects, in Watson H (ed): Paediatric Cardiology. CV Mosby Co, St Louis, 1968, p 376

27. Kaplan S: The treatment of tetralogy of Fallot, in Yu PN, Goodwin JF (eds): Progress in Cardiology. Philadelphia, Lea & Febiger, 1972, p 229

28. Kaplan S, Assali NS: Disorders of circulation, in Assali NS (ed): Pathophysiology of Gestation, vol 3. New York, Academic Press, 1972, p 1

29. Kaplan S, Helmsworth JA, Ahearn EN, Benzing G III, Daoud G, Schwartz DC: Results of palliative procedures for tetralogy of Fallot in infants and young children. Ann Thorac Surg 5:489, 1968

30. Keith JD, Rowe RD, Vlad P: Heart disease in infancy and childhood, New York, The Macmillan Company, 1967

31. Khoury GH, Vectorcardiographic patterns of left ventricular hypertrophy in infancy and childhood, in Hoffman I (ed): Vectorcardiography 2. Philadelphia, Lippincott 1971, p 573

32. Khoury GH, DuShane JW, Ongley PA: The preoperative and postoperative vectorcardiogram in tetralogy of Fallot. Circulation 31:85, 1965

33. Khoury GH, Fowler RS: Normal Frank Vectorcardiogram in infancy and childhood. Br Heart J 29:563, 1967

34. Khoury GH, Fowler RS, Keith JD: The vectorcardiogram in ventricular septal defect. Analysis of 100 cases and correlation with the hemodynamics, in Hoffman I, Taymor RC (eds): vectorcardiography. Philadelphia, Lippincott 1966, p 299

35. Khoury GH, Shaher RM, Fowler RS: The vectorcardiogram in complete transposition of the great vessels: analysis of fifty cases. Circulation 35:178, 1967

36. Kulbertus HE, Coyne JJ, Hallidie-Smith KA: Conduction disturbances before and after surgical closure of ventricular septal defect. Am Heart J 77:123, 1969

37. Lee YC, Scherlis L: Atrial septal defect. Electrocardiographic, vectorcariographic, and catheterization data. Circulation 25:1024, 1962

38. Lev M: The architecture of the conduction system in congenital heart disease. III. Ventricular septal defect. Arch Pathol 70:529, 1960

39. Liebman J, Romberg HG, Downs T, Agusti R: The Frank QRS vectorcardiogram in the premature infant, in Hoffman I, Taymor RC (eds): Vectorcardiography. Philadelphia, Lippincott, 1966, p 256

40. Mair DD, Macartney FJ, Weidman WH, Ritter DG, Ongley PA, Smith RE: The Vectorcardiogram in complete transposition of the great arteries: correlation with anatomic and hemodynamic findings and calculated left ventricular mass, in Hoffman I (ed): Vectorcardiography 2. Philadelphia, Lippincott, 1971, p 610

41. Nadas AS, Gamboa R, Hugenholtz PG: Anomalous left coronary artery originating from the pulmonary artery. Report of two surgically treated cases with a proposal of hemodynamic and therapeutic classification. Circulation 29:167, 1964

42. Namin EP, Arcilla RA, D'Cruz IA, Gasul BM: Evolution of the Frank vectorcardiogram in normal infants. Am J Cardiol 13:757, 1964

43. Neufeld HN, DuShane JW, Wood EH, Kirklin JW, Edwards JE: Origin of both great vessels from the right ventricle. I. Without pulmonary stenosis. Circulation 23:399, 1961

44. Neufeld HN, Titus JL, DuShane JW, Burchell HB, Edwards JE: Isolated ventricular septal defect of the persistent common atrioventricular canal type. Circulation 23:685, 1961

45. Ongley PA, DuShane JW: Counterclockwise superiorly displaced frontal plane loops of the vectorcardiogram in children, in Hoffman I, Taymor RC (eds): Vectorcardiography. Philadelphia, Lippincott, 1966, p 339

46. Paul RN, Megevand RP, Parker J: Tetralogy of fallot with left ventricular hypertrophy. J Pediat 45:672, 1954

47. Pileggi F, Bocanegra J, Tranchesi J, Macruz R, Borges S, Portugal O, Villarinho MG, Barbato E, Décourt LV: The electrocardiogram in tetralogy of Fallot: A study of 142 cases. Am Heart J 59:667, 1960

48. Pryor R, Woodwark GM, Blount JR, SG: Electrocardiographic changes in atrial septal defects: Ostium secundum defect versus ostium primum (Endocardial Cushion) defect. Am Heart J 58:689, 1959

49. Puri PS, Rowe RD, Neill CA: Varying vectorcardiographic patterns in anomalous left coronary artery arising from pulmonary artery. Am Heart J 71:616, 1966

50. Reeve R, Kawamata K, Seltzer A: Reliability of vectorcardiography in assessing the severity of congenital aortic stenosis. Circulation 34:92, 1966

51. Riemenschneider TA, Vincent WR, Ruttenberg HD, Desilets DT: Transposition of the great vessels with hypoplasia of the right ventricle. Circulation 38:386, 1968

52. Rosenbaum MB, Corrado G, Oliveri R, Castellanos A, Elizari MV: Right bundle branch block with left anterior hemiblock surgically induced in tetralogy of Fallot. Am J of Cardiol 26:12, 1970

53. Spach MS, Boineau JP, Long EG, Gabor JB, Gallie TM: Genesis of the vectorcardiogram (Electrocardiogram) in endocardial cushion defects, in Hoffman I, Taymor RC (eds): Vectorcardiography. Philadelphia, Lippincott, 1966, p 307

54. Titus JL, Neufeld HN, Edwards JE: The atrioventricular conduction system in hearts with both great vessels originating from the right ventricle. Am Heart J 67:588, 1964

55. Toscano-Barboza E, Brandenburg RO, Swan HJC: Atrial septal defect. The Electrocardiogram and its hemodynamic correlation in 100 proved cases. Am J Cardiol 2:698, 1958

SECTION III

Exercises in Vectorcardiographic Interpretation and Correlation with the Clinical and Anatomic Findings

In this section 50 vectorcardiograms are presented for the readers to interpret. The conventional electrocardiograms, the author's interpretation, the clinical information, and in most instances, the anatomic findings are given for reference.

Fig. B.1., C.F., 421357

Vectorcardiogram.   The PsÊ loop is abnormally large. The maximum **P** vector in the sagittal and frontal planes exceeds 0.35 mV. From the sagittal plane it can be seen that most of the P loop is located anteriorly. There is a marked displacement of the QRSsÊ loop anteriorly and to the right. The QRS loop is inscribed clockwise in all three planar projections. There is no evidence of a conduction delay. The TsÊ loop is oriented to the left, posteriorly, and slightly superiorly. In the transverse plane the loop is inscribed clockwise.

Vectorcardiographic diagnosis.   Right atrial enlargement. Abnormal right axis deviation. Right ventricular hypertrophy.

Electrocardiographic diagnosis.   Right atrial enlargement. Abnormal right axis deviation. Right ventricular hypertrophy.

Clinical and anatomic findings.   The patient is a 27-year-old woman with severe valvular pulmonic stenosis. During cardiac catheterization a systolic pressure gradient of 120 mm Hg was demonstrated across the pulmonic valve. A small right-to-left shunt was present at the atrial level. At surgery valvular pulmonary stenosis and a patent foramen ovale were found. The right ventricle was markedly enlarged with severe muscular hypertrophy of the outflow tract of the right ventricle. The right atrium was slightly enlarged.

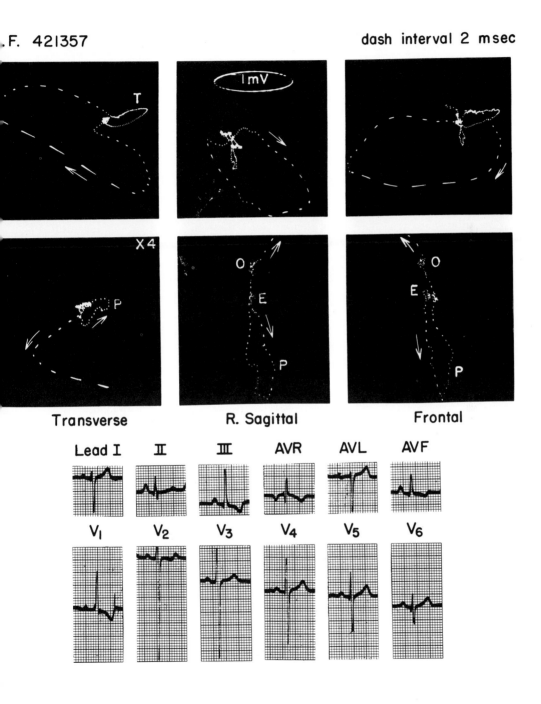

.F. 421357　　　　　　　　　　　dash interval 2 msec

Transverse　　　　　R. Sagittal　　　　　Frontal

Lead I　II　III　AVR　AVL　AVF

V₁　V₂　V₃　V₄　V₅　V₆

Fig. B.2. C.F. 421357

Vectorcardiogram. The QRSsÊ loop is displaced anteriorly and rightward. The duration of the loop is 0.11 sec. There is a slowly inscribed terminal appendage which is directed to the right, anteriorly, and inferiorly. The duration of the terminal slowing is about 0.06 sec. The TsÊ loop is discordant to the terminal **QRS** vectors. In the transverse plane the T loop is inscribed clockwise, and in the right sagittal plane it is inscribed counterclockwise.

Vectorcardiographic diagnosis. Right bundle branch block.

Electrocardiographic diagnosis. Right bundle branch block.

Clinical Information. The tracings were recorded 20 days after surgery from the patient with pulmonary stenosis whose vectorcardiogram and electrocardiogram before operation are illustrated in Fig. B.1. The development of right bundle branch block is probably related to the resection of the hypertrophied muscle of the outflow tract of the right ventricle.

Comment. Anatomic right ventricular hypertrophy was probably still present in this patient at the time of the recording. However, the diagnosis of right ventricular hypertrophy in the presence of right bundle branch block is usually quite difficult. Anterior displacement of the afferent limb of the QRS loop with a figure-of-eight or clockwise inscription of the loop in the transverse plane may be seen in right bundle branch block in the absence of right ventricular hypertrophy. This is particularly true when the duration of the QRS is markedly prolonged. In this case, as the duration of the QRS loop is only 0.11 sec, the rather prominent rightward and anterior QRS forces before the onset of the terminal slowing and the wide frontal plane loop do raise the possibility of right ventricular hypertropy.

C.F. 421357

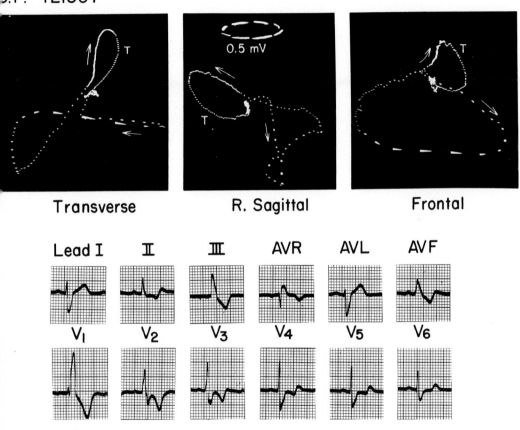

Transverse   R. Sagittal   Frontal

Fig. B.3., J.W., 369171

Vectorcardiogram. The QRSsÊ loop is abnormally large and is displaced posteriorly. The magnitude of the maximum **QRS** vector in all of the three planar projections is about 3 mV. The abnormally large **ST** vector and the TsÊ loop are directed to the right, anteriorly, and superiorly and are about 180° away from the QRSsÊ loop.

Vectorcardiographic diagnosis. Left ventricular hypertrophy.

Electrocardiographic diagnosis. Left ventricular hypertrophy. Left atrial enlargement based on the large negative component of the P wave in lead V_1.

Clinical and anatomic findings. The patient was a 46-year-old man with long-standing hypertensive cardiovascular disease. He died about 6 months after the recording of the illustrated tracings. At autopsy marked left ventricular and mild right ventricular hypertrophy were present. The heart weighed 575 gm. There was no evidence of myocardial infarction.

Comment. The mild right ventricular hypertrophy is not evident on either the vectorcardiogram or the electrocardiogram. It is possible that the clockwise inscription of the front plane QRS loop in the presence of marked left ventricular hypertrophy is significant and suggests the coexistence of right ventricular hypertrophy. The specificity of this sign, however, is still to be proved.

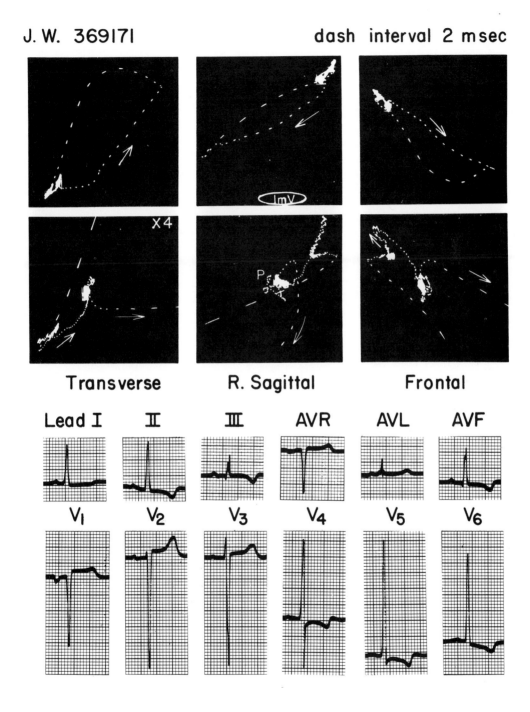

J. W. 369171   dash interval 2 msec

Transverse   R. Sagittal   Frontal

Lead I   II   III   AVR   AVL   AVF

V₁   V₂   V₃   V₄   V₅   V₆

Fig. B.4., A.W.

Vectorcardiogram.   The P loop is normal in its magnitude and orientation in all three planar projections. The direction of inscription of the P loop cannot be determined from the recording. The magnitude and orientation of the QRS loop are within the normal range, with the maximum **QRS** vector being less than 2 mV in each of the three planes. The configuration and direction of inscription of the loop are normal. There is no evidence of a conduction delay. The **ST** vector and T loop are also within normal limits.

Vectorcardiographic diagnosis.   Normal vectorcardiogram.

Electrocardiographic diagnosis.   Normal electrocardiogram.

Clinical findings.   The tracings were recorded from a 38-year-old healthy man. There is no history to suggest cardiovascular disease. Results of his physical examination and chest x-ray are also within normal limits.

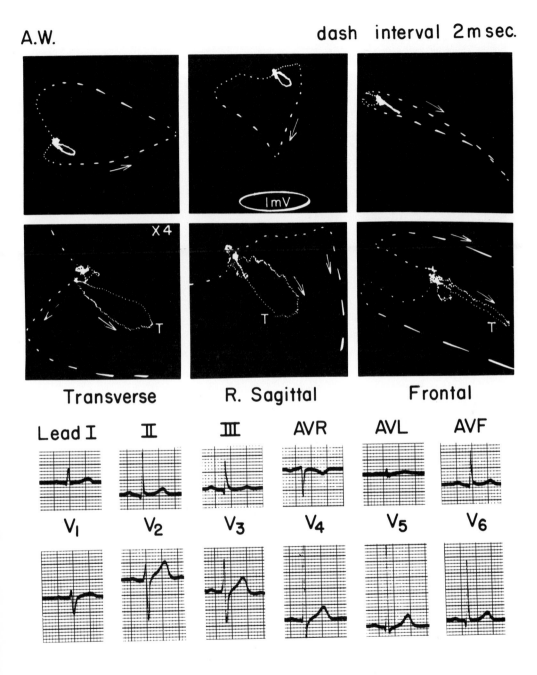

A.W.

dash interval 2 m sec.

X4

1mV

Transverse   R. Sagittal   Frontal

Lead I   II   III   AVR   AVL   AVF

V₁   V₂   V₃   V₄   V₅   V₆

Fig. B.5., L.D., 297110

Vectorcardiogram.   In the transverse plane the vectorcardiogram is essentially normal except for the clockwise inscription of the T loop. In the sagittal and frontal planes the duration of the initial superior QRS forces is at the upper limit of normal. The initial deflection and the efferent limb of the QRS loop in the frontal plane are inscribed clockwise. The magnitude of the maximum left superior **QRS** vector is greater than 0.25 mV. The TsÊ loop is displaced superiorly.

Vectorcardiographic diagnosis.   Inferior myocardial infarction, age undetermined.

Electrocardiographic diagnosis.   Inferior wall myocardial infarction, age undetermined.

Clinical findings.   The patient is a 43-year-old woman who developed an acute myocardial infarction 3 weeks prior to the recording of these tracings. The serial electrocardiograms and enzyme studies were all typical of an acute infarction.

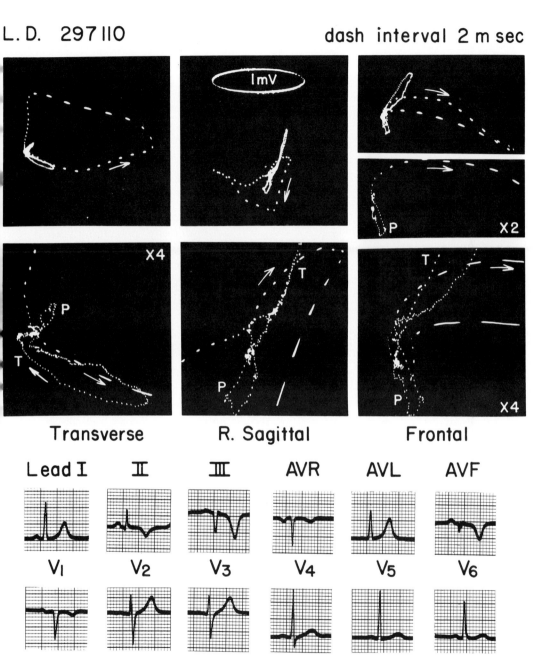

L. D. 297 110   dash interval 2 m sec

Transverse   R. Sagittal   Frontal

Lead I   II   III   AVR   AVL   AVF

V1   V2   V3   V4   V5   V6

Fig. B.6., B.C., 432281

Vectorcardiogram.   The magnitude of the QRSsÊ loop is markedly increased. Its duration is 0.11 sec. The loop is oriented to the left, posteriorly, and inferiorly. In the transverse plane the initial deflection is directed anteriorly and to the right. The loop has a figure-of-eight pattern and its maximum vector measures 5.5 mV. In the sagittal plane the loop is inscribed clockwise and in the frontal plane, counterclockwise. The abnormally large **ST** vector and the T loop are discordant to the maximum **QRS** vector in all of the three planar projections.

Vectorcardiographic diagnosis.   Left ventricular hypertrophy. Intraventricular conduction defect.

Electrocardiographic diagnosis.   Left ventricular hypertrophy. Intranventricular conduction defect.

Clinical and anatomic findings.   The patient was a 17-year-old boy with the clinical diagnoses of rheumatic heart disease, mitral insufficiency, aortic stenosis and insufficiency. He died 10 days after the recording of the tracings. At autopsy the clinical diagnoses were confirmed. The heart weighed 970 gm and was markedly increased in size. There was severe left ventricular hypertrophy and mild right ventricular hypertrophy. The left ventricle measured 2.2 cm in thickness, the right ventricle, 0.4 cm.

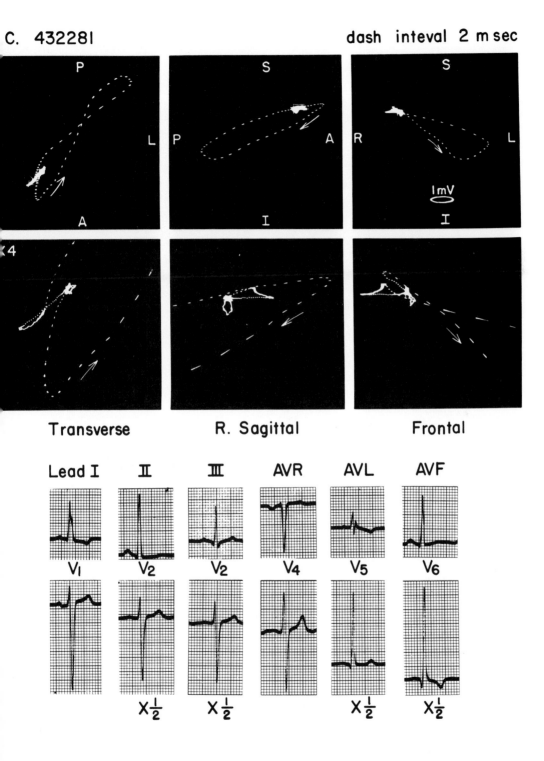

C. 432281

dash inteval 2 m sec

Transverse   R. Sagittal   Frontal

Lead I   II   III   AVR   AVL   AVF

V_1 V_2 V_2 V_4 V_5 V_6

$X\frac{1}{2}$ $X\frac{1}{2}$ $X\frac{1}{2}$ $X\frac{1}{2}$

Fig. B.7., M.M., 436820

Vectorcardiogram. There is an increase in the magnitude of the PsÊ loop, and most of the loop area is located posteriorly. The QRSsÊ loop is normal in size. The duration of the QRSsÊ loop is slightly less than 0.12 sec. There is an overall slight reduction of the speed of inscription of the loop. In the transverse plane the loop inscribes a figure-of-eight pattern mainly attributed to the posterior displacement of the efferent limb. The initial deflection is directed anteriorly and to the left. In the right sagittal plane there is also a figure-of-eight configuration of the QRS loop, and the initial deflection is directed anteriorly and inferiorly. In the frontal plane the loop is inscribed counterclockwise even though the direction of the maximum **QRS** vector is 50°. The abnormally large **ST** vector and the TsÊ loop are directed anteriorly, rightward, and superiorly, and are opposite to the orientation of the QRSsÊ loop. In the sagittal and frontal planes the T loop appears to be quite wide.

Vectorcardiographic diagnosis. Left atrial enlargement. Anterolateral myocardial infarction with intraventricular defect. Possible incomplete left bundle branch block.

Electrocardiographic diagnosis. Incomplete left bundle branch block.

Clinical and anatomic findings. The patient was a 58-year-old man who had arteriosclerotic heart disease with chronic congestive heart failure. He died 8 months after the recording of the tracings. Repeated electrocardiograms taken a few days before death revealed no essential changes from the tracing illustrated. At autopsy there was severe atherosclerosis of the coronary arteries. There were extensive areas of old fibrosed myocardial infarction in the posterior wall and anteroseptal region of the left ventricle. The heart weighed 465 gm. The left ventricle measured 8 to 15 mm in thickness and showed evidence of moderate dilatation and mild hypertrophy. There was moderate right ventricular hypertrophy with the right ventricular wall measuring 6 to 8 mm in thickness.

Comment. In view of the anatomic findings, the posterior displacement of the efferent limb of the QRS loop is most likely caused by the anterior wall myocardial damage rather than incomplete left bundle branch block. The magnitude of the QRS loop is also smaller than in the usual case of incomplete left bundle branch block. Left atrial enlargement as suggested by the vectorcardiogram is often difficult to verify anatomically but is consistent with the rest of the anatomic findings.

I.M. 436820   dash interval 2 msec

Transverse   R. Sagittal   Frontal

Lead I   II   III   AVR   AVL   AVF

V₁   V₂   V₃   V₄   V₅   V₆

Fig. B.8., E.R., 420660

Vectorcardiogram.   The PsÊ loop cannot be identified. There is a rightward displacement of the afferent limb and terminal deflection of the QRSsÊ loop. The duration of the QRSsÊ loop is normal, and there is no evidence of a conduction delay. In the transverse plane the loop is inscribed counterclockwise, but the loop area in the right posterior quadrant exceeds 20 percent of the entire QRS loop. In the frontal plane the loop is inscribed clockwise and is relatively wide. The TsÊ loop is small and irregular in configuration.

Vectorcardiographic diagnosis.   Right ventricular hypertrophy.

Electrocardiographic diagnosis.   Atrial fibrillation. Nonspecific ST-and T-wave abnormalities and/or digitalis effect.

Clinical and anatomic findings.   The patient was a 56-year-old man with rheumatic heart disease, aortic stenosis and insufficiency, mitral stenosis and insufficiency, and tricuspid insufficiency. He died 2 months later, following replacement of the mitral and aortic valves with Starr-Edwards prothesis. At autopsy the heart weighed 680 gm. There were marked dilatation and hypertrophy of the right atrium and right ventricle and mild hypertrophy of the left ventricle. The right ventricular wall measured 6 to 8 mm in thickness and the left ventricular wall, 15 mm.

E.R. 420660

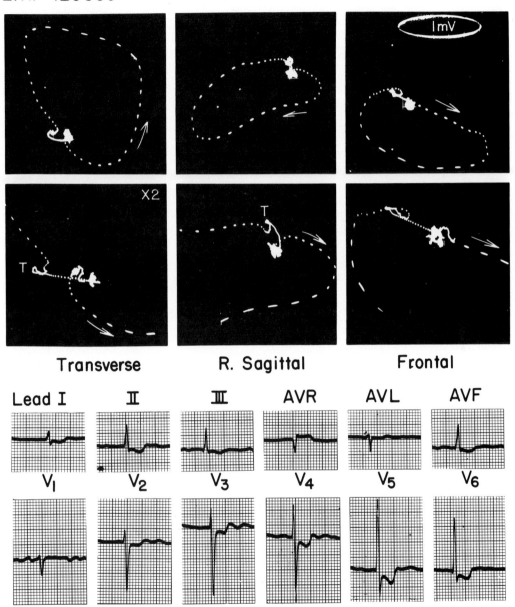

Fig. B.9., L.G., 326665

Vectorcardiogram.   The PsÊ loop is abnormally large. The right sagittal plane reveals that both the anterior and posterior components of the P loop are increased. There is also a marked increase in the magnitude of the QRSsÊ loop. The spatial loop is oriented more posteriorly and superiorly than that of the average normal subject. The abnormally large **ST** vector and the TsÊ loop are oriented to the right, anteriorly and slightly superiorly, and are discordant to the QRSsÊ loop.

Vectorcardiographic diagnosis.   Biatrial enlargement. Left ventricular hypertrophy.

Electrocardiographic Diagnosis.   Left atrial enlargement.Left ventricular hypertrophy.

Clinical and Anatomic findings.   The patient was a 40-year-old man with advanced hypertensive cardiovascular disease and severe congestive heart failure. He died a few days after the recording of the tracings. At autopsy the heart weighed 550 gm. There were marked hypertrophy and dilatation of all the heart chambers. The lumen of the coronary arteries was narrowed by extensive atheromatous lesions, but there was no gross evidence of myocardial infarction.

L.G. 326665

dash interval 2 m sec

Transverse   R. Sagittal   Frontal

Lead I   II   III   AVR   AVL   AVF

V_1 V_2 V_3 V_4 V_5 V_6

$X\frac{1}{2}$ $X\frac{1}{2}$ $X\frac{1}{2}$ $X\frac{1}{2}$ $X\frac{1}{2}$

Fig. B.10., M.J., 327603

Vectorcardiogram. The PsÊ loop is abnormally large, and the magnitude of the maximum **P** vector in the sagittal and frontal planes exceeds 0.2 mV. Most of the loop area is located posteriorly as indicated in the right sagittal plane. The QRSsÊ loop is displaced posteriorly, and in the transverse and sagittal projections the loop appears quite narrow. In the transverse plane, there is a loss of the initial anterior forces. The initial deflection is inscribed briefly posteriorly before it becomes anterior for a very limited course. The 0.02 sec instantaneous vector is directed posteriorly. In the right sagittal plane the posterior course of the initial deflection can also be seen, and the loop is inscribed counterclockwise during that period. The **ST** vector is abnormally large and directed anteriorly. There is also anterior and superior displacement of the TsÊ loop.

Vectorcardiographic diagnosis. Left atrial enlargement. Anteroseptal myocardial infarction, probably acute.

Electrocardiographic diagnosis. Probable acute anterior wall myocardial infarction.

Clincial and antomic findings. The patient was a 70-year-old woman who presented typical clinical features of acute myocardial infarction a few days before the recording of the tracings. A loud pansystolic murmur was heard at the apex. She died 5 days later. At autopsy there was a total occlusion of the anterior descending branch of the left coronary artery with acute infarction of the anterior portion of the interventricular septum and the left anterior ventricular wall. A very small perforation (1 mm in diameter) of the interventricular septum was found. The left ventricle was dilated, and a ventricular aneurysm involving the septum and apex was observed. The heart weighed 365 gm.

M.J. 327603   dash interval 2 m sec

Transverse   R. Sagittal   Frontal

Lead I   II   III   AVR   AVL   AVF

V₁   V₂   V₃   V₄   V₅   V₆

Fig. B.11., B.M., 405541

Vectorcardiogram. The magnitude of the PsÊ loop is increased. The maximum **P** vector in the transverse, sagittal, and frontal planes measures 0.12, 0.3, and 0.3 mV, respectively. Most of the loop area is located posteriorly. The QRSsÊ loop is within normal limits. The TsÊ loop is abnormally small. (The lower panel of the vectorcardiogram displays only the P loop and part of the QRS loop.)

Vectorcardiographic Diagnosis. Left atrial enlargement. Abnormal TsÊ loop.

Electrocardiographic diagnosis. Nonspecific ST-and T-wave changes.

Clinical and anatomic findings. The patient is a 20-year-old woman with rheumatic heart disease and severe mitral stenosis. The diagnosis was confirmed at operation.

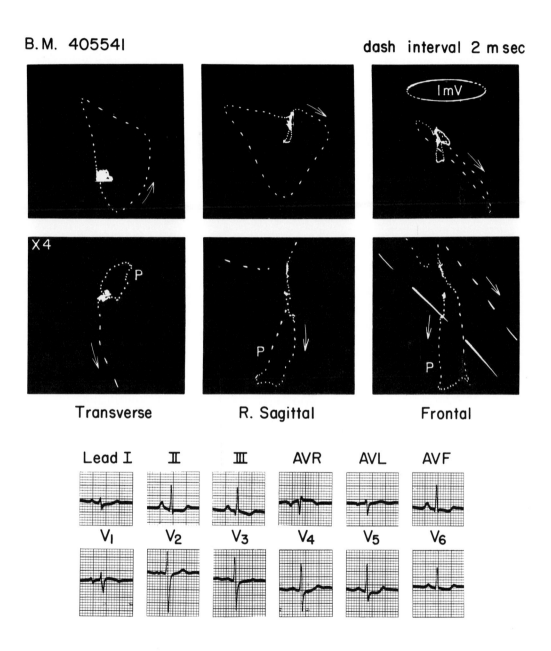

B.M. 405541   dash interval 2 m sec

ImV

X4

P

P

P

Transverse   R. Sagittal   Frontal

Lead I   II   III   AVR   AVL   AVF

V₁   V₂   V₃   V₄   V₅   V₆

Fig. B.12, H.E., 389699

Vectorcardiogram. The magnitude of the QRSsÊ loop is increased. The loop is oriented posteriorly, to the left, and slightly inferiorly. The midportion of the loop is slowly inscribed, and the duration of the QRSsÊ loop is 0.12 sec. In the transverse plane the QRS loop is inscribed in a figure-of-eight pattern with most of the loop being clockwise. The initial deflection is directed anteriorly and to the left. In the right sagittal plane the loop presents a double figure-of-eight pattern and is quite narrow. The frontal plane QRS loop also has a narrow figure-of-eight configuration. The **ST** vector and TsÊ loop are directed anteriorly, to the right and superiorly and are discordant to the QRSsÊ loop.

Vectorcardiographic diagnosis. Complete left bundle branch block.

Electrocardiographic diagnosis. Complete left bundle branch block.

Clinical and anatomic findings. The patient was a 39-year-old man who had rheumatic heart disease with aortic insufficiency and stenosis. He died 2 weeks after the recording of the tracings. At autopsy the heart weighed 975 gm. There were marked dilatation and hypertrophy of the left atrium and left ventricle. The right ventricular wall measured 4 mm in thickness and the left ventricular wall, 18 mm. The bundle of His was found to be replaced by fibrous tissue. Detailed histological examination of the bundle branches was not performed.

Comment. The vectorcardiogram is typical for complete left bundle branch block except the frontal plane QRS loop has a figure-of-eight pattern instead of a counterclockwise inscription. Although the magnitude of the QRSsÊ loop is increased, the diagnosis of left ventricular hypertrophy cannot be made because of the conduction defect. However, the great majority of patients with left bundle branch block do have anatomic left ventricular hypertrophy as in this case.

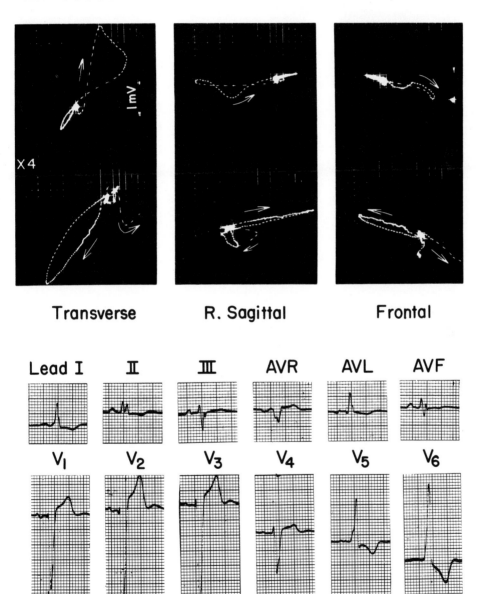

H.E. 389699 dash interval 2.5 m sec

Transverse   R. Sagittal   Frontal

Lead I   II   III   AVR   AVL   AVF

V_1 V_2 V_3 V_4 V_5 V_6

Fig. B.13., H.C., 336961

Vectorcardiogram. The maximum **P** vector in the transverse plane measures 0.12 mV, and most of the P-loop area is located posteriorly. The QRSsÊ loop has a terminal appendage which is directed anteriorly, to the right and slightly superiorly. The terminal appendage is slowly inscribed. In the transverse plane the initial deflection is directed to the left and anteriorly. The maximum **QRS** vector is also so directed with a magnitude of 2.0 mV. In the sagittal and frontal planes the major portion of the QRS loop is inscribed counterclockwise. The TsÊ loop is oriented posteriorly, leftward and inferiorly and is discordant to the terminal appendage of the QRSsÊ loop.

Vectorcardiographic diagnosis. Left atrial enlargement. Right bundle branch block. Probable left ventricular hypertrophy.

Electrocardiographic diagnosis. Right bundle branch block. Probable left ventricular hypertrophy.

Clinical and anatomic findings. The patient was a 78-year-old man known to have hypertensive cardiovascular disease. He died 2.5 months after the recording of these tracings. At autopsy moderate left ventricular hypertrophy was present. The heart weighed 500 gm. The thickness of the left ventricular wall was 20 mm, and the right ventricular wall, 4 mm. The coronary arteries showed mild atherosclerotic changes but no significant narrowing.

Comment. Right bundle branch block usually obscures the vectorcardiographic and electrocardiographic evidence of left ventricular hypertrophy. Since the magnitude of the maximum **QRS** vector is usually reduced when right bundle branch block develops, the relatively large leftward forces in the vectorcardiogram and the tall R wave in the left precordial leads of the electrocardiogram are strongly suggestive of left ventricular hypertrophy. As the body of the QRS loop is displaced superiorly and is inscribed counterclockwise in the frontal plane, one may also suspect the presence of left anterior hemiblock.

H.C. 336961   dash interval 2.5 m sec

Transverse   R. Sagittal   Frontal

Lead I   II   III   AVR   AVL   AVF

V₁   V₂   V₃   V₄   V₅   V₆

X ½   X ½   X ½

Fig. B.14, R.T., 446470

Vectorcardiogram.   The PsÊ loop is abnormally large. The maximum **P** vector measures 0.2, 0.3, and 0.3 mV in the transverse, sagittal, and frontal planes, respectively. The sagittal plane shows the P loop is neither predominantly anterior nor posterior. The QRSsÊ loop is displaced anteriorly and to the right. In the transverse plane the QRS loop has a figure-of-eight pattern with most of the loop inscribed clockwise. In the frontal plane it is wide and is inscribed clockwise with most of the loop area located on the right side. The abnormally large **ST** vector and the TsÊ loop are directed to the left, posteriorly, and inferiorly. The T loop is inscribed clockwise in the transverse plane and counterclockwise in the sagittal plane.

Vectorcardiographic diagnosis.   Atrial enlargement, probably bilateral. Abnormal right axis deviation. Right ventricular hypertrophy.

Electrocardiographic diagnosis.   Abnormal right axis deviation. Right ventricular hypertrophy. Biatrial enlargement.

Clinical and anatomic findings.   The patient is a 25-year-old man with rheumatic heart disease and severe mitral stenosis. X-ray of the chest and fluoroscopy revealed left atrial and right ventricular enlargement. Cardiac catherterization demonstrated high pulmonary arterial and wedge pressures with a mean value of 72 and 20 mm, respectively.

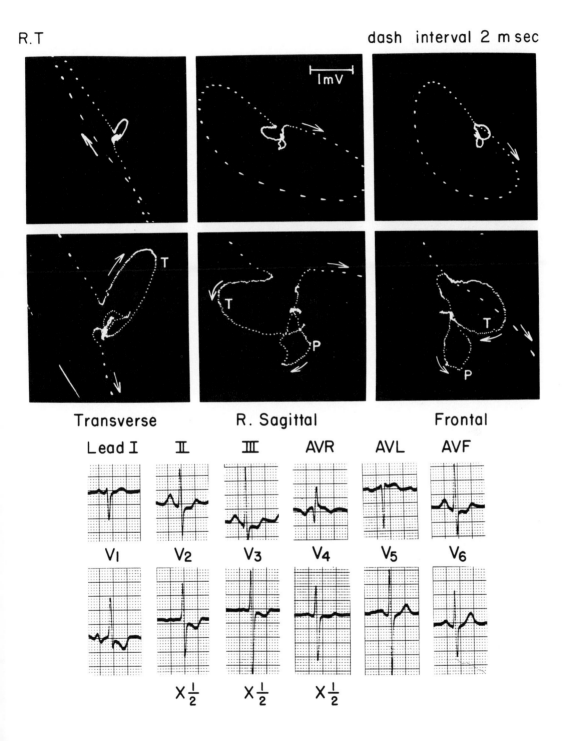

R.T

dash interval 2 m sec

1mV

Transverse   R. Sagittal   Frontal

Lead I   II   III   AVR   AVL   AVF

V₁   V₂   V₃   V₄   V₅   V₆

X½   X½   X½

Fig. B.15., O.U., 443240

Vectorcardiogram.   The QRSsÊ loop is displaced anteriorly. In the transverse plane the great majority of the QRS loop area is located in the left anterior quadrant, and the loop is inscribed counterclockwise. The duration of the anterior QRS forces is 0.05 sec. In the sagittal and frontal planes the QRS loop is inscribed clockwise. The duration of the initial superior QRS forces is 0.026 sec, which is just above the normal upper limit of 0.025 sec. The TsÊ loop is directed anteriorly, leftward and superiorly. The direction of inscription of the T loop in the transverse and sagittal planes is the reverse of the normal.

Vectorcardiographic diagnosis.   Probable inferior and true posterior myocardial infarction.

Electrocardiographic diagnosis.   Probable inferior and true posterior myocardial infarction.

Clinical findings.   The patient is a 55-year-old man who had symptoms suggestive of acute myocardial infarction 17 days prior to the recording of the illustrated tracings. The diagnosis was supported by serum enzyme elevation. Serial electrocardiograms showed progressive T wave inversion in the inferior leads and increased amplitude of the T wave in the right precordial leads. There was also gradual diminution of the amplitude and eventual disappearance of the S wave in lead V_2.

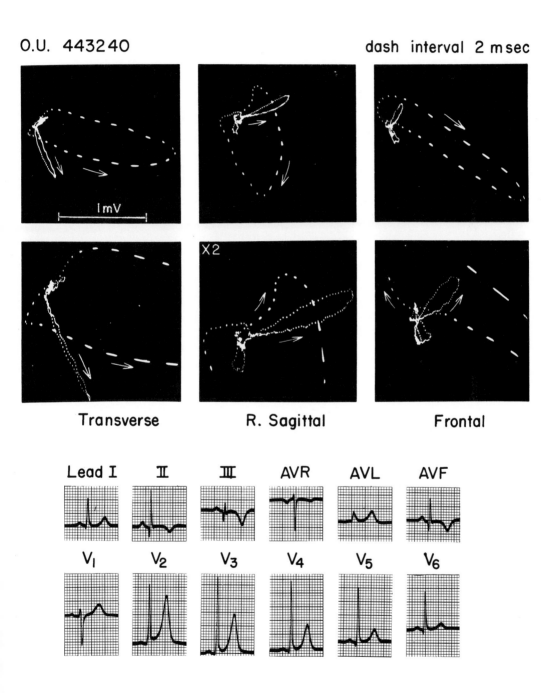

O.U. 443240   dash interval 2 msec

1 mV

X2

Transverse   R. Sagittal   Frontal

Lead I   II   III   AVR   AVL   AVF

V_1 V_2 V_3 V_4 V_5 V_6

Fig. B.16., E.D., 416369

Vectorcardiogram.   The spatial QRS loop is displaced anteriorly and to the right. There is no evidence of a conduction delay. In the transverse plane the QRS loop is inscribed clockwise. In the right sagittal plane it is inscribed counterclockwise. The loop has a figure-of-eight pattern in the frontal plane, and nearly all of the loop area is located inferiorly. The **ST** vector and the TsÊ loop are directed posteriorly, leftward and inferiorly. The direction of inscription of the T loop in the transverse and sagittal planes is the reversal of the normal.

Vectorcardiographic diagnosis.   Right axis deviation. Right ventricular hypertrophy.

Electrocardiographic diagnosis.   Right axis deviation. Incomplete right bundle branch block. Right ventricular hypertrophy.

Clinical and anatomic findings.   The patient was a 32-year-old man with the ostium secundum type of atrial septal defect and severe pulmonary hypertension. He died 6 days after surgical repair of the atrial septal defect. The illustrated tracings were recorded before surgery. At autopsy the heart weighed 480 gm. The left ventricular wall measured 10 mm in thickness, and the right ventricular wall, 7 mm. Except for the right ventricular hypertrophy, the myocardium was normal. There was marked dilatation of the pulmonary arterial system in which severe atherosclerosis was present. The coronary arteries revealed minimal atherosclerosis.

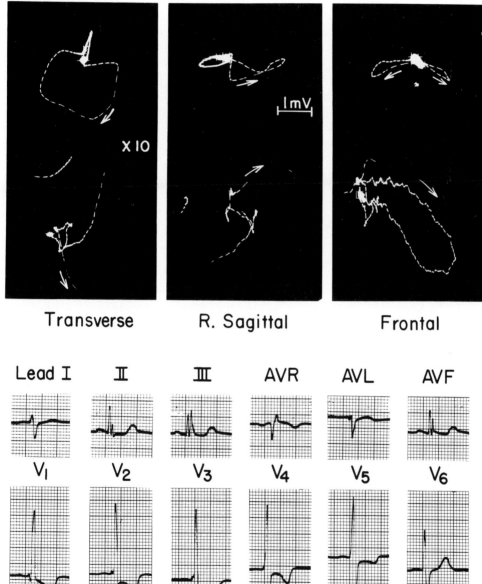

E.D. 416369   dash interval 2.5 m sec

Transverse   R. Sagittal   Frontal

Lead I   II   III   AVR   AVL   AVF

V_1 V_2 V_3 V_4 V_5 V_6

$X\frac{1}{2}$ $X\frac{1}{2}$ $X\frac{1}{2}$

Fig. B.17., J.C., 207156

Vectorcardiogram.   The magnitude of the maximum **P** vector in the transverse plane exceeds the normal upper limit. Most of the loop area is located posteriorly. The spatial QRS loop has a terminal appendage which is slowly inscribed and is directed anteriorly, rightward and superiorly. The duration of the QRSsÊ loop is increased. The initial deflection and the efferent limb of the QRS loop in all the planar projections remain normal. The TsÊ loop is directed posteriorly, to the left and inferiorly and is opposite to the direction of the terminal appendage of the QRSsÊ loop. The direction of inscription of the T loop in the transverse and right sagittal planes is the reverse of the normal.

Vectorcardiographic diagnosis.   Left atrial enlargement. Complete right bundle branch block.

Electrocardiographic diagnosis.   Abnormal P wave. Complete right bundle branch block.

Clinical and anatomic findings.   The patient was a 77-year-old man with chronic lymphocytic leukemia. He was also treated for mild congestive heart failure which was believed to be due to arteriosclerotic heart disease. He died about 7 months later because of severe lobular pneumonia. Repeated electrocardiograms taken shortly before his death showed no significant change from the illustrated tracing. At autopsy the heart weighed 400 gm. with an increase of the thickness of the left ventricular wall to 17 mm. The right ventricular wall was normal in thickness. The myocardium of the interventricular septum showed small areas of focal fibrosis. There were moderate atherosclerotic changes in the coronary arteries without significant narrowing of the lumen.

Comment.   The absence of vectorcardiographic and electrocardiographic evidence of left ventricular hypertrophy demonstrated at autopsy is not surprising. The right bundle branch block may be related to the focal fibrosis of the interventricular septum even though special studies of the conduction tissue were not done. It is usually difficult to correlate the vectorcardiographic or electrocardiographic diagnosis of left atrial enlargement with the anatomic findings. Dilatation of the atrium during life may not be observed at postmortem examination. A slight or moderate degree of atrial hypertrophy is also difficult to demonstrate. However, the presence of left ventricular hypertrophy in this case does support associated left atrial involvement.

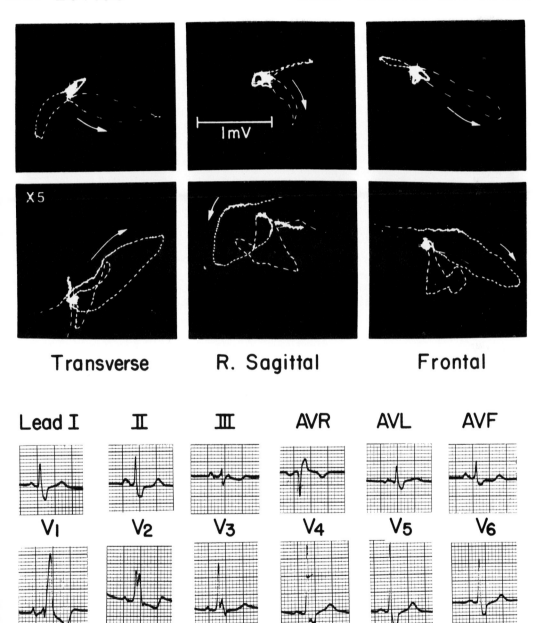

J.C. 207156   dash interval 2.5 m sec

X5

Transverse   R. Sagittal   Frontal

Lead I   II   III   AVR   AVL   AVF

V₁   V₂   V₃   V₄   V₅   V₆

Fig. B.18., J.S., 435674

Vectorcardiogram. The magnitude of the QRSsÊ loop is increased. The loop is directed to the left, slightly posteriorly and superiorly. In the transverse plane the initial deflection is written to the left and posteriorly and the great majority of the QRS loop is inscribed clockwise. In the sagittal plane the initial deflection is directed inferiorly, at first slightly anteriorly and then posteriorly. (The small initial anterior forces are not seen in the transverse plane. They are obscured by the P loop.) The 0.02 sec instantaneous **QRS** vector is directed posteriorly. The majority of the loop is inscribed clockwise. In the frontal plane it is inscribed counterclockwise. The large **ST** vector and the TsÊ loop are oriented to the right, anteriorly, and inferiorly and are essentially opposite to the direction of the QRSsÊ loop.

Vectorcardiographic diagnosis. Left ventricular hypertrophy. Incomplete left bundle branch block. An anteroseptal myocardial infarction cannot be ruled out.

Electrocardiographic diagnosis. Left ventricular hypertrophy. Incomplete left bundle branch block. An anteroseptal myocardial infarction cannot be ruled out.

Clinical and anatomic findings. The patient was a 39-year-old man with severe aortic insufficiency caused by perforation of the aortic cusps as a result of subacute bacterial endocarditis. He died shortly after surgery for the replacement of the aortic valve with a Starr-Edwards prothesis. The tracings were recorded the day before surgery. At autopsy the heart weighed 720 gm. The right ventricular wall measured 5 mm in thickness, and the left ventricular wall, 18 mm. The left ventricle was markedly dilated and moderately hypertrophied. The right ventricle was slightly hypertrophied and dilated. Dilatation and hypertrophy of the right atrium were also observed. The coronary arteries were normal and there was no evidence of myocardial infarction.

Comment. This case serves to emphasize the difficulty in the diagnosis of anteroseptal myocardial infarction when left ventricular hypertrophy is present. The incomplete left bundle branch block further reduces the initial anterior QRS forces.

S.   435674   dash interval 2 msec

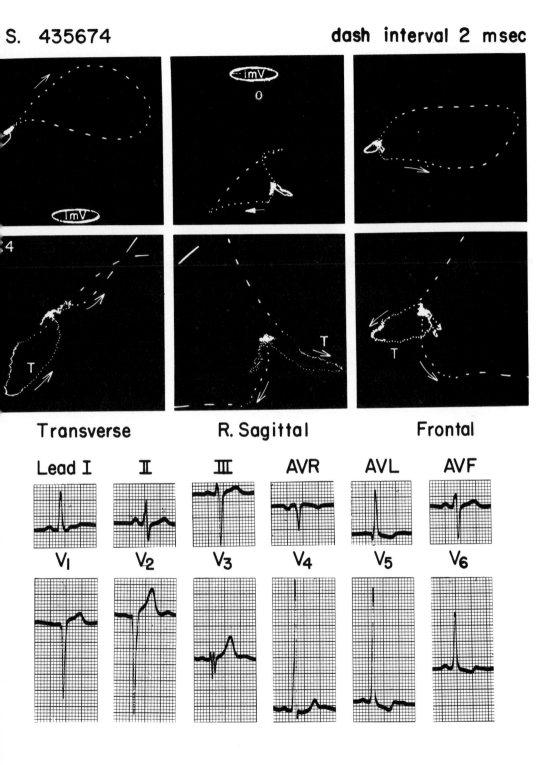

Transverse   R. Sagittal   Frontal

Lead I   II   III   AVR   AVL   AVF

V₁   V₂   V₃   V₄   V₅   V₆

Fig. B.19., L.D., 379223

Vectorcardiogram. In the transverse plane the efferent limb of the QRS loop is markedly displaced to the right side of the isoelectric point. The loop is inscribed clockwise. The T loop is also displaced to the right and posteriorly and is inscribed clockwise. There is some loss of the normal slow inscription of the outgoing portion of the T loop. In the right sagittal plane the QRS loop is displaced posteriorly and superiorly. The direction of inscription remains clockwise. The T loop is small and directed superiorly and posteriorly. It is inscribed counterclockwise. In the frontal plane most of the QRS loop is located on the right and the loop is inscribed clockwise. The T loop is oriented rightward and superiorly.

Vectorcardiographic diagnosis. Anterolateral myocardial infarction, age undetermined. The superior orientation of the T loop also suggests inferior myocardial ischemia. Left anterior hemiblock.

Electrocardiographic diagnosis. Anterolateral myocardial infarction, age undetermined. Inferior wall myocardial ischemia. Left anterior hemiblock.

Clinical findings. The tracings were recorded from a 47-year-old man 10 days after the onset of an acute myocardial infarction. The diagnosis was documented by serial electrocardiographic changes and elevation of serum enzymes.

Comment. The vectorcardiographic diagnosis of left anterior hemiblock was made in spite of the frontal plane QRS loop being displaced rightward and inscribed clockwise. These atypical findings are attributed to the anterolateral myocardial infarction.

.D. 379223

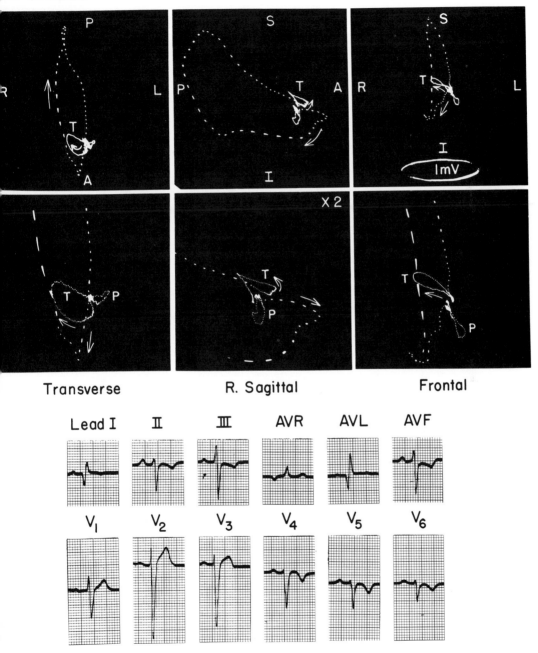

Transverse   R. Sagittal   Frontal

Lead I   II   III   AVR   AVL   AVF

V_1 V_2 V_3 V_4 V_5 V_6

Fig. B.20., R.B., 420296

Vectorcardiogram.   The magnitude of the maximum **P** vector in the transverse plane slightly exceeds the normal upper limit, and most of the loop area is located posteriorly. The QRSsÊ loop is abnormally large and is oriented to the left, posteriorly, and more or less horizontally. There is an increase of the duration of the loop with slow inscription of its mid and late portions. In the transverse plane the initial deflection is directed anteriorly, and the rest of the QRS loop inscribes a figure-of-eight pattern with most of the loop being clockwise. In the sagittal plane the QRS loop is inscribed clockwise and in the frontal plane, essentially counter-clockwise. The TsÊ loop is 180° discordant to the QRSsÊ loop.

Vectorcardiographic diagnosis.   Left atrial enlargement. Complete left bundle branch block.

Electrocardiographic diagnosis.   Probable left atrial enlargement. First degree AV block. Complete left bundle branch block.

Clinical and anatomic findings.   The patient was a 63-year-old man who was thought to have left ventricular failure attributed to rheumatic and arteriosclerotic heart disease. He died about 11 months later. Electrocardiograms taken shortly before death showed no significant change from the one illustrated. At autopsy the heart weighed 580 gm., and the left ventricular wall was 2 cm in thickness. Left ventricular hypertrophy was present. The mitral valve was thickened and partially calcified, resulting in both stenosis and insufficiency. The coronary arteries were narrowed to a slight degree by atherosclerotic plaques. Focal fibrosis of the myocardium was found with microscopic examination.

R.B. 420296   dash interval 2.5 m sec

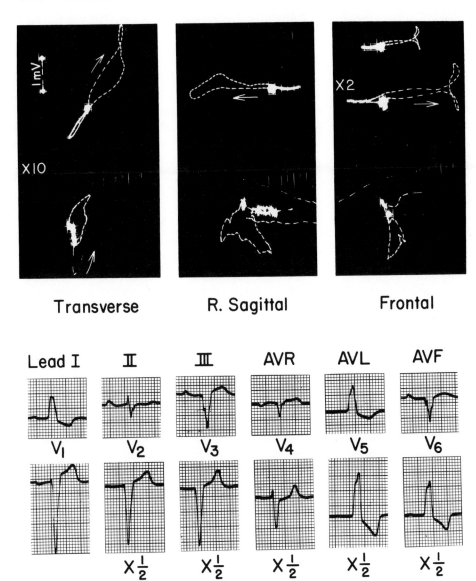

Transverse   R. Sagittal   Frontal

Lead I   II   III   AVR   AVL   AVF

V₁   V₂   V₃   V₄   V₅   V₆

X½   X½   X½   X½   X½

Fig. B.21., M. H., 314867

Vectorcardiogram. The P loop is small. Its orientation is within normal limits. There is marked anterior displacement of the QRS loop. The initial deflection is slowly inscribed and is directed anteriorly and superiorly. The T loop is within normal limits.

Vectorcardiographic diagnosis. Wolff-Parkinson-White syndrome, type A.

Electrocardiographic diagnosis. Posteroinferior lateral myocardial infarction versus atypical Wolff-Parkinson-White syndrome, type A.

Clinical findings. The patient is a 62-year-old man who for more than 20 years has had a history of paroxysmal supraventricular tachycardia which was documented by electrocardiogram. He has no history suggestive of coronary artery disease. Physical examination revealed moderate hypertension. The findings are otherwise within normal limits. The chest x-ray was also normal.

Comment. The diagnosis of Wolff-Parkinson-White syndrome is supported by the history of paroxysmal supraventricular tachycardia. The atypical feature is the normal P-R interval. The delta wave is not prominent in the electrocardiogram although a definite slowing of the speed of inscription of the early QRS loop is present. This case also illustrates the pseudoinfarction pattern often seen in patients with the WPW syndrome. The differentiation is often quite difficult when the P-R interval is within the normal limits in the atypical case.

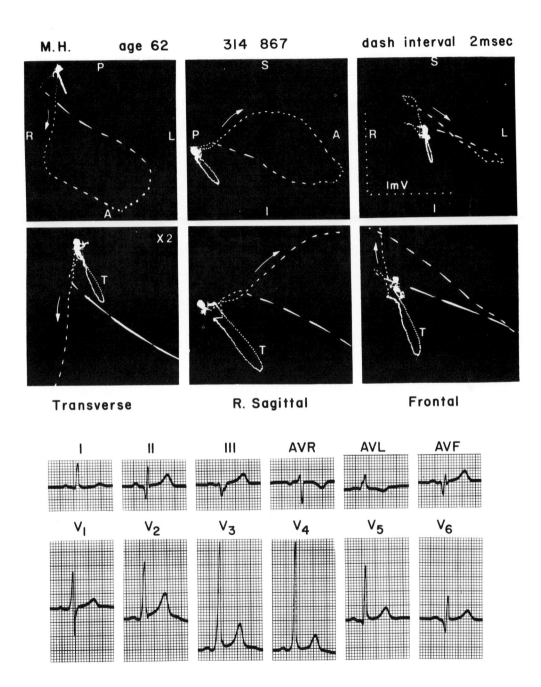

M.H.   age 62   314 867   dash interval 2msec

Transverse   R. Sagittal   Frontal

Fig. B.22., R.B., 228732

Vectorcardiogram.   The PsÊ loop cannot be identified. There is an anterior displacement of the QRSsÊ loop. In the transverse plane the anterior and rightward QRS loop area exceeds 70 percent of the total. In the frontal plane the loop is inscribed clockwise and more than 20 percent of the loop area is located in the right inferior quadrant. There is no evidence of a conduction delay and the duration of the QRS loop is normal. The TsÊ loop is small and abnormal in configuration. It is directed posteriorly, superiorly, and to the right.

Vectorcardiographic diagnosis.   Right ventricular hypertrophy. Abnormal TsÊ loop.

Electrocardiographic diagnosis.   Atrial fibrillation. Probable right ventricular hypertrophy. Nonspecific ST- and T-wave changes.

Clinical and anatomic findings.   The patient was a 37-year-old woman with rheumatic heart disease, severe mitral stenosis, and moderate tricuspid insufficiency. She had recurrent episodes of pulmonary embolism. She died 1 month after the recording of the illustrated tracings. At autopsy the heart weighed 530 gm. There was moderate dilatation and hypertrophy of the right ventricle and moderate degree of left atrial dilatation. The right ventricle measured 6 to 7 mm in thickness and the left ventricle, up to 16 mm. No significant left ventricular hypertrophy or dilation was thought to be present. Extensive, multiple, organized and organizing stenosing pulmonary emboli were observed.

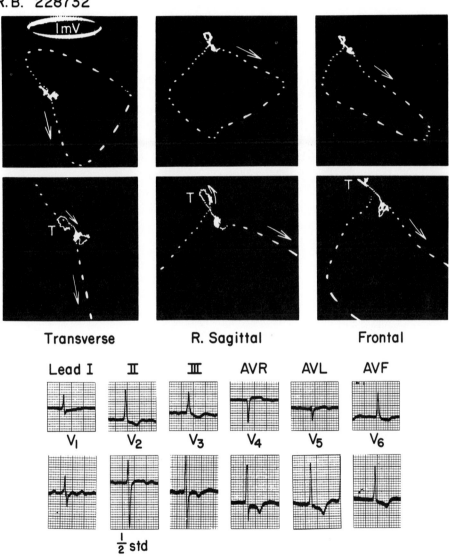

R.B. 228732

Transverse   R. Sagittal   Frontal

Lead I   II   III   AVR   AVL   AVF

V₁   V₂   V₃   V₄   V₅   V₆

½ std

Fig. B.23., G.C., 358609

Vectorcardiogram. The magnitude of the PsÊ loop is increased and the maximum **P** vector in all of the planar projections exceeds the upper normal limits. Most of the PsÊ loop is located posteriorly. There is also marked increase in the magnitude of the QRSsÊ loop. The duration of the QRSsÊ loop slightly exceeds 0.10 sec, but there is no evidence of a conduction delay. The loop is displaced posteriorly and slightly superiorly but remains leftward. In both the transverse and sagittal planes the QRS loop inscribes a figure-of-eight pattern, and in the transverse plane the initial deflection is directed anteriorly and to the left. The direction of inscription of the loop in the frontal plane is counterclockwise. The abnormally large ST vector and the TsÊ loop are directed anteriorly, rightward, and are discordant to the QRSsÊ loop.

Vectorcardiographic diagnosis. Left atrial enlargement. Left ventricular hypertrophy. Incomplete left bundle branch block.

Electrocardiograhpic diagnosis. Left atrial enlargement. Left ventricular hypertrophy. Possible old anterior myocardial infarction.

Clinical and anatomic findings. The patient was a 51-year-old man with severe calcific aortic stenosis. Cardiac catheterization demonstrated a systolic pressure gradient of 100 mm Hg across the aortic valve. The patient died 2 months later just before the scheduled date of surgery. At autopsy the heart weighed 860 gm. There was marked left ventricular hypertrophy with the left ventricular wall measuring 22 mm in thickness. A mild-to-moderate degree of right ventricular hypertrophy was also present. The coronary arteries showed mild atherosclerosis. The myocardium was unremarkable on gross examination. Microscopic examination showed widespread small areas of fibrosis.

G.C. 358609

dash interval 2 m sec

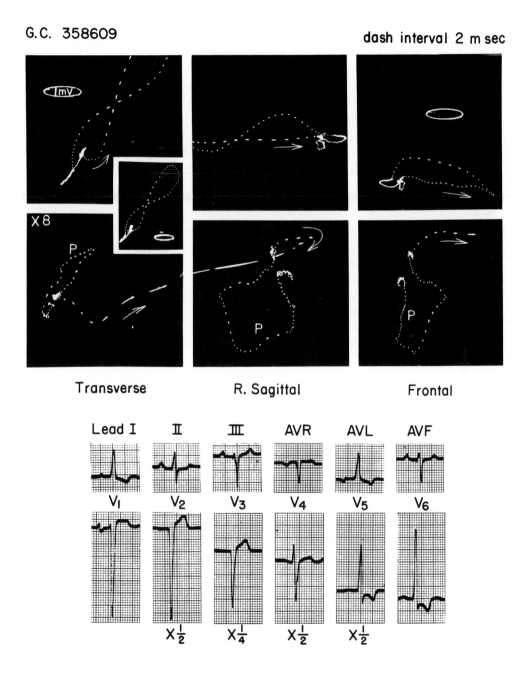

Transverse   R. Sagittal   Frontal

Lead I   II   III   AVR   AVL   AVF

V₁   V₂   V₃   V₄   V₅   V₆

$X\frac{1}{2}$ $X\frac{1}{4}$ $X\frac{1}{2}$ $X\frac{1}{2}$

Fig. B.24., G.P., 023036

Vectorcardiogram. The PsÊ loop is small and difficult to analyze because of insufficient magnification. The magnitude of the QRSsÊ loop is abnormally increased. The loop is displaced posteriorly, to the right and superiorly. The late portion of the loop is slowly inscribed and suggests conduction abnormalities. In the transverse plane the initial deflection is directed anteriorly and to the left. The QRS loop is inscribed mainly clockwise with most of the loop area located in the right posterior quadrant. The loop is inscribed clockwise in the sagittal plane and is superiorly displaced. The direction of inscription of the QRS loop in the frontal plane is essentially clockwise and most of the loop is located to the right. The abnormally large **ST** vector and the TsÊ loop are directed anteriorly, leftward and inferiorly and are discordant to the QRSsÊ loop.

Vectorcardiographic diagnosis. Atypical left bundle branch block. Right axis deviation. Possible right ventricular hypertrophy.

Electrocardiographic diagnosis. First-degree AV block. Intraventricular conduction defect. Indeterminate axis.

Clinical, physiologic and surgical findings. The patient is a 44-year-old man with the ostium primum type of atrial septal defect. Cardiac catheterization revealed normal pulmonary artery pressure. At surgery a huge ostium primum type of defect was found and repaired.

Comment. This is an unusual vectorcardiogram and electrocardiogram in a patient with atrial septal defect. The rightward displacement of the QRS loop which has otherwise the characteristics of a left bundle branch block pattern may be caused by right ventricular hypertrophy secondary to volume overload of the right ventricle. Several other cases with similar vectorcardiographic findings have been observed by the author which are also associated with anatomical right ventricular hypertrophy or pulmonary hypertension. (Chou TC, Helm RA: The diagnosis of right ventricular hypertrophy in the presence of left bundle branch block. Proc. XIth Int Vectorcardiogr symp. Amsterdam, North-Holland, 1971, p 289.)

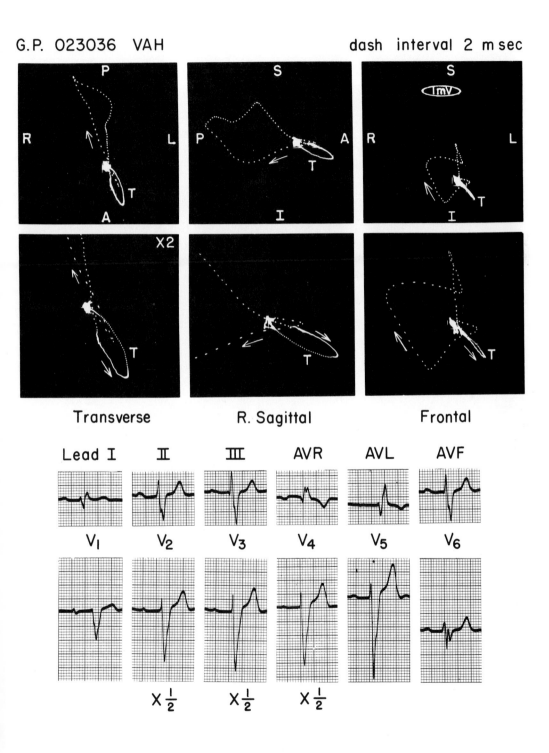

G.P. 023036 VAH   dash interval 2 m sec

Transverse   R. Sagittal   Frontal

Lead I   II   III   AVR   AVL   AVF

V₁   V₂   V₃   V₄   V₅   V₆

X½   X½   X½

Fig. B.25. O.S., 448522

Vectorcardiogram. The PsÊ loop is normal. The QRSsÊ loop is displaced posteriorly. The maximum **QRS** vector measures 2.3 mV in both the transverse and sagittal planes. In the transverse plane there is an indentation of the efferent limb of the QRS loop. The **ST** vector and TsÊ loop are directed anteriorly, rightward, and superiorly.

Vectorcardiographic diagnosis. Left ventricular hypertrophy. The indentation of the QRS loop seen in the transverse plane suggests the possibility of lateral wall myocardial damage.

Electrocardiographic diagnosis. Nonspecific ST- and T-wave abnormalities or digitalis effect, or both. Possible anterolateral myocardial infarction.

Clinical and anatomical findings. The patient is a 55-year-old man with aortic stenosis. He has frequent attacks of angina pectoris. During cardiac catheterization a systolic gradient of 85 mm Hg was demonstrated across the aortic valve. Coronary arteriogram revealed narrowing and irregularity of the right coronary artery. However, the major branches of the left coronary artery appeared normal. The diagnosis of aortic stenosis was confirmed during surgery, and the left ventricle was found to be moderately hypertrophied.

O.S. 448522

dash interval 2 msec.

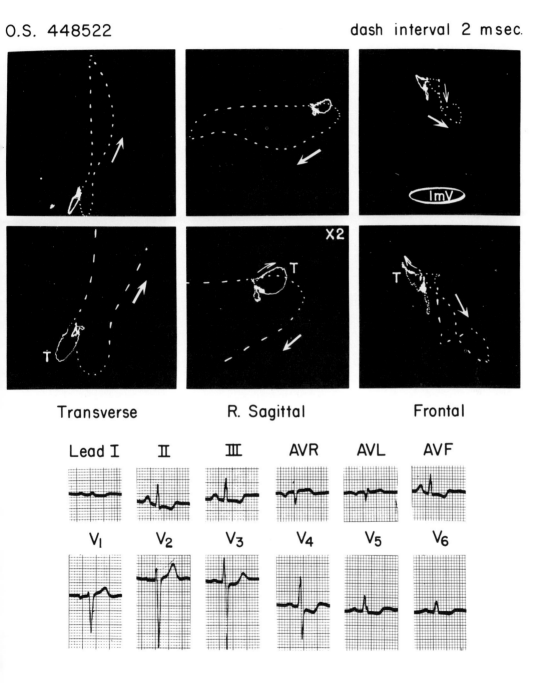

Transverse R. Sagittal Frontal

Lead I   II   III   AVR   AVL   AVF

V_1 V_2 V_3 V_4 V_5 V_6

Fig. B.26., E.E., 433938

Vectorcardiogram. There is a marked reduction of the initial anterior QRS forces as demonstrated in the transverse and sagittal planes. There is also an abnormal increase in the duration and magnitude of the initial superior forces as seen in the sagittal and frontal planes. The QRS loop is inscribed counterclockwise in the right sagittal plane and at first clockwise and then counterclockwise in the frontal plane. A relatively large area of the QRS loop is located on the right in both the transverse and the frontal planes. The large spatial **ST** vector is directed anteriorly and inferiorly. The T loop is displaced slightly to the right and is inscribed clockwise in the transverse plane.

Vectorcardiographic diagnosis. Acute anteroseptal and inferior myocardial infarction. The increase of the late right posterior QRS forces suggests the possibility of right ventricular hypertrophy.

Electrocardiographic diagnosis. Acute anteroseptal and inferior myocardial infarction.

Clinical and anatomic findings. The patient was a 77-year-old woman whose serial electrocardiograms were typical of acute anteroseptal and inferior myocardial infarction. The above tracings were recorded 10 days after the onset of her illness. She died 1 week later. At autopsy severe coronary atherosclerosis was found with complete occlusion of the right coronary artery and recent thrombosis of the anterior descending branch of the left coronary artery at its proximal third. The myocardium revealed extensive infarction of the inferior wall of the left and right ventricles and the interventricular septum as well as a small portion of the anterior left ventricular wall. Ventricular hypertrophy was not found, but there was moderate right ventricular dilatation. Multiple and extensive embolization of the pulmonary arteries was observed. Both recent and organized emboli were present. the prosector's conclusion was that the extensive recurrent pulmonary embolism was the immediate cause of death.

Comment. Since right ventricular hypertrophy was not demonstrated anatomically, right ventricular dilatation secondary to extensive pulmonary embolism was probably responsible for the increase of the late right posterior QRS forces.

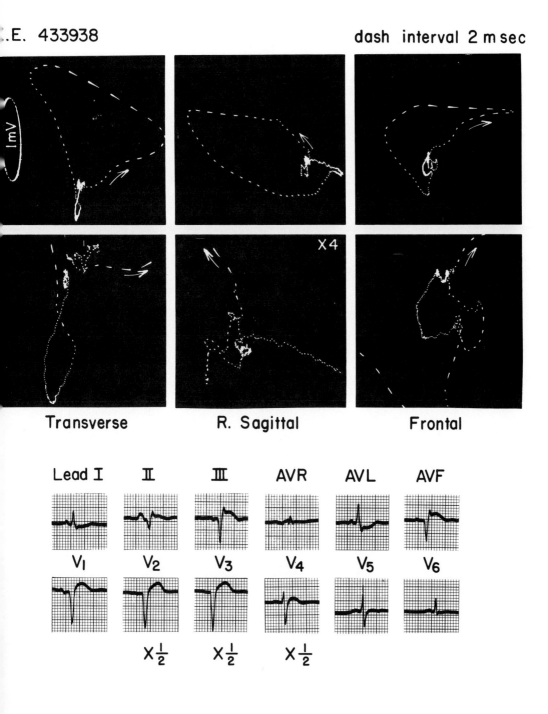

.E. 433938

dash interval 2 m sec

1 mV

Transverse   R. Sagittal   Frontal

Lead I   II   III   AVR   AVL   AVF

V₁   V₂   V₃   V₄   V₅   V₆

X½   X½   X½

Fig. B.27., L.W., 222667

Vectorcardiogram. The PsÊ loop is abnormally large and both the anterior and the posterior components are prominent. The late portion of the QRSsÊ loop is displaced posteriorly, rightward, and superiorly. In the transverse plane the area of the QRS loop in the right posterior quadrant is about 50 percent of the entire loop. In the frontal plane the loop is inscribed clockwise and is wide with most of the loop area located on the right side. The TsÊ loop is displaced slightly posteriorly.

Vectorcardiographic diagnosis. Atrial enlargement, probably bilateral. Abnormal right axis deviation. Right ventricular hypertrophy.

Electrocardiographic diagnosis. Right atrial enlargement. Abnormal right axis deviation. Right ventricular hypertrophy.

Clinical and anatomic findings. The patient was a 25-year-old extremely obese woman (400 lbs) who was believed to have the Pickwickian syndrome with chronic cor pulmonale and repeated pulmonary emboli. She died about 22 months after the recording of the above tracings. Repeated electrocardiograms up to 2 days before her death did not show any significant changes from the one illustrated. At autopsy the heart weighted 615 gm. There was marked right ventricular hypertrophy and mild to moderate left ventricular hypertrophy. The right ventricular wall measured 9 mm in thickness, the left ventricular wall, 19 mm. There was considerable right atrial hypertrophy and dilatation. Multiple bilateral pulmonary emboli and infarctions were present.

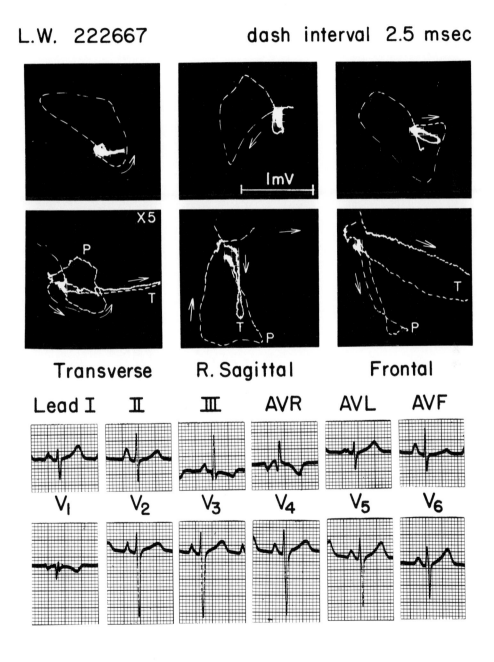

L.W. 222667   dash interval 2.5 msec

Transverse   R. Sagittal   Frontal

Lead I   II   III   AVR   AVL   AVF

V₁   V₂   V₃   V₄   V₅   V₆

Fig. B.28., I.J., 297842

Vectorcardiogram.   The PsÊ loop is within normal limits. The efferent limb of the QRSsÊ loop is displaced posteriorly and superiorly. In the transverse plane the QRS loop is narrow and inscribed essentially clockwise. In the sagittal plane it is inscribed counterclockwise. The duration of its initial superior forces is increased. The TsÊ loop is oriented rightward, posteriorly, and superiorly. In the transverse and sagittal planes the T loop is inscribed clockwise (the T loop is not shown in the magnified sagittal projection).

Vectorcardiographic diagnosis.   Anterolateral and inferior myocardial infarction.

Electrocardiographic diagnosis.   Anterior myocardial infarction. Inferior myocardial ischemia.

Clinical and anatomic findings.   The patient was a 55-year-old woman with diabetes and severe hypertension. She had a history of acute myocardial infarction 3 and 4 years ago. See Fig. B.29 for later tracings and anatomic findings.

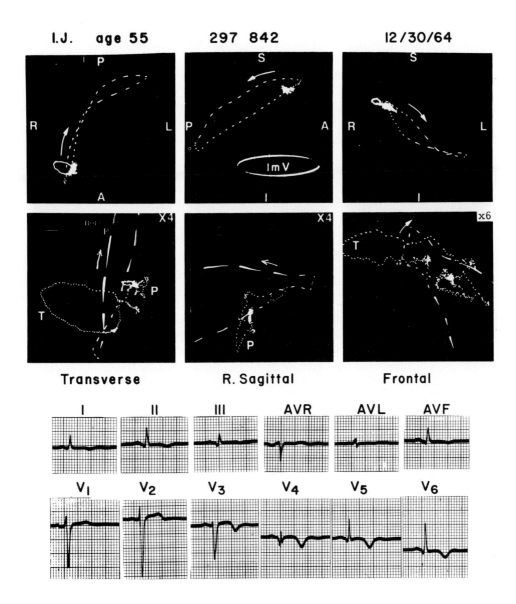

Fig. B.29., I.J., 297842

Vectorcardiogram. The initial deflection of the spatial QRS loop is directed leftward, anteriorly, and inferiorly. The efferent limb is displaced to the right, posteriorly, and superiorly. In the transverse plane most of the QRS loop is inscribed clockwise; in the sagittal plane, counterclockwise. In the frontal plane the maximum **QRS** vector is directed at 70° which is abnormal. The QRS loop has an irregular configuration. The T loop is displaced anteriorly, rightward, and superiorly.

Vectorcardiographic diagnosis. Lateral wall myocardial infarction. Possible inferior wall myocardial infarction.

Electrocardiographic diagnosis. Intraventricular conduction defect or atypical incomplete left bundle branch block.

Clinical and anatomic findings. These tracings were obtained almost 6 years after Fig. B.28 from the same patient. She suffered another episode of severe chest pain accompanied by enzyme elevation 2 weeks prior to the present recordings. She died 4 days later. Autopsy revealed a heart weight of 390 gm with combined ventricular hypertrophy. The right coronary artery was completely occluded 4 cm distal to its origin. About 80 percent narrowing was found in the anterior descending branch of the left coronary artery 5 cm from its orifice. Two areas of old myocardial infarction were present involving the anterolateral and inferior wall of the left ventricle. An extensive recent myocardial infarct was found in the posterolateral wall of the left ventricle.

Comment. It is reasonable to assume the changes depicted in Fig. B.28 are attributed to the two old myocardial infarcts demonstrated at autopsy. The addition of the recent posterolateral myocardial infarction is responsible for the anterior and further rightward displacement of the efferent limb of the QRS loop. The transverse plane QRS loop correlates well with the combined effect of the anterolateral and posterolateral damage. The signs of inferior myocardial infarction have been mostly obscured after the development of the new infarct. The electrocardiogram is no longer diagnostic of infarction of any location by the usual criteria. Neither the vectorcardiogram nor the electrocardiogram show any evidence of combined ventricular hypertrophy.

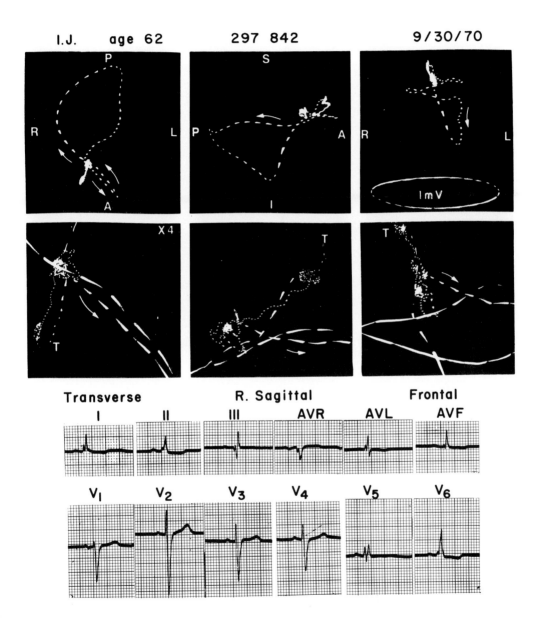

I.J.　age 62　　297 842　　9/30/70

Transverse　　R. Sagittal　　Frontal

I　II　III　AVR　AVL　AVF

V_1　V_2　V_3　V_4　V_5　V_6

Fig. B.30., C.D., 304474

Vectorcardiogram. There is a reversal of the orientation and direction of inscription of the P, QRS, and T loops in the transverse and frontal planes. They present a mirror-image pattern of the normal vectorcardiogram. In the right sagittal plane the vectorcardiogram is normal.

Vectorcardiographic diagnosis. Mirror-image dextrocardia.

Electrocardiographic diagnosis. Mirror-image dextrocardia.

Clinical findings. The patient is a 15-year-old girl who has mirror-image dextrocardia associated with situs inversus of the other organs. There is no evidence of other congenital malformation of the heart.

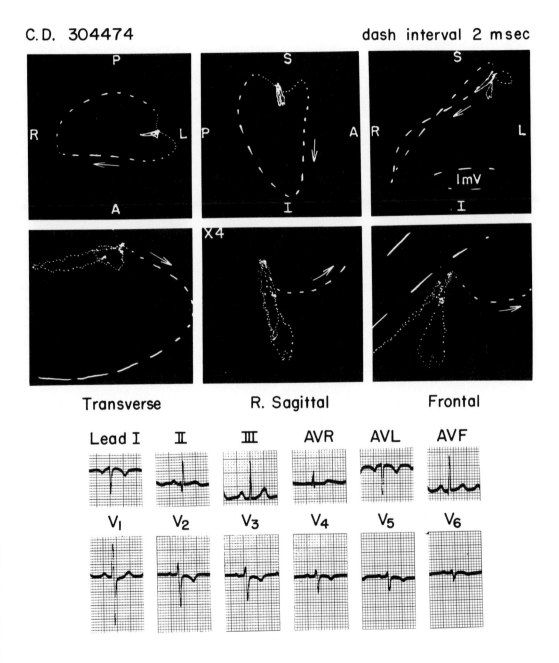

C.D. 304474   dash interval 2 msec

Transverse   R. Sagittal   Frontal

Lead I   II   III   AVR   AVL   AVF

V₁   V₂   V₃   V₄   V₅   V₆

Fig. B.31., P.A., 265670

Vectorcardiogram. There is a marked superior displacement of the PsÊ loop as seen in the sagittal and frontal planes. The QRSsÊ loop showed a loss of its initial anterior forces as demonstrated in the transverse and sagittal planes. In the transverse plane the efferent limb of the QRS loop is displaced to the right and posteriorly, and the loop is inscribed clockwise. In the right sagittal plane the QRS loop has a figure-of-eight pattern with most of the loop being inscribed counterclockwise. In the frontal plane the loop is inscribed counterclockwise, and the duration of the initial rightward forces is 0.024 sec, which exceeds the normal upper limit of 0.022 sec. The direction of the **ST** vector is normal. However, its magnitude in the transverse and sagittal planes is slightly increased. The TsÊ loop is abnormally wide and is directed to the right and inferiorly. It is inscribed at a rather uniform speed. The direction of inscription is clockwise in all the three planar projections.

Vectorcardiographic diagnosis. Ectopic atrial pacemaker. Extensive anterior myocardial infarction, the age of which is uncertain; it may be acute in view of the large anteriorly directed **ST** vector.

Electrocardiographic diagnosis. Anteroseptal myocardial infarction, probably with some lateral wall involvement. The age of the infarct is uncertain and may be acute.

Clinical findings. The patient is a 56-year-old woman who had an acute anterior myocardial infarction 7 years ago. Repeated electrocardiograms in the past few years show essentially the same pattern as depicted in the illustrated tracing. X-ray examination reveals that the heart size is normal, and there was no demonstrable evidence of a ventricular aneurysm.

Comment. The orientation of the PsÊ loop does not correlate well with the P-wave pattern in the electrocardiogram. Even though the vectorcardiogram was recorded immediately after the electrocardiogram, there was probably a shifting of the atrial pacemaker during that interval. The vectorcardiogram reveals more extensive changes in the QRS forces than the electrocardiogram. This case also illustrates that serial tracings are necessary to determine the age of an infarction. Both the vectorcardiogram and electrocardiogram are consistent with the diagnosis of an acute infarction.

P.A. 265670   dash interval 2 m sec

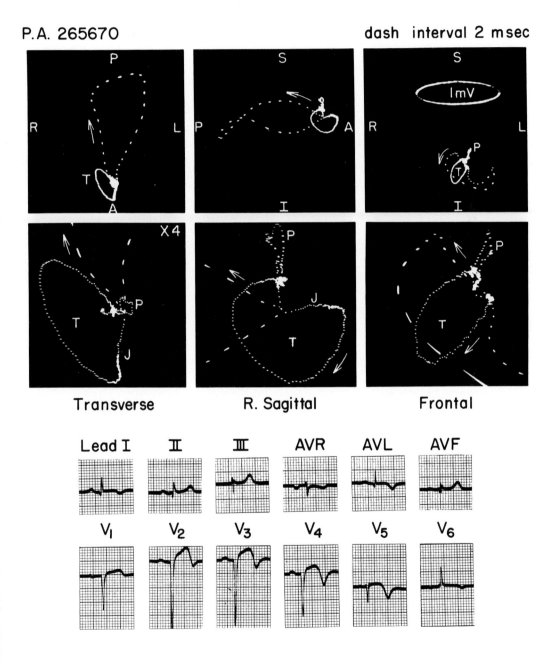

Transverse   R. Sagittal   Frontal

Lead I   II   III   AVR   AVL   AVF

V_1 V_2 V_3 V_4 V_5 V_6

Fig. B.32., E. H., 459643

Vectorcardiogram. The maximum **P** vector in the transverse plane exceeds 0.1mV and is directed posteriorly. There is an increase in the duration of the initial rightward QRS forces which is 0.03 sec. There is also a superior displacement of the QRS loop. In the right sagittal plane the loop has a figure-of-eight pattern with its early portion inscribed counterclockwise. In the frontal plane the maximum **QRS** vector is directed at 5°. The initial deflection and efferent limb are inscribed clockwise. There is also a marked upward convexity of the terminal part of the QRS loop. The T loop is displaced rightward.

Vectorcardiographic diagnosis. Left atrial enlargement. Inferior and lateral myocardial infarction.

Electrocardiographic diagnosis. Anterolateral myocardial infarction.

Clinical and anatomic findings. The patient was a 72-year-old man with a history of hypertension, coronary artery disease, and congestive heart failure. He died of massive cerebral hemorrhage 20 days after the recording of the tracings. At autopsy the heart weighed 800 gm with combined ventricular hypertrophy. A healed myocardial infarction measuring $4 \times 2 \times 1$ cm was found in the inferior wall of the left ventricle. A small healed anterolateral infarct measuring $0.6 \times 0.6 \times 0.3$ cm was also identified. In the posterobasal wall of the left ventricle a subacute infarct measuring $1 \times 1 \times 0.3$ cm was present.

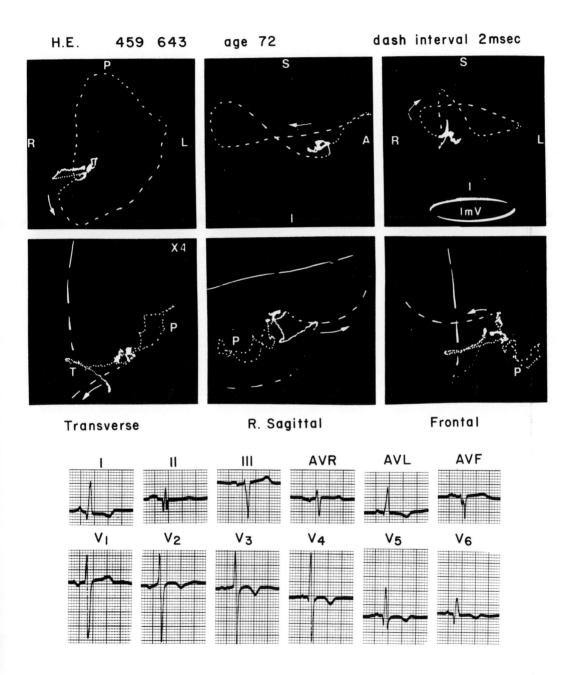

H.E.   459 643   age 72   dash interval 2msec

Transverse   R. Sagittal   Frontal

Fig. B.33., W.B., 385192

Vectorcardiogram. The QRSsÊ loop is small and the magnitude of the maximum **QRS** vector in the transverse plane is 0.85 mV which is at the lower limit of normal. In the transverse plane there is a posterior displacement of the QRS loop and the entire loop is rotated counterclockwise. The 0.02-sec vector is directed posteriorly. In the frontal plane the loop becomes more vertical in position, and the direction of the maximum **QRS** vector is 65° which is at the upper limit of normal. The **ST** vector and the T loop are normal.

Vectorcardiographic diagnosis. The vectorcardiogram is consistent with pulmonary emphysema.

Electrocardiographic diagnosis. The small complexes in lead I, the leftward displacement of the transitional zone in the precordial leads, and the relatively small amplitude of the R wave in the left precordial leads are consistent with pulmonary emphysema.

Clinical findings. The patient is a 59-year-old man with inactive pulmonary tuberculosis. The chest x-ray shows evidence of pulmonary emphysema. There are no symptoms or signs suggestive of cardiac disease.

Comment. This is an example to illustrate that the reduction of the anterior QRS forces and the posterior orientation of the 0.02-sec **QRS** vector may be the result of pulmonary emphysema rather than anterior myocardial infarction.

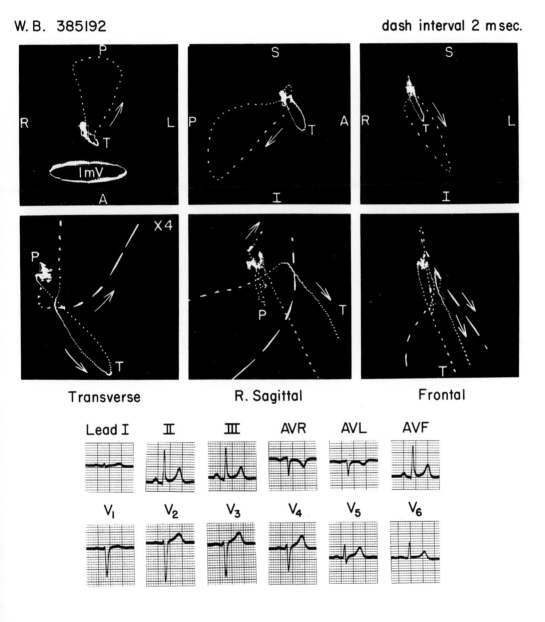

W. B. 385192   dash interval 2 m sec.

Transverse   R. Sagittal   Frontal

Lead I   II   III   AVR   AVL   AVF

V₁   V₂   V₃   V₄   V₅   V₆

Fig. B.34., G.K., 437343

Vectorcardiogram. The QRSsÊ loop is normal in magnitude. It is, however, displaced posteriorly and superiorly. The duration of the loop exceeds 0.12 sec, and the entire loop is slowly inscribed, especially in its last portion. In the transverse plane there is an absence of the initial anterior forces, and the QRS loop is inscribed clockwise. In the frontal plane the superiorly displaced loop is inscribed counter-clockwise except for its early portion which is clockwise. The abnormally large **ST** vector and the TsÊ loop are directed anteriorly, rightward, and inferiorly and are more or less discordant to the QRSsÊ loop.

Vectorcardiographic diagnosis. Anterior and inferior myocardial damage. Left anterior hemiblock. Additional intraventricular conduction defect.

Electrocardiographic diagnosis. Anterior and inferior wall myocardial damage. Left anterior hemiblock. Additional intraventricular conduction defect. First-degree AV block.

Clinical and anatomic findings. The patient was a 75-year-old man with severe congestive heart failure. He died shortly after admission. At autopsy the heart weighed 505 gm. The right ventricular wall measured 4 mm in thickness, and the left ventricular wall, 14 mm. A moderate degree of left ventricular hypertrophy was present. The coronary arteries showed a mild degree of atherosclerosis. There was no evidence of myocardial infarction on gross examination. Microscopic examination revealed widespread filled-out areas of fibrosis. There were also scanty small areas of recent necrosis. The findings were believed to be consistent with primary myocardial disease.

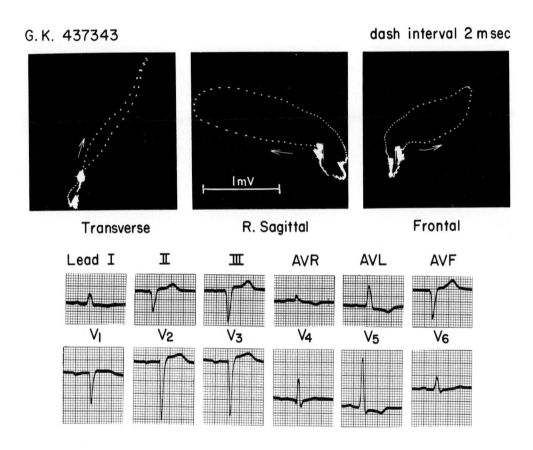

G.K. 437343　　　　　　　　　　　　　　dash interval 2 m sec

Transverse　　　　R. Sagittal　　　　Frontal

Lead I　　II　　III　　AVR　　AVL　　AVF

V1　　V2　　V3　　V4　　V5　　V6

Fig. B.35., E.M., 248158

Vectorcardiogram. The PsÊ loop cannot be identified. The magnitude of the QRSsÊ loop is increased with the maximum **QRS** vector measuring 3 mV or more in each of the three planar projections. The orientation of the spatial loop is normal. The anterior QRS forces are quite prominent. The **ST** vector and TsÊ loop are directed to the right, superiorly, and slightly posteriorly.

Vectorcardiographic diagnosis. Left ventricular hypertrophy. Possible coexisting right ventricular hypertrophy based on the prominent anterior QRS forces in the presence of left ventricular hypertrophy. The posterior orientation of the **ST** vector and TsÊ loop suggest additional abnormalities other than those related to left ventricular hypertrophy.

Electrocardiographic diagnosis. Atrial fibrillation. Left ventricular hypertrophy. Possible right ventricular hypertrophy due to the tall R wave in lead V_2. Digitalis effect.

Clinical and anatomic findings. The patient was a 24-year-old woman with rheumatic heart disease, mitral insufficiency and stenosis. She underwent surgery for the replacement of the mitral valve with a prothesis shortly after the tracings were recorded, and the clinical diagnosis was confirmed. She died 40 days later. At autopsy the heart weighed 590 gm. There was severe dilatation of the left atrium and moderate degree of hypertrophy and dilatation of the left ventricle. The right atrium and right ventricle were dilated, but there was no significant right ventricular hypertrophy. The left ventricular wall measured 1.5 to 1.6 cm in thickness and the right ventricular wall, 0.3 to 0.5 cm in thickness. The coronary arteries were normal.

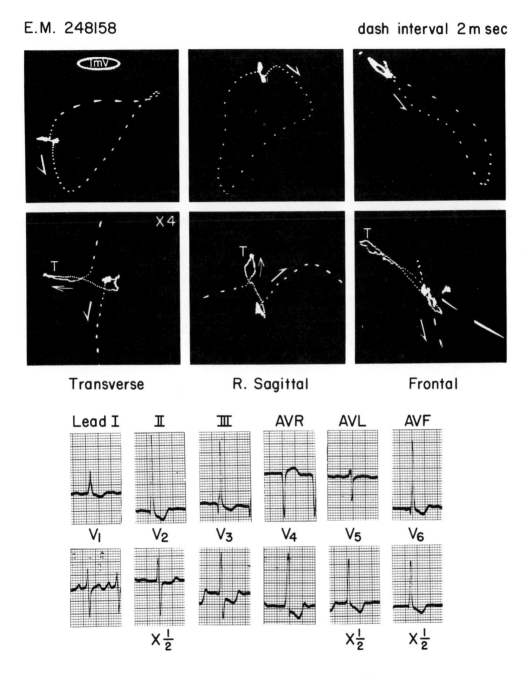

E.M. 248158

dash interval 2 m sec

Fig. B.36., M.M., 442262

Vectorcardiogram. The PsÊ loop is normal. There is a loss of the initial anterior QRS forces. In the transverse plane the initial deflection is inscribed posteriorly, and there is also a posterior and medial displacement of the efferent limb of the QRS loop. In the sagittal plane the loop is displaced somewhat superiorly. In the frontal plane the loop is inscribed counterclockwise even though the direction of the maximum **QRS** vector is 45°. The **ST** vector is oriented anteriorly, superiorly, and to the right. Its magnitude is increased. The TsÊ loop is wide and is inscribed at a uniform speed. It is oriented to the right and inferiorly with part of it anterior and part of it posterior to the isoelectric point.

Vectorcardiographic diagnosis. Anteroseptal myocardial infarction with probably some involvement of the lateral wall. The age of the infarction is undetermined but may be acute.

Electrocardiographic diagnosis. Anteroseptal myocardial infarction with probably some lateral extension. The age of the infarction is uncertain but may be acute.

Clinical findings. The patient is a 63-year-old man who suffered an acute myocardial infarction recently. The diagnosis was supported by serial electrocardiographic changes and elevation of serum enzymes.

M.M. 442262

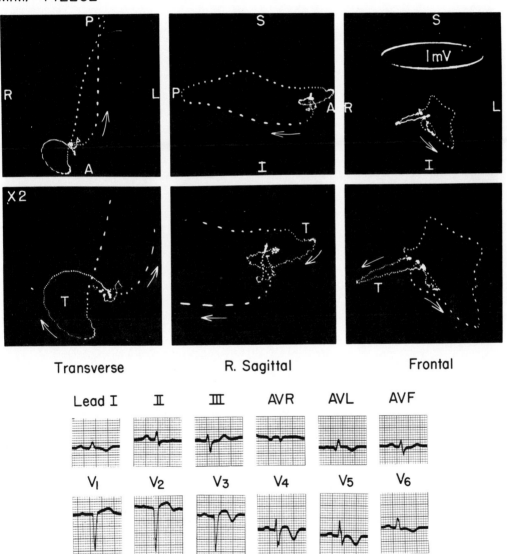

Transverse   R. Sagittal   Frontal

Fig. B.37., J.S., 04402

Vectorcardiogram. The PsÊ loop is abnormally large, and the magnitude of the maximum **P** vector in the sagittal and frontal planes is 0.2 and 0.25 mV, respectively. The majority of the P loop is located posteriorly. The magnitude of the QRSsÊ loop is also markedly increased. The loop is displaced posteriorly and superiorly. There is no evidence of a conduction delay. In the transverse plane the initial deflection and the efferent limb of the QRS loop are displaced rightward and posteriorly. The early portion of the loop is inscribed clockwise. In the right sagittal plane there is a superior displacement of the initial deflection and the efferent limb. The loop is at first inscribed counterclockwise and then clockwise. In the frontal plane the abnormal increase in the duration of the initial superior QRS forces can also be seen clearly. The first half of the loop is inscribed clockwise and the remainder, counterclockwise. The direction of the maximum **QRS** vector is −5°. The spatial **ST** vector is abnormally large and is directed anteriorly, inferiorly and slightly to the left. The orientation of the TsÊ loop is discordant to that of the QRSsÊ loop.

Vectorcardiographic diagnosis. Left atrial enlargement. Left anterior hemiblock. Left ventricular hypertrophy. Anterior and inferior myocardial infarction.

Electrocardiographic diagnosis. Left anterior hemiblock. Left ventricular hypertrophy. Anterior and inferior myocardial infarction.

Clinical findings. The patient is a 44-year-old man with symptoms and signs suggestive of hypertrophic subaortic stenosis. X-ray examination of the chest revealed mild left ventricular preponderance. Cardiac catheterization demonstrated a systolic pressure gradient of 50 mm Hg between the left ventricular cavity and the outflow tract.

Comment. In view of the clinical and physiologic findings, the accuracy of the vectorcardiographic and electrocardiographic diagnosis of anterior and inferior myocardial infarction is highly questionable. The presence of an infarction pattern in idiopathic hypertrophic subaortic stenosis in the absence of coronary artery disease has been well recognized. In 56 percent of the 123 cases reported by Frank and Braunwald, an abnormal Q wave was observed (Circulation 37:759, 1968). Four of the ten cases reported by Estes et al had both the electrocardiographic and vectorcardiographic signs suggestive of previous myocardial infarction (Amer Heart J 65:155, 1963). The abnormal initial QRS forces have been attributed to massive septal hypertrophy.

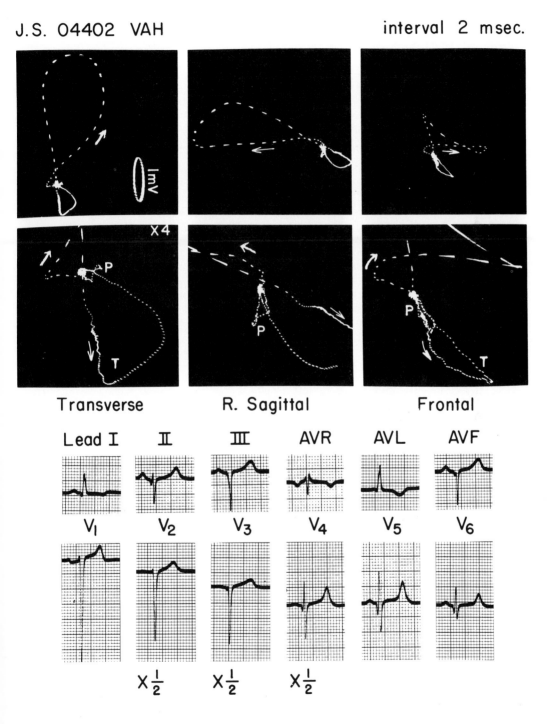

J.S. 04402 VAH   interval 2 msec.

Transverse   R. Sagittal   Frontal

Lead I   II   III   AVR   AVL   AVF

V_1 V_2 V_3 V_4 V_5 V_6

$X\frac{1}{2}$ $X\frac{1}{2}$ $X\frac{1}{2}$

Fig. B.38., I.K., 148706

Vectorcardiogram.   The magnitude of the maximum **P** vector in the transverse plane exceeds the normal upper limit of 0.1 mV. Most of the P loop is located posteriorly. The QRSsÊ loop is displaced posteriorly and superiorly. The duration of the QRSsÊ loop is 0.12 sec. The later portion of the loop is slowly inscribed and suggests conduction delay. In the transverse plane most of the QRS loop is inscribed clockwise. This is also true for the initial portion of the loop. In the sagittal plane there is a downward concavity of the afferent limb of the QRS loop which is otherwise inscribed clockwise. The frontal plane QRS loop is inscribed counterclockwise. The large **ST** vector and the TsÊ loop are directed to the right, anteriorly, and slightly inferiorly.

Vectorcardiographic diagnosis.   Left atrial enlargement. Atypical left bundle branch block. The initial clockwise inscription of the QRS loop in the transverse plane is suggestive of septal infarction. The concavity in the sagittal plane QRS loop may also be due to myocardial damage.

Electrocardiographic diagnosis.   Abnormal P wave, probably caused by left atrial enlargement. Complete left bundle branch block.

Clinical findings.   The patient is a 74-year-old woman with diabetes mellitus who developed typical symptoms of acute myocardial infarction 2.5 weeks prior to the date of the illustrated tracings. There was a definite rise of the serum transaminase level. The patient also has a history of myocardial infarction 5 months previously. X-ray of the chest revealed cardiomegaly.

Comment.   The diagnosis of myocardial infarction in the presence of left bundle branch block is generally considered difficult. Certain features which are atypical for left bundle branch block may indicate the presence of myocardial damage. (The reader may refer to Chapter 11 for the discussion of this subject.) The counterclockwise, superiorly displaced frontal plane QRS loop is also consistent with left anterior hemiblock. Whether this additional diagnosis is justifiable in a patient with left bundle branch block, however, is controversial.

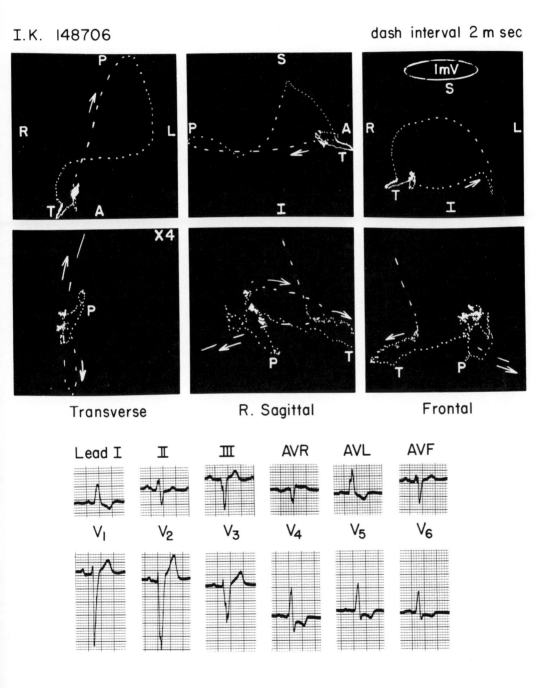

I.K. 148706

dash interval 2 m sec

Transverse   R. Sagittal   Frontal

Lead I   II   III   AVR   AVL   AVF

V_1 V_2 V_3 V_4 V_5 V_6

Fig. B.39., J.M., 127598

Vectorcardiogram. The PsÊ loop is long and narrow. The magnitude of the maximum **P** vector in the sagittal and frontal planes exceeds the normal upper limits. All of the loop area is located anteriorly. In the frontal plane the P loop is vertical in position. The QRSsÊ loop is small. The magnitude of the maximum **QRS** vector in the three planar projections is either at or below the lower limits of normal. In the transverse plane there is a reduction of the initial anterior QRS forces, and the QRS loop is displaced posteriorly. In the right sagittal plane there is an abnormal initial counterclockwise inscription of the QRS loop.

Vectorcardiographic diagnosis. Right atrial enlargement. The vectorcardiogram is consistent with pulmonary emphysema. Possible anterior wall myocardial damage.

Electrocardiographic diagnosis. Right atrial enlargement. The tracing is consistent with pulmonary emphysema. Possible old anterior myocardial damage.

Clinical and anatomic findings. The patient was a 62-year-old man with chronic osteomyelitis. Physical examination and x-ray of the chest revealed findings suggestive of pulmonary emphysema. The heart was normal in size. He died about 10 months later of a cerebral vascular accident. The electrocardiogram taken 1 week prior to his death was essentially the same as the one illustrated. At autopsy the heart weighed 305 gm, and there was no evidence of either left or right ventricular hypertrophy. The anterior descending branch of the left coronary artery exhibited atheromatous plagues narrowing the vessel at various points up to 40 percent. The right coronary artery appeared unaffected. There was no evidence of myocardial infarction reported on gross examination but microscopic examination showed several areas of myocardial fibrosis. The right atrium appeared moderately dilated. The presence or absence of pulmonary emphysema was not mentioned in the pathology report.

Comment. It is known that electrocardiographic pseudoinfarction pattern is often observed in patients with pulmonary emphysema. This is such an example. It is very doubtful the microscopic area of fibrosis have any significant effect on the electrocardiogram.

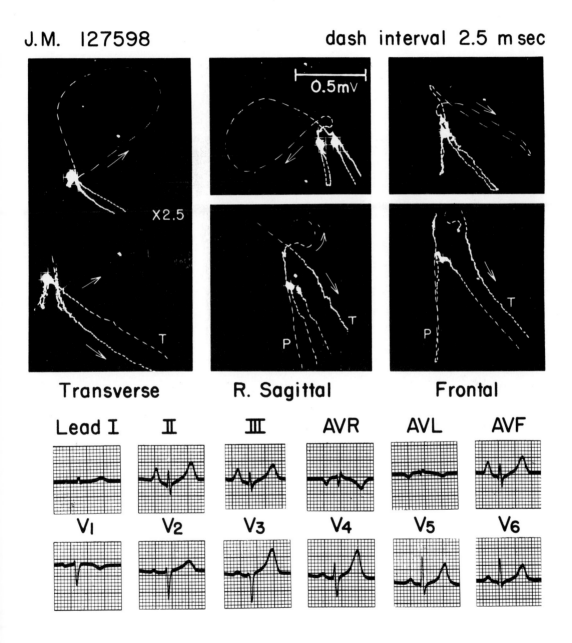

J.M. 127598

dash interval 2.5 m sec

0.5mv

X2.5

Transverse   R. Sagittal   Frontal

Lead I   II   III   AVR   AVL   AVF

V1   V2   V3   V4   V5   V6

Fig. B. 40., H.W., 285233

Vectorcardiogram. The magnitude of the QRSsÊ loop is within the normal range. There is a superior displacement of the efferent limb of the QRS loop as seen in the sagittal and frontal projections. The initial superior forces have a duration of over 0.05 sec. The loop has a figure-of-eight pattern in the sagittal and frontal planes. In the right sagittal plane the great majority of the loop is inscribed counterclockwise. In the frontal plane the efferent limb is inscribed clockwise and the direction of the maximum **QRS** vector is − 10°. Both the **ST** vector and the TsÊ loop are directed to the right, anteriorly, and inferiorly.

Vectorcardiographic diagnosis. Inferior wall myocardial infarction. Nonspecific **ST** vector and T-loop abnormalities.

Electrocardiographic diagnosis. Left ventricular hypertrophy based on the large QRS complexes in the limb leads and the ST- and T-wave changes. Inferior wall myocardial infarction.

Clinical and anatomic findings. The patient was a 74-year-old woman with diabetes mellitus and hypertensive cardiovascular disease. At autopsy, which was done about 6 months after the recording of the illustrated tracings, there was moderate left ventricular hypertrophy. The heart weighed 520 gm with the free wall of the left and right ventricles measuring 16 and 4 mm in thickness, respectively. Atherosclerosis was present in the coronary arteries with a moderate degree of luminal constriction, most pronounced on the left. There was diffuse scarring of the anterior portion of the left ventricle.

Comment. This is an example of a false-negative vectorcardiographic diagnosis of left ventricular hypertrophy. Although both the vectorcardiogram and electrocardiogram show evidence of myocardial infarction, there is rather poor anatomical correlation as to the location of the damage.

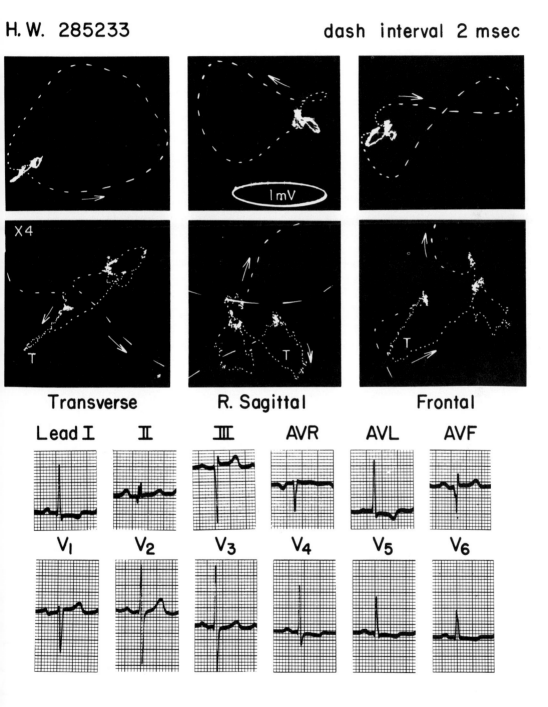

H.W. 285233   dash interval 2 msec

Transverse   R. Sagittal   Frontal

Lead I   II   III   AVR   AVL   AVF

V₁   V₂   V₃   V₄   V₅   V₆

Fig. B.41., D.T., 393490

Vectorcardiogram. A distinct PsÊ loop cannot be identified. There is a posterior displacement of the QRSsÊ loop. In the transverse plane the magnitude of the maximum **QRS** vector is 1.8 mV, which is slightly below the upper limit of normal. Its direction is −60°. The time of occurrence of the maximum **QRS** vector is 0.06 sec, which is delayed. The maximum posterior force exceeds 1.2 mV. The spatial **ST** vector is displaced to the right, superiorly and anteriorly. The TsÊ loop is small and abnormal in configuration.

Vectorcardiographic diagnosis. Left ventricular hypertrophy.

Electrocardiographic diagnosis. Left ventricular hypertrophy. Atrial fibrillation.

Clinical and anatomic findings. The patient was a 41-year-old woman who had rheumatic heart disease with insufficiency and stenosis of the mitral and aortic valves. Replacement of the mitral valve with a Starr-Edwards prothesis was done a few days after the recording of the tracings. She died 6 months later. At autopsy the heart weighed 525 gm. There was a moderate degree of right ventricular hypertrophy. The left ventricle was hypertrophied and markedly dilated. There was also some mild dilatation and moderate hypertrophy of the left atrium. The coronary arteries were normal, and there was no evidence of myocardial infarction.

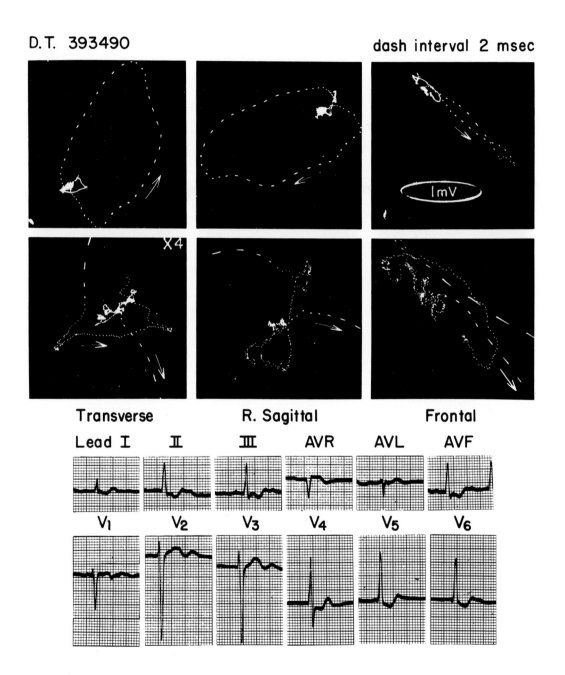

Fig. B.42., P.S., 427741

Vectorcardiogram. The magnitude of the PsÊ loop appears to be increased although the exact measurement of the voltage is difficult because of insufficient magnification. The anterior and posterior atrial forces are of approximately equal strength. The QRSsÊ loop is oriented to the left but is displaced more posteriorly and superiorly. The duration of the loop is 0.11 sec. In the transverse plane the QRS loop has a double figure-of-eight pattern. Its initial deflection is directed anteriorly and slightly to the left. In each of the three planar projections the **ST** vector is abnormally large and has a direction opposite to that of the maximum **QRS** vector. The T loop is similarly oriented.

Vectorcardiographic diagnosis. Probable biatrial enlargement. Left ventricular hypertrophy. Incomplete left bundle branch block.

Electrocardiographic diagnosis. Probable left atrial enlargement. Left ventricular hypertrophy. Intraventricular conduction defect.

Clinical and anatomic findings. The patient is a 47-year-old man with history and physical findings suggestive of idiopathic hypertrophic subaortic stenosis. During left heart catheterization a systolic pressure gradient of 95 mm Hg was demonstrated between the left ventricular cavity and the outflow tract. The diagnosis was later verified at surgery.

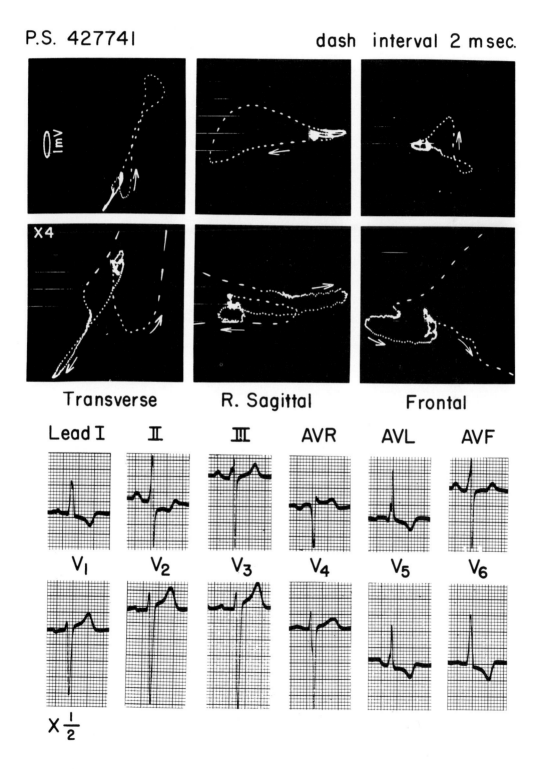

P.S. 427741 dash interval 2 msec.

1mV

X4

Transverse   R. Sagittal   Frontal

Lead I   II   III   AVR   AVL   AVF

V₁   V₂   V₃   V₄   V₅   V₆

X ½

Fig. B.43., T.C., 514937

Vectorcardiogram.   The P loop is within normal limits. There is a marked anterior and some rightward displacement of the QRS loop. In the transverse plane the direction of inscription of the loop remains counterclockwise. In the frontal projection the loop is inscribed counterclockwise even though the maximum **QRS** vector is directed at 65°. The T loop is small and is directed at 80° in the transverse plane and 70° in the frontal plane.

Vectorcardiographic diagnosis.   Posterolateral myocardial damage versus right ventricular hypertrophy or rightward displacement of the heart.

Electrocardiographic diagnosis.   Posterior myocardial damage versus right ventricular hypertrophy or rightward displacement of the heart.

Clinical and Anatomic findings.   The patient was a 28-year-old man with stage IV Hodgkin's disease. He had a complete collapse of his right lung with rightward displacmeent of the heart. The patient died about 1 month after the recording of the tracings. At autopsy the diagnosis was confirmed. The heart weight was normal and there was no evidence of ventricular hypertrophy or myocardial damage.

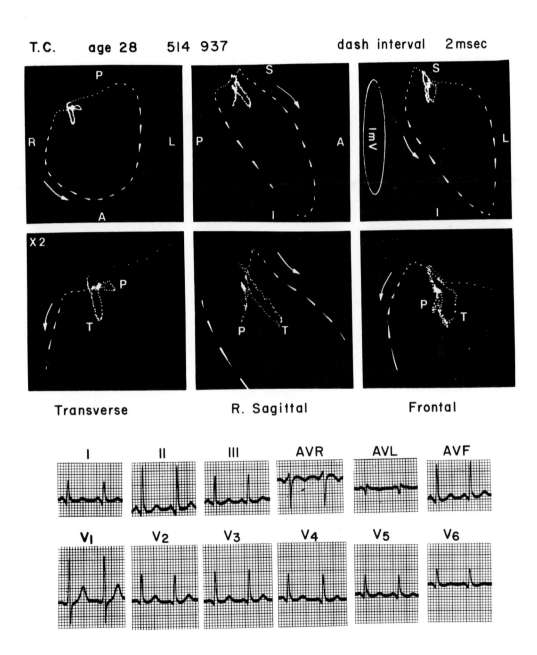

T.C.   age 28   514 937   dash interval   2 msec

Transverse   R. Sagittal   Frontal

I   II   III   AVR   AVL   AVF

V₁   V₂   V₃   V₄   V₅   V₆

Fig. B.44., E.Mc., 439289

Vectorcardiogram.   The PsÊ loop cannot be identified. There is a posterior and rightward displacement of the QRSsÊ loop. The duration of the QRSsÊ loop is increased and exceeds 0.13 sec. The afferent limb of the loop is slowly inscribed. In the transverse plane the initial deflection is directed anteriorly and to the left, and the loop is inscribed clockwise. In the right sagittal plane the loop is inscribed clockwise, and in the frontal plane it presents a figure-of-eight pattern. The **ST** vector and TsÊ loop are discordant to the QRSsÊ loop.

Vectorcardiographic diagnosis.   Atypical left bundle branch block. The rightward displacement of the QRSsÊ loop suggests possible right ventricular hypertrophy.

Electrocardiographic diagnosis.   Abnormal right axis deviation. Intraventricular conduction defect. Atrial fibrillation.

Clinical and anatomic findings.   The patient was a 64-year-old woman with a large traumatic arteriovenous fistula and aneurysm involving the right renal artery and vein. She had marked cardiomegaly and refractory congestive heart failure and died approximately 1 month after the recording of the tracings. At autopsy the heart weighed 608 gm. The right ventricle and right atrium were massively dilated and hypertrophied. Hypertrophy of the left-sided chambers was present but less severe. Left ventricular dilatation was only moderate. The coronary arteries were normal and patent. The myocardium was slightly flabby but exhibited no specific lesions. Multiple pulmonary emboli, both recent and old, were observed.

Comment.   The massive right ventricular hypertrophy is probably responsible for the rightward displacement of the QRSsÊ loop which is otherwise consistent with left bundle branch block. The augmentation of the right ventricular forces which ordinarily are insignificant may in this instance "pull" the QRS loop toward the right even though left bundle branch block is present. This case is quite similar to the one illustrated in Fig. B.24.

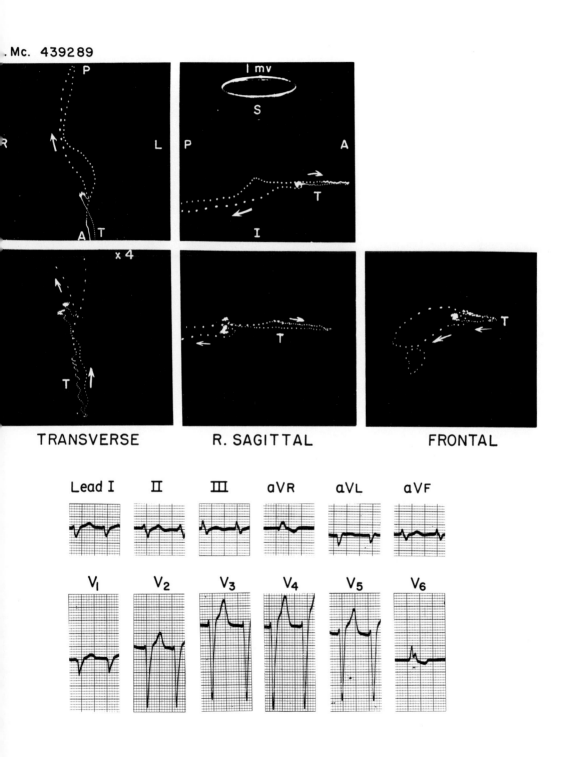

Mc. 439289

TRANSVERSE   R. SAGITTAL   FRONTAL

Lead I   II   III   aVR   aVL   aVF

V_1 V_2 V_3 V_4 V_5 V_6

Fig. B.45., R.E., 187721

Vectorcardiogram. The magnitude of the PsÊ loop is increased. The maximum **P** vector in the sagittal and frontal planes measures 0.4 and 0.3 mV, respectively. The sagittal plane reveals that most of the loop area is located anteriorly. There is a marked rightward displacement of the QRSsÊ loop. In the transverse plane the QRS loop is narrow and is inscribed clockwise. In the frontal plane the loop is wide and most of the loop area is located to the right. There is no evidence of a conduction delay and the duration of the QRSsÊ loop is normal.

Vectorcardiographic diagnosis. Right atrial enlargement. Abnormal right axis deviation. Right ventricular hypertrophy.

Electrocardiographic diagnosis. Right atrial enlargement. Abnormal right axis deviation. Right ventricular hypertrophy.

Clinical and anatomic findings. The patient was a 28-year-old woman with congenital polycystic disease of the lung and chronic cor pulmonale. The diagnoses were confirmed at autopsy. The heart weighed 275 gm. The weight of the free wall of the right ventricle was about twice the free wall of the left ventricle.

R.E. 187721   dash interval 2 m sec

Transverse   R. Sagittal   Frontal

Lead I   II   III   AVR   AVL   AVF

V₁   V₂   V₃   V₄   V₅   V₆

½ std   ½ std

Fig. B.46., E.C., 419599

Vectorcardiogram. The magnitude of the maximum **P** vector exceeds the normal upper limit in both the transverse and frontal planes. Its direction in the frontal plane is 15°. The magnitude of the QRSsÊ loop is within the normal limit. However, the loop is displaced posteriorly and becomes less leftward. In the right sagittal plane there is a figure-of-eight pattern. In the frontal projection there is an upward convexity of the midportion of the QRS loop which is abnormal. Both the spatial **ST** vector and the TsÊ loop are displaced to the right.

Vectorcardiographic diagnosis. Probably left atrial enlargement. The upward displacement of the efferent limb of the QRS loop in the sagittal plane and the upward convexity seen in the frontal plane QRS loop are suggestive of inferior wall myocardial damage. The decrease of the leftward QRS forces in the transverse plane may be due to some involvement of the lateral wall of the left ventricle. The rightward deviation of the T loop is consistent with lateral myocardial ischemia.

Electrocardiographic diagnosis. Possible left atrial enlargement in view of the relatively large negative component of the P wave in lead V_1. Intraventricular conduction defect. Anterolateral myocardial ischemia.

Clinical findings. The patient is a 32-year-old woman with essential hypertension. She had an acute inferior myocardial infarction 2 years previously. The diagnosis was supported by typical symptoms, enzyme elevation and serial electrocardiographic changes. One day before the recording of the illustrated tracings, she had another episode of chest pain which was followed by definite enzyme elevation. The subsequent electrocardiograms, however, showed only T-wave changes.

Comment. The notching of the QRS complex in the inferior leads is the counterpart of the upward convexity seen in the frontal plane QRS loop. The rather low voltage of the R wave in leads I and V_6 is consistent with, but not diagnostic of, lateral wall myocardial damage

E.C. 419599   dash interval 2 m sec

Transverse   R. Sagittal   Frontal

Lead I   II   III   AVR   AVL   AVF

V₁   V₂   V₃   V₄   V₅   V₆

Fig. B.47., J.B., 410485

Vectorcardiogram.   The magnitude of the maximum **P** vector in the transverse plane appears to be slightly above the normal upper limit although the exact voltage is difficult to determine because of insufficient magnification. Most of the P loop area is located posteriorly. The QRSsÊ loop is markedly increased in magnitude. The spatial loop is oriented to the left, posteriorly, and is displaced superiorly. In the transverse plane the initial deflection of the QRS loop is directed anteriorly and to the left, and the loop inscribes a figure-of-eight pattern. In the frontal plane the loop is wide and inscribed counterclockwise. The abnormally large **ST** vector and the TsÊ loop are approximately 180° discordant to the QRSsÊ loop.

Vectorcardiographic diagnosis.   Possible left atrial enlargement. Left ventricular hypertrophy. Left anterior hemiblock. Incomplete left bundle branch block.

Electrocardiographic diagnosis.   Possible left atrial enlargement. Left ventricular hypertrophy. Left anterior hemiblock.

Clinical findings.   The patient, a 51-year-old man, has severe syphilitic aortic insufficiency with probable eversion of one of the aortic cusps. His blood pressure was recorded as 184/0. X-ray examination of the chest reveals cardiomegaly.

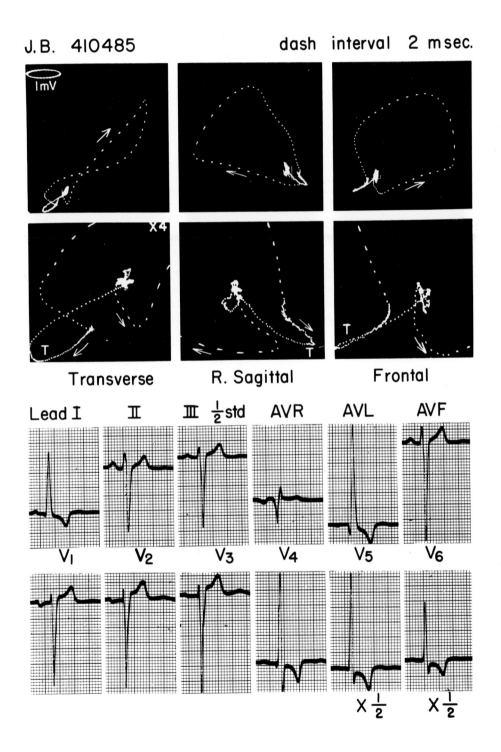

J.B. 410485   dash interval 2 msec.

Transverse   R. Sagittal   Frontal

Lead I   II   III ½std   AVR   AVL   AVF

V₁   V₂   V₃   V₄   V₅   V₆

Fig. B.48., J.C., 438356

Vectorcardiogram.   There is an anterior displacement of the afferent limb of the QRSsÊ loop which is best seen in the transverse plane projection. In that projection the QRS loop has a double figure-of-eight pattern. There is no evidence of a conduction delay. The TsÊ loop is directed to the right, posteriorly and superiorly, and is opposite to the orientation of the normal TsÊ loop. There is some loss of the normal initial slowing in the inscription of the loop. The T loop is inscribed clockwise in the transverse plane and counterclockwise in the right sagittal plane.

Vectorcardiographic diagnosis.   The TsÊ loop changes are consistent with pericarditis, myocarditis or myocardial ischemia. The anterior displacement of the afferent limb of the QRS loop is consistent with myocardial damage of the posterior wall or right ventricular hypertrophy.

Electrocardiographic diagnosis.   The T-wave changes are consistent with pericarditis, myocarditis or myocardial ischemia.

Clinical findings.   The patient is a 17-year-old boy who has acute pericarditis, probably caused by histoplasmosis. During the course of his illness, he developed pericardial effusion with tamponade. The tracings were recorded 2 weeks after the onset of the illness when the amount of the effusion began to decrease.

Comment.   The abnormal QRS loop as displayed in the transverse plane of the vectorcardiogram remains unexplained. The abnormality is less distinct in the conventional electrocardiogram and manifests itself only as a notching of the relatively tall R wave in lead V_1.

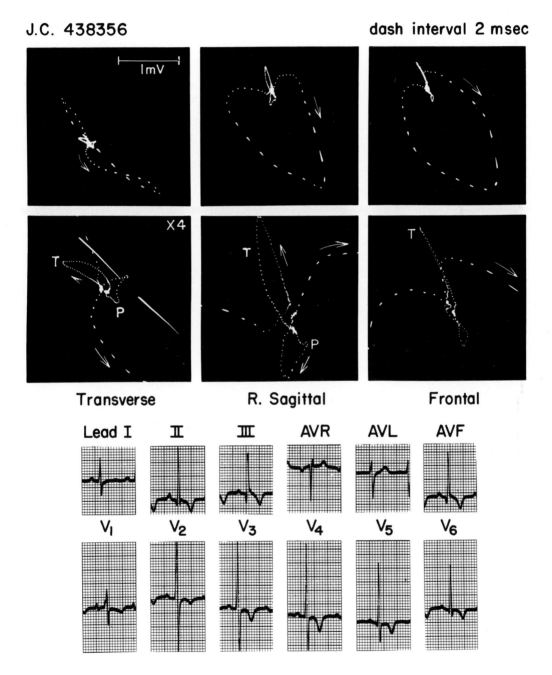

J.C. 438356

dash interval 2 msec

ImV

X4

T

P

T

P

T

Transverse

R. Sagittal

Frontal

Lead I   II   III   AVR   AVL   AVF

V₁   V₂   V₃   V₄   V₅   V₆

Fig. B.49., J.F., 371292

Vectorcardiogram. In the transverse plane the initial deflection and the efferent limb of the QRS loop are displaced posteriorly. The loop is inscribed clockwise at first and then counterclockwise. The T loop is displaced to the right, and a portion of the loop area is located posteriorly. It is inscribed clockwise. In the right sagittal plane the absence of the initial anterior QRS forces is also well demonstrated. The QRS loop has a figure-of-eight pattern with the initial portion inscribed counterclockwise. In the frontal plane the efferent limb of the QRS loop is displaced superiorly and is inscribed clockwise. The remainder of the loop is inscribed counterclockwise. The entire loop is located superiorly. The rightward displacement of the T loop is also seen in this projection.

Vectorcardiographic diagnosis. Anterior and inferior myocardial infarction, age undetermined. Left anterior hemiblock.

Electrocardiographic diagnosis. Anterior wall myocardial infarction. Possible inferior myocardial infarction. Left anterior hemiblock.

Clinical findings. The patient is a 74-year-old man with a history of well-documented myocardial infarction 8 months before the tracings were recorded.

J.F. 371292   dash interval 2 msec

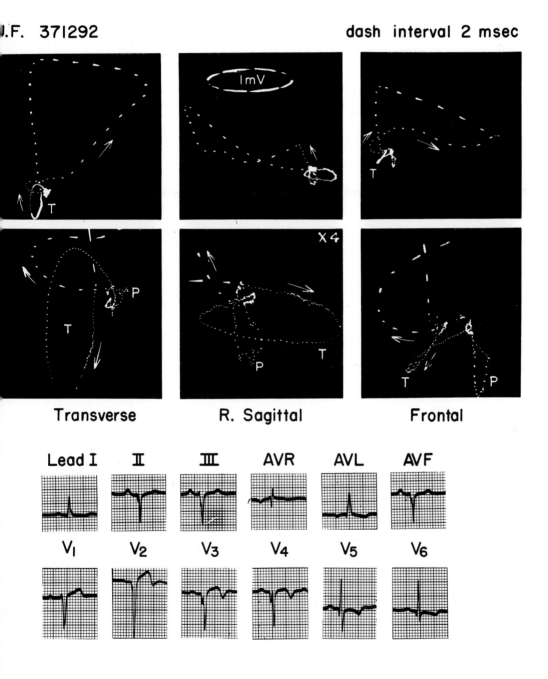

Transverse   R. Sagittal   Frontal

Lead I   II   III   AVR   AVL   AVF

V_1 V_2 V_3 V_4 V_5 V_6

Fig. B.50., R.N., 502716

Vectorcardiogram. The P loop is within normal limits. The duration of the QRS loop is increased to 0.016 sec. The main body of the QRS loop is normal. There is however a terminal appendage which is slowly inscribed and is directed leftward, anteriorly, and inferiorly. This is probably the so-called J loop. The **ST** vector is displaced rightward and superiorly. The T loop is within normal limits.

Vectorcardiographic diagnosis. The tracing is suggestive of profound hypothermia.

Electrocardiographic diagnosis. The tracing is suggestive of profound hypothermia.

Clinical findings. The patient was a 24-year-old man who sustained a head injury and became comatose. His rectal temperature fell to 85°F at the time of the recording of these tracings. The heart rate was 53/min. Both the vectorcardiogram and electrocardiogram gradually returned to normality after his body temperature was brought back to normal.

Comment. The "J loop" in the vectorcardiogram which is the equivalent of the "J deflection" in the electrocardiogram is a characteristic finding in profound hypothermia. Its electrophysiological basis, however, is not yet understood. (Emslie-Smith D: The spatial vectorcardiogram in hypothermia. Brit Heart J 20:175, 1958. Trevino A, Razi F, Beller BM: The characteristic electrocardiogram of accidental hypothermia. Arch Int Med 127:470, 1971)

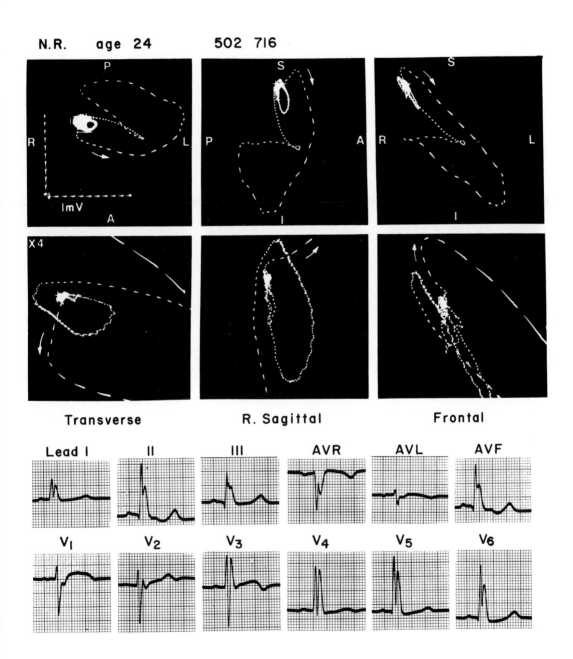

N.R.   age 24   502 716

Transverse   R. Sagittal   Frontal

Lead I   II   III   AVR   AVL   AVF

V₁   V₂   V₃   V₄   V₅   V₆

Index